Smart Sensing Technologies for Personalised Coaching

Smart Sensing Technologies for Personalised Coaching

Editors

Oresti Banos
Hermie Hermens
Christopher Nugent
Hector Pomares

MDPI • Basel • Beijing • Wuhan • Barcelona • Belgrade • Manchester • Tokyo • Cluj • Tianjin

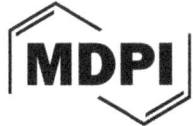

Editors

Oresti Banos
Department of Computer Architecture and Computer Technology
University of Granada
Granada
Spain

Hermie Hermens
Biomedical Signals and Systems
University of Twente
Enschede
The Netherlands

Christopher Nugent
School of Computing and Mathematics
Ulster University
Ulster
Spain

Hector Pomares
Department of Computer Architecture and Computer Technology
University of Granada
Granada
Spain

Editorial Office
MDPI
St. Alban-Anlage 66
4052 Basel, Switzerland

This is a reprint of articles from the Special Issue published online in the open access journal *Sensors* (ISSN 1424-8220) (available at: www.mdpi.com/journal/sensors/special_issues/personalised_coaching).

For citation purposes, cite each article independently as indicated on the article page online and as indicated below:

LastName, A.A.; LastName, B.B.; LastName, C.C. Article Title. *Journal Name* **Year**, *Volume Number*, Page Range.

ISBN 978-3-0365-1790-2 (Hbk)
ISBN 978-3-0365-1789-6 (PDF)

© 2021 by the authors. Articles in this book are Open Access and distributed under the Creative Commons Attribution (CC BY) license, which allows users to download, copy and build upon published articles, as long as the author and publisher are properly credited, which ensures maximum dissemination and a wider impact of our publications.

The book as a whole is distributed by MDPI under the terms and conditions of the Creative Commons license CC BY-NC-ND.

Contents

About the Editors vii

Preface to "Smart Sensing Technologies for Personalised Coaching" ix

Oresti Banos, Hermie Hermens, Christopher Nugent and Hector Pomares
Smart Sensing Technologies for Personalised e-Coaching
Reprinted from: *Sensors* **2018**, *18*, 1751, doi:10.3390/s18061751 1

Talko B. Dijkhuis, Frank J. Blaauw, Miriam W. Van Ittersum, Hugo Velthuijsen and Marco Aiello
Personalized Physical Activity Coaching: A Machine Learning Approach
Reprinted from: *Sensors* **2018**, *18*, 623, doi:10.3390/s18020623 5

Michel C. A. Klein, Adnan Manzoor and Julia S. Mollee
Active2Gether: A Personalized m-Health Intervention to Encourage Physical Activity
Reprinted from: *Sensors* **2017**, *17*, 1436, doi:10.3390/s17061436 21

Daniel Aranki, Gao Xian Peh, Gregorij Kurillo and Ruzena Bajcsy
The Feasibility and Usability of RunningCoach: A Remote Coaching System for Long-Distance Runners
Reprinted from: *Sensors* **2018**, *18*, 175, doi:10.3390/s18010175 37

Javier Medina Quero, María Rosa Fernández Olmo, María Dolores Peláez Aguilera and Macarena Espinilla Estévez
Real-Time Monitoring in Home-Based Cardiac Rehabilitation Using Wrist-Worn Heart Rate Devices
Reprinted from: *Sensors* **2017**, *17*, 2892, doi:10.3390/s17122892 57

Kee-Hoon Kim and Sung-Bae Cho
Modular Bayesian Networks with Low-Power Wearable Sensors for Recognizing Eating Activities
Reprinted from: *Sensors* **2017**, *17*, 2877, doi:10.3390/s17122877 73

Gustavo López, Iván González, Elitania Jimenez-Garcia, Jesús Fontecha, Jose A. Brenes, Luis A. Guerrero and José Bravo
Smart Device-Based Notifications to Promote Healthy Behavior Related to Childhood Obesity and Overweight
Reprinted from: *Sensors* **2018**, *18*, 271, doi:10.3390/s18010271 89

Chris Baber, Ahmad Khattab, Martin Russell, Joachim Hermsdörfer and Alan Wing
Creating Affording Situations: Coaching through Animate Objects
Reprinted from: *Sensors* **2017**, *17*, 2308, doi:10.3390/s17102308 111

Avgoustinos Filippoupolitis, William Oliff, Babak Takand and George Loukas
Location-Enhanced Activity Recognition in Indoor Environments Using Off the Shelf Smart Watch Technology and BLE Beacons
Reprinted from: *Sensors* **2017**, *17*, 1230, doi:10.3390/s17061230 129

Muhammad Fahim, Thar Baker, Asad Masood Khattak, Babar Shah, Saiqa Aleem and Francis Chow
Context Mining of Sedentary Behaviour for Promoting Self-Awareness Using a Smartphone
Reprinted from: *Sensors* **2018**, *18*, 874, doi:10.3390/s18030874 155

Daniel H. De La Iglesia, Juan F. De Paz, Gabriel Villarrubia González, Alberto L. Barriuso, Javier Bajo and Juan M. Corchado
Increasing the Intensity over Time of an Electric-Assist Bike Based on the User and Route: The Bike Becomes the Gym
Reprinted from: *Sensors* **2018**, *18*, 220, doi:10.3390/s18010220 . . . . **171**

Randy Klaassen, Kim C. M. Bul, Rieks Op den Akker, Gert Jan Van der Burg, Pamela M. Kato and Pierpaolo Di Bitonto
Design and Evaluation of a Pervasive Coaching and Gamification Platform for Young Diabetes Patients
Reprinted from: *Sensors* **2018**, *18*, 402, doi:10.3390/s18020402 . . . . **193**

About the Editors

Oresti Banos

Oresti Baños is a tenured professor of computational behavior modelling at the University of Granada (Spain, 2019–present). He is also a senior research scientist affiliated with the Centre for Information and Communication Technologies at the University of Granada (CITIC-UGR). He is a research collaborator at Kyung Hee University (South Korea, 2016–present) and at the University of Twente (The Netherlands, 2018–present). He is a former assistant professor at the University of Twente (2016–2018); postdoctoral fellow at Kyung Hee University (2014–2016); predoctoral fellow at CITIC-UGR (2010–2014); and visiting scholar at the Technical University of Eindhoven (the Netherlands, 2012), the Swiss Federal Institute of Technology Zurich (Switzerland, 2011), and the University of Alabama (USA, 2011). His research includes work on the intersection of wearable, ubiquitous, and mobile computing with data mining and artificial intelligence for digital health and wellness applications.

Hermie Hermens

Prof. Dr. Ir. Hermie J. Hermens studied biomedical engineering at the University of Twente and then became head of the research group at Roessingh, Centre for Rehabilitation. In 1990, he was a co-founder and first director of RRD. He studied his PhD on surface EMG, became a professor in neuromuscular control (2001), and later (2010) became a professor of telemedicine. Currently, he supervises 15 PhD students, and 26 PhD students have finished their studies under his (co)supervision.

Christopher Nugent

Christopher Nugent is currently the head of the School of Computing at Ulster University and leads the Pervasive Computing Research Centre. Chris was awarded a first class honors in BEng electronic systems and a PhD in biomedical engineering, both from the University of Ulster in 1995 and 1998, respectively. He became a fellow of the Higher Education Academy in 2015. He has held a visiting professorship at Halmstad University (Sweden) and the University of Florence (Italy) and is currently a visiting professor at Lulea Technical University (Sweden). In 2016, he was awarded a Senior Distinguished Research Fellowship by Ulster University. His research addresses the themes of the development and evaluation of technologies to support pervasive healthcare within smart environments. Specifically, this has involved research in the topics of mobile-based reminding solutions, activity recognition, and behavior modelling and, more recently, in technology adoption modelling.

Hector Pomares

Hector Pomares (MSc in electrical engineering in 1995, MSc in physics in 1997, and PhD from the University of Granada in 2000, all of them with honors) is currently a full professor at the University of Granada. He has published more than 60 articles in the most prestigious scientific journals and contributed to more than 150 papers in international conferences. He has been a visiting researcher at the University of Dortmund (Germany), the University of California at Berkeley (USA), the University of Texas A&M (USA), the University of Applied Sciences Muenster (Germany), the Technical University of Graz (Austria), and the University of Amsterdam (Netherlands). Currrently, he is the director of the doctoral program in Information and Communication Technologies at the University of Granada.

Preface to "Smart Sensing Technologies for Personalised Coaching"

People living in both developed and developing countries face serious health challenges related to sedentary lifestyles. It is therefore essential to find new ways to improve health so that people can live longer and can age well. With an ever-growing number of smart sensing systems developed and deployed across the globe, experts are primed to help coach people toward healthier behaviors. The increasing accountability associated with app- and device-based behavior tracking not only provides timely and personalized information and support but also gives us an incentive to set goals and to do more. This book presents some of the recent efforts made towards automatic and autonomous identification and coaching of troublesome behaviors to procure lasting, beneficial behavioral changes.

Oresti Banos, Hermie Hermens, Christopher Nugent, Hector Pomares
Editors

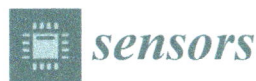

Editorial

Smart Sensing Technologies for Personalised e-Coaching

Oresti Banos [1,2,*], **Hermie Hermens** [1,3], **Christopher Nugent** [4] **and Hector Pomares** [2]

1. Biomedical Signals and Systems Group, University of Twente, 7522 NB Enschede, The Netherlands; H.Hermens@rrd.nl
2. CITIC-UGR, University of Granada, E-18015 Granada, Spain; hector@ugr.es
3. Telemedicine Group, Roessingh Research and Development, 7500 AH Enschede, The Netherlands
4. Smart Environments Research Group, Ulster University, Newtownabbey BT37 0QB, UK; cd.nugent@ulster.ac.uk
* Correspondence: o.banoslegran@utwente.nl; Tel.: +31-543-895329

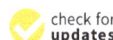

Received: 25 May 2018; Accepted: 28 May 2018; Published: 29 May 2018

Abstract: People living in both developed and developing countries face serious health challenges related to sedentary lifestyles. It is therefore essential to find new ways to improve health so that people can live longer and age well. With an ever-growing number of smart sensing systems developed and deployed across the globe, experts are primed to help coach people to have healthier behaviors. The increasing accountability associated with app- and device-based behavior tracking not only provides timely and personalized information and support, but also gives us an incentive to set goals and do more. This paper outlines some of the recent efforts made towards automatic and autonomous identification and coaching of troublesome behaviors to procure lasting, beneficial behavioral changes.

Keywords: e-coaching; wearable sensors; smartphones; smart objects; activity recognition; context-awareness; behavior change

1. Introduction

Lifestyle choices can have a tremendous impact on people's health and wellness. Avoiding unhealthy habits is nowadays a priority, and to achieve this goal, ground-breaking mechanisms are required to automatically and autonomously identify and eventually change people's behaviors. An increasing number of smart, ubiquitous sensing technologies are being developed all over the world to coach people on healthier and more responsible behavior, providing them with timely personalized information and support. This Special Issue aims at bringing together the latest experiences, findings, and developments on smart sensing, modeling, and understanding of human behavior for the provision of personalized coaching and support services.

2. Contributions

This special issue has collected eleven outstanding papers touching upon different aspects of smart sensing for e-coaching applications. In the following, a brief summary of the scope and main contributions of each of these papers is provided as a teaser for the interested reader.

As it has been pointed out in the introduction of this editorial, sedentary lifestyles are one of the major causes of health problems in our society. In "Personalized Physical Activity Coaching: A Machine Learning Approach" [1], the authors report their experiences with different machine learning algorithms to timely estimate the probability for a given subject of achieving a personalized step goal. They integrated this model into a web app that helps the expert predict, with a level of certainty, whether the subject will be able to achieve their goal based on their most immediate prior performance.

Not only is it important to detect or predict the activity patterns of a given user, but also to ensure that the users are properly informed and to encourage people to change at the point of need. In "Active2Gether: A Personalized m-Health Intervention to Encourage Physical Activity" [2], the authors present a system that monitors young adults' physical behavior by using wearable and mobile sensors, facilitates social comparison, and provides personalized intelligent feedback. The authors share interesting lessons learned during the design, implementation, and evaluation of the system, such as the difficulties encountered while directly accessing the data of commercially available activity trackers.

Promoting or encouraging people to exercise is normally positive. In some cases, like sports, it is also important to provide tailored instructions to avoid possible injuries. In "The Feasibility and Usability of RunningCoach: A Remote Coaching System for Long-Distance Runners" [3], the authors propose a mobile system that monitors running cadence levels, which are shown to be strongly associated with running-related injuries. The system uses this information to estimate the optimal cadence for the runner, which can in turn modulate their running style while reducing the risk of injuries.

Minimizing risks is of utmost importance to ensure a plentiful life, especially when it comes to more serious heart-related aspects. In "Real-Time Monitoring in Home-Based Cardiac Rehabilitation Using Wrist-Worn Heart Rate Devices" [4], the authors present a system that facilitates the continuous monitoring of heart-rate activity during home-based rehabilitation sessions. The approach leverages existing clinical guidelines for monitoring the heart rate of the patient. The registered data is then modeled through fuzzy techniques in order to realize remote cardiac rehabilitation sessions.

The recognition of physical activities has been widely explored during recent years. However, not much effort has been put into the detection of rather complex activities such as eating. In "Modular Bayesian Networks with Low-Power Wearable Sensors for Recognizing Eating Activities" [5], the authors propose an approach combining wearable and mobile sensors to detect such complex activity. The approach builds on a probabilistic Bayesian network with a modular and tree-structured form to reduce time complexity and increase scalability. Their results show that good detections can be made even when some of the sensor values have a very heterogeneous pattern or are missing.

Recognizing eating patterns turns to be quite useful when trying to understand dietary habits. Thus, it is necessary to provide recommendations and feedback to users, to support them in improving their routines. In "Smart Device-Based Notifications to Promote Healthy Behavior Related to Childhood Obesity and Overweight" [6], the authors present a prototype targeted at parents to increase their awareness towards nutrition and exercise. The system is based on smart objects that can be attached to the fridge to remind parents visually to prepare a healthy snack or to bring the necessary sports equipment. According to the authors, the system has been rated positively by both nutritionists and physical therapists.

The popularity of the internet-of-things is making smart objects quite an interesting technology for e-coaching. In "Creating Affording Situations: Coaching through Animate Objects" [7], the authors explore the use of these devices to cue actions in everyday activities. Patients with neurological disorders can often struggle with such activities, for example, by confusing the sequence in which tasks should be performed or forgetting which action can be realized using a given object. This work presents a set of prototypes that exploit the use of lights and audio on animated objects to influence activity by reducing uncertainty, which in turn can challenge pre-learned action sequences.

Smart objects are typically confined to indoor environments. Understanding how people behave in such environments is—next to other reasons such as energy management, security, and safety—of much relevance. In "Location-Enhanced Activity Recognition in Indoor Environments Using Off the Shelf Smart Watch Technology and BLE Beacons" [8], the authors propose a system that uses commercial off-the-shelf smartwatches and Bluetooth low energy beacons. By combining these two technologies, the authors show clear improvements in the recognition of activities with respect to prior works that exclusively rely on either device.

Detecting the activity a user is performing is as important as understanding the context around such activity. In "Context Mining of Sedentary Behaviour for Promoting Self-Awareness Using a Smartphone" [9], the authors exploit sensors embedded into regular smartphones to mine the temporal context of passive behaviors. The proposed system uses the inertial sensors to first differentiate between active or still; if the person is categorized into the latter, then environmental audio is captured and processed to identify the specific context. This information is then used to trigger a coaching action to interrupt such a sedentary behavior and stimulate an active one.

People often attribute their sedentariness to being extremely occupied over the day. Thus, finding ways to introduce exercise into their lives has become of much relevance. In "Increasing the Intensity over Time of an Electric-Assist Bike Based on the User and Route: The Bike Becomes the Gym" [10], the authors present an application that increases the pedaling intensity for an electric pedal-assist-bike. The system personalizes the "extra effort" a person has to put into their normal cycling based on the user's strength and the route's characteristics. A social component also motivates interaction and competition between users, based on a scoring system that shows the level of their performances.

There is a great realm of solutions for e-coaching building on smart technologies as can be seen from the examples outlined above. However, as coaching on healthy behaviors is a broad challenge, not only is it important to develop individual solutions but also infrastructures that can accommodate and combine several of them. In "Design and Evaluation of a Pervasive Coaching and Gamification Platform for Young Diabetes Patients" [11], the authors describe a platform that integrates mobile digital coaching systems connected with wearable sensors, serious games, and patient web portals to personal health records, with the aim to support patients with chronic conditions and their caregivers in realizing the ideality of self-management. This work shows how behavioral change theories can be engrained in the design of e-coaching technologies, with the aim of developing successful and long-lasting interventions in healthcare.

Acknowledgments: The authors are grateful to the anonymous reviewers and want to thank the editorial staff of Sensors for the kind co-operation, patience, and committed engagement. The authors also want to acknowledge received funding from the European Union's Horizon 2020 research and innovation programme under Grant Agreement #769553. This result only reflects the author's view and the EU is not responsible for any use that may be made of the information it contains.

Conflicts of Interest: The authors declare no conflict of interest.

References

1. Dijkhuis, T.B.; Blaauw, F.J.; van Ittersum, M.W.; Velthuijsen, H.; Aiello, M. Personalized Physical Activity Coaching: A Machine Learning Approach. *Sensors* **2018**, *18*, 623, doi:10.3390/s18020623.
2. Klein, M.C.A.; Manzoor, A.; Mollee, J.S. Active2Gether: A Personalized m-Health Intervention to Encourage Physical Activity. *Sensors* **2017**, *17*, 1436, doi:10.3390/s17061436.
3. Aranki, D.; Peh, G.X.; Kurillo, G.; Bajcsy, R. The Feasibility and Usability of RunningCoach: A Remote Coaching System for Long-Distance Runners. *Sensors* **2018**, *18*, 175, doi:10.3390/s18010175.
4. Medina Quero, J.; Fernández Olmo, M.R.; Peláez Aguilera, M.D.; Espinilla Estévez, M. Real-Time Monitoring in Home-Based Cardiac Rehabilitation Using Wrist-Worn Heart Rate Devices. *Sensors* **2017**, *17*, 2892, doi:10.3390/s17122892.
5. Kim, K.H.; Cho, S.B. Modular Bayesian Networks with Low-Power Wearable Sensors for Recognizing Eating Activities. *Sensors* **2017**, *17*, doi:10.3390/s17122877.
6. López, G.; González, I.; Jimenez-Garcia, E.; Fontecha, J.; Brenes, J.A.; Guerrero, L.A.; Bravo, J. Smart Device-Based Notifications to Promote Healthy Behavior Related to Childhood Obesity and Overweight. *Sensors* **2018**, *18*, 271, doi:10.3390/s18010271.
7. Baber, C.; Khattab, A.; Russell, M.; Hermsdörfer, J.; Wing, A. Creating Affording Situations: Coaching through Animate Objects. *Sensors* **2017**, *17*, 2308, doi:10.3390/s17102308.

8. Filippoupolitis, A.; Oliff, W.; Takand, B.; Loukas, G. Location-Enhanced Activity Recognition in Indoor Environments Using Off the Shelf Smart Watch Technology and BLE Beacons. *Sensors* **2017**, *17*, 1230, doi:10.3390/s17061230.
9. Fahim, M.; Baker, T.; Khattak, A.M.; Shah, B.; Aleem, S.; Chow, F. Context Mining of Sedentary Behaviour for Promoting Self-Awareness Using a Smartphone. *Sensors* **2018**, *18*, 874, doi:10.3390/s18030874.
10. De La Iglesia, D.H.; De Paz, J.F.; Villarrubia González, G.; Barriuso, A.L.; Bajo, J.; Corchado, J.M. Increasing the Intensity over Time of an Electric-Assist Bike Based on the User and Route: The Bike Becomes the Gym. *Sensors* **2018**, *18*, 220, doi:10.3390/s18010220.
11. Klaassen, R.; Bul, K.C.M.; op den Akker, R.; van der Burg, G.J.; Kato, P.M.; Di Bitonto, P. Design and Evaluation of a Pervasive Coaching and Gamification Platform for Young Diabetes Patients. *Sensors* **2018**, *18*, 402, doi:10.3390/s18020402.

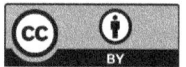

© 2018 by the authors. Licensee MDPI, Basel, Switzerland. This article is an open access article distributed under the terms and conditions of the Creative Commons Attribution (CC BY) license (http://creativecommons.org/licenses/by/4.0/).

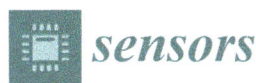

Article
Personalized Physical Activity Coaching: A Machine Learning Approach

Talko B. Dijkhuis [1,2,*], Frank J. Blaauw [1,3], Miriam W. van Ittersum [4], Hugo Velthuijsen [2] and Marco Aiello [1]

1. Johann Bernoulli Institute for Mathematics and Computer Science, Faculty of Science and Engineering (FSE), University of Groningen, Nijenborgh 9, 9747 AG Groningen, The Netherlands; f.j.blaauw@rug.nl (F.J.B.); m.aiello@rug.nl (M.A.)
2. Institute of Communication, Hanze University of Applied Sciences, Media and ICT, Zernikeplein 11, 9746 AS Groningen, The Netherlands; h.velthuijsen@pl.hanze.nl
3. Developmental Psychology, University of Groningen, Grote Kruisstraat 2/1, 9712 TS Groningen, The Netherlands
4. School for Health Care Studies, Hanze University of Applied Sciences, Petrus Driessenstraat 3, 9714 CA Groningen, The Netherlands; m.w.van.ittersum@pl.hanze.nl
* Correspondence: t.dijkhuis@rug.nl; Tel.: +31-06-4777-6769

Received: 7 February 2018; Accepted: 15 February 2018; Published: 19 February 2018

Abstract: Living a sedentary lifestyle is one of the major causes of numerous health problems. To encourage employees to lead a less sedentary life, the Hanze University started a health promotion program. One of the interventions in the program was the use of an activity tracker to record participants' daily step count. The daily step count served as input for a fortnightly coaching session. In this paper, we investigate the possibility of automating part of the coaching procedure on physical activity by providing personalized feedback throughout the day on a participant's progress in achieving a personal step goal. The gathered step count data was used to train eight different machine learning algorithms to make hourly estimations of the probability of achieving a personalized, daily steps threshold. In 80% of the individual cases, the Random Forest algorithm was the best performing algorithm (mean accuracy = 0.93, range = 0.88–0.99, and mean F1-score = 0.90, range = 0.87–0.94). To demonstrate the practical usefulness of these models, we developed a proof-of-concept Web application that provides personalized feedback about whether a participant is expected to reach his or her daily threshold. We argue that the use of machine learning could become an invaluable asset in the process of automated personalized coaching. The individualized algorithms allow for predicting physical activity during the day and provides the possibility to intervene in time.

Keywords: physical activity; machine learning; coaching; sedentary lifestyle

1. Introduction

Unhealthy lifestyles lead to increased premature mortality and are a risk factor for sustaining noncommunicable diseases (NCDs) such as cardiovascular diseases, cancers, chronic respiratory diseases, and diabetes [1]. NCDs caused 63% of all deaths that occurred globally in 2008 [1]. There are four behavioral factors that have a significant influence on the prevention of NDCs: healthy nutrition, not smoking, maintaining a healthy body weight, and sufficient physical activity. Insufficient physical activity is one of the leading risk factors for the major NCDs and not meeting the recommended level of physical activity is associated with approximately 5.3 million deaths that occurred globally in 2008 [2].

A high amount of sedentary time without sufficient daily physical activity leads to a higher rate of all-cause mortality [3]. Besides the increased risk of premature mortality in the long term, the short-term quality of life, being able to work, and social participation is also threatened by insufficient physical activity [4]. Fortunately, these risks are eliminated when this sedentary time is compensated for with sufficient physical activity of moderate intensity [3].

In Western civilization, living a sedentary lifestyle is the rule rather than the exception, as many people work in office environments. In pursuance of preventing the negative effects of insufficient physical activity in the workplace, the Hanze University of Applied Sciences Groningen (HUAS), a large university in the northern part of the Netherlands, started a novel initiative named (in Dutch): 'Het Nieuwe Gezonde Werken' (The New Healthy Way of Working; HNGW). With HNGW, the HUAS aims to promote a healthy lifestyle and physical activity during the workday. HNGW consists of providing participants with educational group meetings, food boxes with healthy recipes, and individual coaching sessions supplemented with an activity tracker. Despite the fact that participants are coached every two weeks and measured continuously, it remains difficult for a coach to provide timely personalized feedback. The manual task of creating personalized feedback is time consuming, and as such it is not always possible for the participants to get in-depth and timely daily feedback on their progression. Furthermore, current activity trackers do not provide a prediction for reaching the daily goal.

In order to fill this gap, we propose a novel, personalized, and flexible machine-learning-based procedure that can automate a part of the coaching process and serve as a source of information on a participant's progress with physical activity during the day. The personalized model provides, throughout the day, information on the probability of the participant meeting his or her daily physical activity goal. We demonstrate the accuracy and effectiveness of this solution in practice by training different machine learning algorithms and evaluating their performance using a train-test split dataset from the HNGW data. We apply techniques like grid search and cross-validation to optimize each model in order to find their best configuration. To show the applicability of this research in practice, we developed a proof of concept Web application, which has, to the best of our knowledge, not been done before. With the personalized actionable information the application provides, we demonstrate that machine learning automating is feasible as a part of the coaching process. The techniques described in this work could serve two goals in the field of personalized coaching. Firstly, we envision how coaches can use such applications and how these applications can provide them with detailed insight about the participants' activity during the day. Secondly, the tool could be used as a self-support tool, in which the participants' engagement with their lifestyle might increase as a result of the extra feedback.

2. Related Work

A number of studies have been performed on physical activity over days, where the sources of variance in activity is related to the subject, the day of the week, the season, and occupational and non-occupational days [5]. Tudor-Locke et al. (2005) showed that the individual is the main source of variability in physical activity next to the difference between the Sunday and the rest of the week [6]. Another study identified physical inactivity being lower on weekend days, and Saturday was the most active day of the week for both men and women [5].

To reduce sedentary time and increase physical activity levels, individuals need to change their behavior and daily routines. This is hard to achieve because of various reasons, and requires interventions and coaching strategies that use well-established techniques to induce a behavior change. A review by Gardner et al. (2016) found that self-monitoring, problem solving, and restructuring the social or physical environment were the most promising behavior change strategies, and—although the evidence base is quite weak—advises environmental restructuring, persuasion, and education to enhance self-regulatory skills [7]. Interventions aimed at increasing physical activity levels or reducing sedentary time varies widely in content and in effectiveness. For example, studies focusing on exercise training and behavioral approaches have demonstrated conflicting results, whereas interventions focusing on reducing sedentary time seem to be more promising [8–12]. The use of active video games seems to be effective in increasing physical activity, but has inconsistent findings on whether they are suitable to meet the recommended levels [13]. Also, interventions targeting recreational screen time reduction might be effective when using health promotion curricula or counseling [14]. Web- or app-based interventions to improve diet, physical activity, and sedentary behavior can be effective. Multi-component interventions appear to be more effective than stand-alone app interventions, although the optimal number and combination of app features and level of participant contact needed remain to be confirmed [15,16]. The workplace is often used for health promotion interventions. Recent reviews on workplace interventions for reducing sitting at work found initial evidence that the use of alternative workstations (sit-stand desks or treadmills) can decrease workplace sitting by thirty minutes to two hours. In addition, one review found that interventions promoting stair use and personalized behavioral interventions increase physical activity, while the other found no considerable or inconsistent effects of various interventions [17,18].

Step counters provide an objective measure of activity levels and enable self-monitoring. Furthermore, most modern consumer-based activity trackers already contain several behavior change models or theories [19,20]. Therefore, based on the aforementioned, using activity trackers in interventions to promote healthy lifestyles is promising. From meta-analyses by Qiu et al. and Stephenson et al. it was concluded that step counter use was indeed associated with small but significant effects in reducing sedentary time [21,22]. Adding an activity tracker to physical therapy or counseling was effective in some populations [23–25]. Besides collecting activity data for therapy or counseling, it is known that the Fitbit itself also serves as an intervention mechanism [26]. The mere fact of wearing an activity tracker (even without any form of coaching) could motivate physical activity and improve health-related quality of life [27,28]. On the other hand, studies on workplace interventions using activity trackers report conflicting results [29–33].

There are several studies that use sensor or activity tracker data to build a custom-made application to support research. An example is the social computer game, Fish'n'Steps, which connects the daily steps of an employee to the growth and activity of the individual avatar fish in a virtual fish tank. The more one is active, the faster the fish grows and prospers [34]. Another example is the study on increased physical activity as the effect of social support groups using pedometers and an app [35].

Although applying machine learning to coaching is new, machine learning techniques in combination with sensors have been applied before to identify the type of activity. Identifying human activity using machine learning and sensor data have been studied, for example, by Wang et al. for recognizing human daily activities from an accelerometer signal [36], by Li et al. on the quantification of the lifetime circadian rhythm of physical activity [37], or by Catal et al. on the use of an ensemble of classifiers for accelerometer-based activity recognition [38]. Only a few studies have investigated the use of actionable, data-driven predictive models. A study on creating a predictive physical fatigue model based on sensors identified relevant features for predicting physical fatigue, however the model was not proven to be predictive enough to be applied [39].

In order to improve physical activity in combination with activity trackers, a coaching feature is helpful, but only when the messages are personal and placed in context [40]. Perceiving the coaching information as personal and relevant is crucial for the effectiveness of (e)Coaching [41]. Such tailored (e)Coaching has many aspects, two of which are personalization and timing [42]. Timeliness of information is important for participants to be able to process the information and apply the advice while it is still relevant for them. In order to provide such advice, access to real-time predictions is vital, as it allows for timing the moment of coaching, either virtual or in real life and as flexible as needed. To the best of our knowledge, no studies exist about the use of sensor data combined with machine learning techniques for creating validated and individualized predictive models on physical activity. The individualized models could help the coach and the participant in the process of behavior change and increased physical activity.

3. Materials and Methods

The present work revolves around the HNGW project. This project was started in 2015 and focuses on promoting a healthy lifestyle. We describe the design of this study and how the resulting data is used in the present work. Next we describe our analysis pipeline. We describe the conversion of the raw data set into a feature set, the evaluation methods of the predictive models, and the choice of the algorithms. Finally we shed light on the proof of concept application we created to demonstrate how these techniques could be used in practice.

3.1. Study Design

The goal of the workplace health promotion intervention HNGW at the HUAS was to increase physical activity during workdays, by improving both physical and mental health, and several work-related variables. In the study, several performance-based tests and self-reported questionnaires were used to assess its effectiveness on a group level.

Forty-eight eligible participants from the HUAS were randomized into two groups, stratified according to age, gender, BMI, and baseline self-reported health. One group followed a twelve-week workplace health promotion intervention; the other served as a control during the first twelve weeks and thereafter received the twelve-week workplace health promotion intervention.

During the study, minutely step count data of the participants was collected. Step count was measured using a wrist-worn activity tracker, the Fitbit Flex. The Fitbit Flex has been shown to be a reliable and valid device for step count and suitable for health enhancement programs [13]. Further details of the trial design on HNGW at the HUAS are represented in the manuscript of van Ittersum et al. [43].

3.2. Data Set

The anonymized data used in the present study was collected from participants during their participation in the HNGW health promotion program. All participants provided informed consent for participation in the HNGW study and for the use of their anonymized data for research purposes.

We used the steps per minute of each participant, resulting in a total of 349,920 measurements across all participants. We only considered the step data collected during the intervention period. That is, for both the intervention and the control group, we used the last twelve weeks of available step data. By focusing on the intervention period, we have a more homogeneous sample than we would have when including both the intervention and control data.

While the Fitbit platform provides us with several minutely measures (e.g., steps, metabolic equivalent of tasks [METs], calories, and distance), in our analysis we only included the steps variable. We used the steps variable as we expect it to be the most accurate and relevant, as all other variables are by-products derived using approximation algorithms.

3.3. Data Processing, Transformation, and Performance

To prepare the available minutely step data as input for training the algorithms, we first performed a data cleaning, reformatting, and pre-processing step. First, we removed incomplete days from the data set. We also removed all days with zero steps and weekend days. We then converted all provided variables in a format that could be used by our algorithms, by augmenting our initial data set with several new augmented variables, such as hour of the workday, the number of steps for that hour, and a cumulative sum of the number of steps till that hour.

Note that we define a workday as the weekdays Monday to Friday. The normal working hours at the university are between 8:00 AM and 5:00 PM. The HNGW tried to motivate the participants to walk at least a part of the distance they commute daily. As a consequence, the hours of interest are the combination of the working hours and the period of commuting. Therefore we only considered the number of steps per hour between 7:00 AM and 6:00 PM. As features for training the algorithms, we used the hour per workday (ranged from 7:00 AM to 6:00 PM), the number of steps of that hour, and the cumulative sum of the number of steps till that hour.

As the outcome measure, we calculated the average number of steps for all workdays over all weeks. That is, for each individual, we calculated one average for all workdays. We considered the number of steps between 7:00 AM and 6:00 PM. Note that this outcome measure is not used as input in the training process. We constructed a binary outcome variable represented by the indicator variable $Y_j = (s_j \geq \theta_j)$, in which s_j refers to the number of steps on a workday for individual j, and θ_j refers to the specific step goal for that j. The indicator function returns one (the 'true' label) when the inside condition holds, and zero (the 'false' label) otherwise.

Three days of repeated measures are necessary to represent adults' usual activity levels with an 80% confidence [6]. Forty-four participants met the criteria. The processing and transformation for these forty-four participants resulted in a total of 120,480 data blocks (for the number of steps, mean = 9031, median = 8543, range = 0–47,121). The total number of positives when the threshold is met at 6:00 PM, is 1528. The total number of negatives when the threshold is not met at 6:00 PM, is 1879.

Note that we did not include any of the group level/baseline variables like age or gender, as we only considered personalized models. Although these variables might affect the outcome, they do not vary within the individual and as such do not add information.

3.4. Evaluation of the Performance of Algorithms and Models

We trained eight different machine learning algorithms. To compare their performance, we used a method known as 'confusion matrices'. The confusion matrices give an overview of the true positives (TP; the model predicted a 'true' label and the actual data contained a 'true' label), true negatives (TN; the model predicted a 'false' label and the actual data turned out to have a 'false' label), false positives (FP; the model predicted a 'true' label, but the actual data contained a 'false' label), and false negatives (FN; the model predicted a 'false' label, but in fact the data contained a 'true' label) of a model. An example of a confusion matrix is provided in Table 1. These confusion matrices served as a basis for the calculation of two other performance measures: The accuracy and the F1-score [15].

Table 1. Confusion matrix.

		True Class	
		Yes	No
Predicted class	Yes	True Positives (TP)	False Negatives (FN)
	No	False Positives (FP)	True Negatives (TN)

True Positive: the threshold of daily steps was met and predicted; True Negative: the threshold of daily steps was not met and predicted; False Negative: the threshold of daily steps was met and not predicted; False Positive: the threshold of daily steps was not met and not predicted.

Accuracy is a metric to determine the nearness of the prediction to the true value. A value of the accuracy close to one indicates the best performance. It calculates the ratio between the correctly classified cases and all cases as Accuracy = $\frac{TP+TN}{TP+TN+FP+FN}$.

Besides the accuracy metric, we calculated the F1-score for each model. Similar to the accuracy metric, the F1-score takes its values from between zero and one, one corresponding to the best performance. To calculate the F1-score, we use two other metrics known as the precision and the recall of the model. Precision is the proportion of the true positives and the false negatives, and is calculated as Precision = $\frac{TP}{TP+FN}$.

Recall is the true positive rate, which is calculated as Recall = $\frac{TP}{TP+FP}$.

Using these definitions of precision and recall, the F1-score can be calculated as F1-score = $2 \times \frac{Precision \times Recall}{Precision + Recall}$.

3.5. Computing the Personalized Predictive Model

We aim to predict (throughout the day) whether or not an individual will meet his or her daily step goal. Prediction of meeting a set goal is a supervised two-class classification problem. Nowadays, many different algorithms for performing such classifications are available. Unfortunately, it is generally considered impossible to determine *a priori* which algorithm will perform best on any given data set [44]. Although distinct algorithms are better suited for different types of data and problems, the type of algorithm is merely an indication of the most suitable algorithm. Currently, the preferred way to find the best-performing algorithm is by empirically testing each of them [45]. Nevertheless, there exist general guidelines to direct the search for specific algorithms for the problem at hand. One of the leading organizations on open source machine learning library, scikit-learn.org, offers a flowchart about which algorithms can be chosen in which situation [46]. Also, Microsoft provides a 'cheat sheet' on their Azure machine learning platform [47]. The flow chart and ´cheat sheet´ served as a basis for our selection process and we chose the following machine learning classification algorithms: (i) AdaBoost (ADA), (ii) Decision Trees (DT), (iii) KNeighborsClassifier (KNN), (iv) Logistic Regression (LR), (v) Neural Networking(NN), (vi) Stochastic Gradient Descent (SGD), (vii) Random Forest (RF), and (viii) Support Vector Classification (SVC). The performance of each of these algorithms was first determined for seventy percent of the whole dataset including five-fold cross-validation with scaling of the factors for KNN, NN, SGD, and SVC. Subsequently, for every participant we individualized the algorithms with five-fold cross-validation and grid search on selected hyperparameters. Seventy percent of the available individual data was used as training data. After training the algorithms, the algorithms were turned into persistent predictive models per participant. We used the individual models to construct confusion matrices, which in turn served as a basis for the F1-score and the accuracy per individual predictive model. To compare the performance of the machine learning models, we included a baseline model. This baseline model checks the cumulative step count. If this cumulative step count equals or exceeds the average personalized goal, the model returns true and false otherwise. We ranked all machine learning models (including the baseline model) using the average of the F1-score and the accuracy.

3.6. Proof of Concept

We designed and implemented a Web application to demonstrate how the personalized prediction based on machine learning and activity tracker data could be used in practice. We developed this application as a Web application, which can be accessed on http://personalized-coaching.compsy.nl/. In this application, the user can input the values 'Hour of the day', 'Steps previous hour', 'Total steps till the Hour', combined with the participant's ID and the algorithm to use. The Web application then uses the individualized model and input data to predict the outcome together with the probability thereof.

3.7. Implementation Details

We used scikit-learn (v0.18, [48]) to establish the best predictive model for the individual. Scikit-learn is an open-source Python module integrating a wide range of machine learning algorithms. Scikit learn was integrated in Anaconda (v4.2.13, [49]) and Jupyter Notebooks (4.0.6, [50]) was used in combination with Python (v3.5.2, [49]) for creating the data processing and machine learning pipeline. Jupyter Notebooks is an interactive method to write and run various programming languages, such as Python. The participants, their physical activity data, and the results of the performance of the algorithms and models were saved in an Oracle database (v11g2 XE; [51]). The Oracle database management system is a widely-used SQL-based system for persisting data. The source code and corresponding notebooks of the machine learning procedure is available as open-source software on Github (https://github.com/compsy/personalized-coaching-ml).

For the Web application, we used Flask (Version 0.10.1, [52]), a Python-based Web application microframework for developing Web applications. We used a PostgreSQL database to store information regarding the models and the participants. The machine learning models resulting from the pipeline are exported as Python Pickle files, which were imported into the Web application. The infrastructure-as-a-service provider Heroku is used to host a demo version of the Web application. This Web application is available at http://personalized-coaching.compsy.nl. The Web application is available as open-source software on Github (https://github.com/compsy/personalized-coaching-app).

4. Results

After optimizing our machine learning models by applying grid search in combination with cross-validation, we assessed the models using the test set. The results are presented here.

4.1. Accuracy and F1-Score on Group Level

Table 2 presents the F1-score and accuracy of the eight different algorithms at the group level. The top three group algorithms based on the mean accuracy and F1-score are:

Table 2. Algorithms and their scores for the whole dataset.

Algorithm Name	Mean Accuracy (Standard Deviation)	Mean F1 (Standard Deviation)	Rank
AdaBoost (ADA)	0.776623 (0.002080)	0.854157 (0.001626)	1
Neural Networking (NN)	0.777774 (0.001545)	0.852797 (0.002938)	2
Support Vector Classifier (SVC)	0.770728 (0.002505)	0.856341 (0.002405)	3
Stochastic Gradient Descent (SGD)	0.767623 (0.005490)	0.853575 (0.004574)	4
KNeighborsClassifier (KNN)	0.749171 (0.005683)	0.829826 (0.005544)	5
Logistic Regression (LR)	0.742125 (0.009821)	0.825725 (0.008487)	6
Random Forest (RF)	0.737451 (0.003210)	0.819065 (0.003840)	7
Decision Tree (DT)	0.720535 (0.004787)	0.804220 (0.003006)	8

AdaBoost, Neural Networking, and Support Vector Classifier.

We visualized the accuracy and F1-score per algorithm using boxplots in Figures 1 and 2. The box represents the second and third quartile groups and the red line indicates the median. The upper whisker visualizes the fourth quartile group and the lower whisker visualizes the first quartile group. Finally, the plus sign indicates outliers on either side of both whiskers.

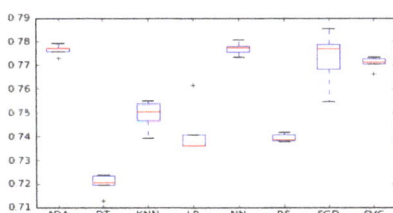

Figure 1. Algorithm accuracy comparison.

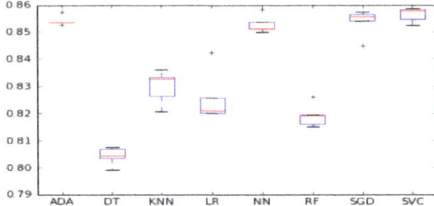

Figure 2. Algorithm F1-score comparison.

4.2. Individual Algorithms

We trained all algorithms on the training set of each individual and performed cross-validation to tune the hyperparameters. Table 3 lists the used machine learning algorithms, the set of tested hyperparameters, and the selected grid search values.

Table 3. Algorithms, used parameters, and grid search values.

Algorithm name	Hyperparameters	Values
AdaBoost (ADA)	n_estimators: number of decision trees in the ensemble	[10,50]
	learning rate: the shrink of the contribution of each successive decision tree in the ensemble	[0.1, 0.5, 1.0, 10.0]
Decision Tree (DT)	criterion: the algorithm to use to decide on split	['gini', 'entropy']
	max_features: the number of features to consider when to split	['auto','sqrt','log2']
KNeighborsClassifier (KNN)	metrics: the distance metric to use	['minkowski','euclidean','manhattan']
	weights: weight function used	['uniform','distance']
	n_neighbors: number of neighbors to use for queries	[5, 6, 7, 8, 9]
Neural Networking (NN)	learning_rate_init: the control of the step-size in updating the weights	['constant', 'invscaling', 'adaptive']
	activation: the activation function for the hidden layer	['identity', 'logistic', 'tanh', 'relu']
	learning_rate: the rate for the weight of the updates	[0.01, 0.05, 0.1, 0.5, 1.0]
Logistic Regression (LR)	C: regularization strength	[0.001, 0.01, 0.1, 1, 10, 100, 1000]
	penalty: whether to use Lasso (L1) or Ridge (L2) regularization	['l1', 'l2']
	fit_intercept: whether or not to compute the intercept of the linear classifier	[True, False]
Stochastic Gradient Descent (SGD)	fit_intercept: whether or not the intercept should be computed	[True, False]
	l1_ratio: the penalty is set to L1 or L2	[0,0.15,1]
	loss: quantification of the loss	['log','modified_huber']
Support Vector Classifier (SVM)	kernel: the kernel type to be used in the algorithm	['linear','rbf']
Random Forest (RF)	n_estimators:number of decision trees	[10, 50, 100, 500]
	max_features: the number of features to consider when to split	[0.1, 0.25, 0.5, 0.75, 'sqrt', 'log2', None]
	criterion: which algorithm should be used to decide on split	['gini', 'entropy']

The accuracy and F1-score of the individual algorithms differ. Figure 3 visualizes the results of the average of the individual scores.

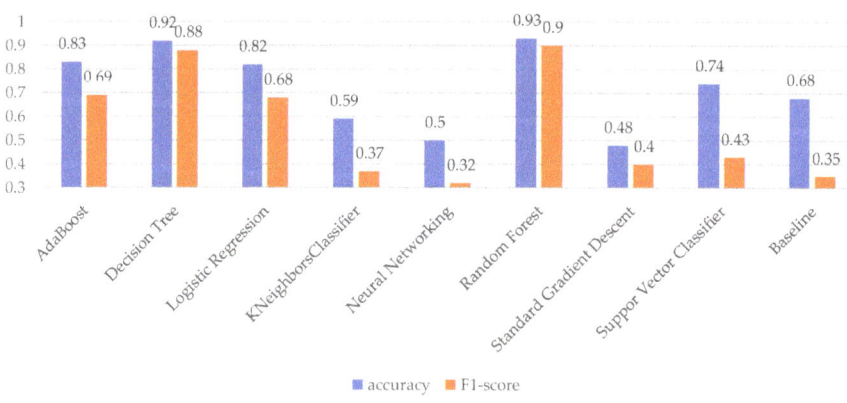

Figure 3. Average accuracy and F1-score per model.

For thirty-five subjects, the best-performing individual model was the Random Forest algorithm, in eight cases this was the Decision Tree algorithm, and for one subject the AdaBoost algorithm performed best. The average accuracy of the Random Forest algorithm is 0.93 (range 0.88–0.99). Thus, in terms of accuracy, the individual Random Forest models score better than its counterpart that was generalized over all individuals (mean personalized accuracy = 0.93 versus mean generalized accuracy = 0.82). The average accuracy of the Decision Tree model is 0.93 (range 0.91–0.97) and outperforms the generalized, group-based Decision Tree accuracy of 0.75. The accuracy of the single AdaBoost model is 0.98, which outperforms the group accuracy of 0.85.

The mean F1-score of the Random Forest model is 0.90 (range 0.87–0.94). The mean F1-score of the Decision Tree model based on the eight best performing models is 0.90 (range 0.87–0.93). Finally, the best AdaBoost model has an F1-score of 0.92, while the group accuracy for the AdaBoost algorithm was 0.77.

The use of grid search to tune the hyperparameters of the algorithms led to several optimized models per individual. To demonstrate the difference this optimization operation can have, we present an example of two individual models with different hyperparameter configurations in Table 4. Table 5 gives an overview of the number of occurrences of a value for the Random Forest hyperparameters.

Table 4. Example of different tuned personalized Random Forest models.

Participant	Parameters	Values
	criterion	gini
1119	max_features	sqrt
	n_estimators	50
	criterion	entropy
1121	max_features	log2
	n_estimators	50

Table 5. The number of different values per Random Forest hyperparameter.

Hyperparameter	Value	Number of Occurrences
criterion	entropy	7
	gini	37
max_features	0.1	4
	0.25	5
	0.5	7
	0.75	15
	log2	2
	sqrt	2
	null	9
n_estimators	10	3
	100	17
	50	16
	500	6

The accuracy and F1-score of the various machine learning algorithms increase slightly during the day. The size of this increase differs slightly per machine learning algorithm. For instance, the F1-score of Random Forest increases with 10% during the day, starting with an F1-score of 0.89 at 7:00 AM and ending with an F1-score of 0.97 at 6:00 PM. Both Figures 4 and 5 also show the increase in accuracy and F1-score of the baseline algorithm during the day. Its accuracy starts with 0.55 and ends at 1 at the end of the workday, while the F1-score starts at 0 and ends at 1. The accuracy increases for Random Forest, Logistic Regression, and AdaBoost, whereas the accuracy of Neural Networking is best at 11:00 AM and Stochastic Gradient Descent remains the same.

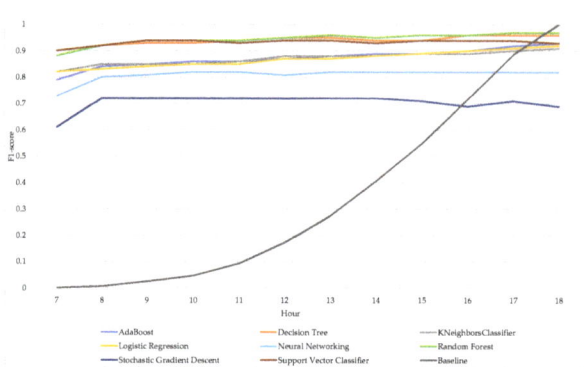

Figure 4. Average F1-Score per algorithm, per hour based on the individual scores.

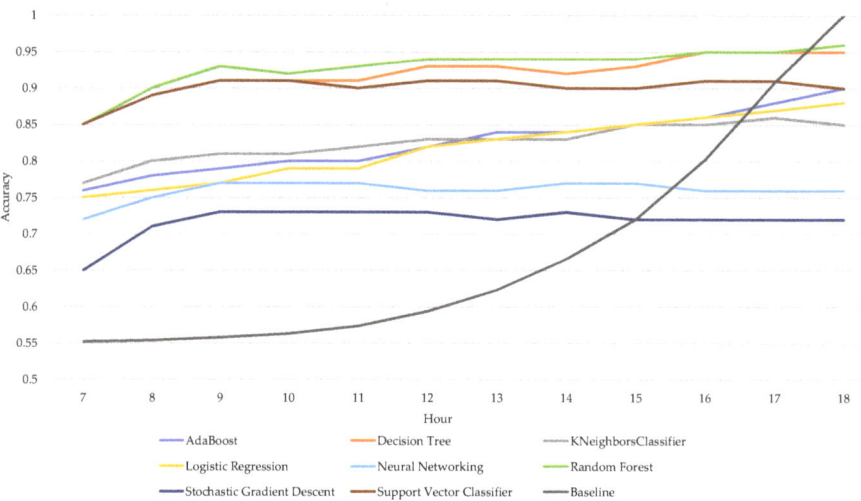

Figure 5. Average accuracy per algorithm, per hour based on the individual scores.

4.3. The Web Application

The Web application is a demonstration of how the aforementioned machine learning techniques could be used in practice, from the perspective of both the coach and the participant. The application allows the user to determine whether a participant will achieve his or her goal for the day, during the day, by applying the individualized algorithms. The procedure for predicting this goal is as follows. First, the user selects a participant identifier from the dropdown menu. After this selection had been made, the application selects the best and personalized machine learning algorithm for this specific participant. Then the user can fill out a form, providing the necessary details to base the prediction on (hour of day, the number of steps so far, and the number of steps in the past hour). Finally, when the user submits the form, the application returns advice personalized for the individual selected from the dropdown menu. The demo application is available at http://personalized-coaching.compsy.nl/. Figure 6 provides a screenshot of both the input fields of the application and the generated prediction and advice.

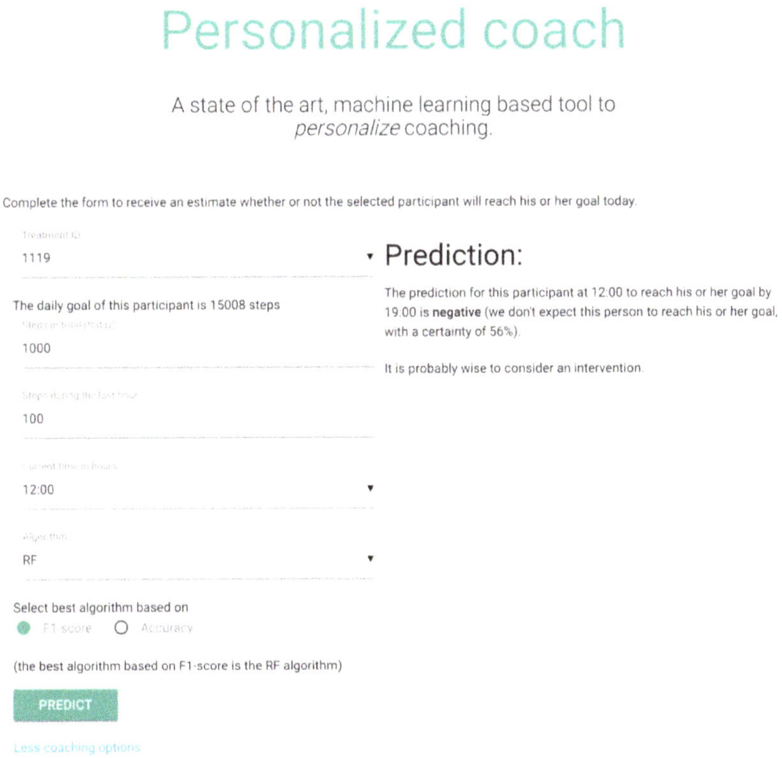

Figure 6. Screenshot of the Personalized Coach Web Application.

5. Discussion

We investigated machine learning as a means to support personalized coaching on physical activity. We demonstrated that for our particular data sets, the tree algorithms and tree-based ensemble algorithms performed especially well. To demonstrate how the results of machine learning techniques could be used in practice, an application was used to aid the coaching of the physical activity process. Furthermore, the analysis shows that selecting the right algorithm, using the dataset of the individual participant, and tuning its individual algorithm parameters, can lead to significant improvements in predictive performance and is a critical step in machine learning application. All source code, including the different notebooks and the proof-of-concept Web application is available online as open-source software. The source code can serve as a blueprint for other researchers when aiming to apply machine learning for coaching.

Although Random Forest outperformed most of the other algorithms, it is problematic to provide a generalized recommendation for specific algorithms, parameters, or parameter settings [44]. Presumably due to individually different physical activity patterns, different algorithms and parameters have to be considered. As a starting point, we selected the algorithms based on well-established sources [41,42], applied cross-validation, and grid-searched the values of the selected parameters. Nevertheless, it's important to note that these algorithms, parameters, and grid search values might not work best on all individual physical patterns, and the algorithms, parameters, and grid search values should only be used as starting points. Future work might consist of investigating the underlying mechanisms to be able to choose the best algorithm beforehand.

We based the prediction solely on the hour of the day and the number of steps. These steps are naturally increasing over the day, and as such, not independent from each other. By including the cumulative number of steps for each block of data, and by including the number of steps made in the past hour, we assume each block to be independent from the other blocks, and as such, are still able to use the regular machine learning methods.

A limitation of the present work is that all participants included in this study participated in an intervention. This intervention might have made the participants more aware and engaged with the project, and as such, the individualized models might be biased towards the best scenario. When people are not extrinsically motivated to meet their daily physical activity goal, and lower their physical activity, the predictive power of the models and therefor the effect of automated intervention will lessen. On the other hand, when an intervention like the health promotion program ends, the individualized models check the participant on his or her performance as if the program is supporting the participant.

As presented in the state of the art literature, the total number of steps differ significantly between Sunday and rest of the weekdays [5,6,48]. Within this health promotion program, the focus was on improving physical activity during working hours and commuting. Therefore, the machine learning models were trained based on the normal workweek. Only one model per participant, based on the five weekdays, is adequate to predict whether or not a participant will meet his or her threshold. It may be necessary to conduct different models for the weekend and weekdays when a health promotion program is expanded to weekends. A reason to establish more than one or two models per participant is found in the variances between weekdays [5]. Examples of different factors that could influence the level of physical activity are weekly sport obligations, weekly meetings, or lunch walks on certain days. Constructing a model per weekday might establish an even more personalized and precise prediction.

In the present work, we only train our machine learning algorithms on variables provided by the activity tracker, extending this set of variables with other (exogenous) variables from other data sources. For example, the data can be extended to include information on the changes in the weather conditions and/or season, which are known to correlate with the day-to-day activity [5,53], or non-working time during weekdays like national holidays and free time, or part-time working schedule, for the activity level differs between non-occupational and occupational time, or the influence and effectiveness of coaching and interventions. Adding the mentioned factors to the dataset might improve the predictive accuracy of the model and might increase the effectiveness of the coaching process.

To apply the personalized machine learning models effectively, they have to become a part of a larger ecosystem. An ideal coaching process is fully tailored to the individual participant. One of the most important characteristics of the personalization of a coaching strategy consists in the timing and ease to execute triggers to change behavior [54]. To support these two aspects of coaching, timely information on the participant and the effectiveness of the coaching strategy are needed. Coaching might not be limited to a personal real life coach but also may include virtual coaching. An example of a possible use of the system is: at the moment the participant doesn't score a 'yes' for two hours in a row on the prediction of meeting his threshold, a notification is sent out to both the participant and the coach. On the basis of this notification, the participant and the coach can take action; the coach can timely intervene to stimulate his client to become physically active and the participant can become instantly more active. Blok et al. proposed a system which combines the real-time analysis of activity tracker data and other personal streaming data as well as the evaluation of virtual coaching strategies, which enables it to tune the coaching to the person [55]. The present work could serve as a central component of a virtual coach system like that envisioned by Blok et al. [55].

To make the information even more personal and relevant, a promising direction for future work is to include a prediction of the actual number of steps at the end of the day. Adding more (and personalized) information might strengthen the effectiveness of the system. To do so, we could apply a similar procedure to the one presented in this study, but instead replace our classification algorithms with regression machine learning algorithms. The predicted number of steps could be a valuable extension in addition to the currently implemented classification of the step goal.

To conclude, machine learning is a viable asset to automate personalized daily physical activity prediction. Coaching can provide accurate and timely information on the participants' physical activity, even early in the day. This is the result of applying machine learning to the behavior of the individual participant as precisely and frequently measured by wearable sensors. The prediction of the participant meeting his goal in combination with the probability of such achievement allows for early intervention and can be used to provide support for personalized coaching. Also, the motivation for self-coaching might be increased, while every model is personalized and the results are better fitted to the situation. Furthermore, machine learning techniques empower automated coaching and personalization.

Acknowledgments: We thank the Hanze University Health Program for providing the physical activity data of the Health Program and all the participants in the experiment.

Author Contributions: Miriam van Ittersum conceived and designed the study of the health promotion program; Talko Dijkhuis developed the database, notebooks and performed the experiments; Talko Dijkhuis analyzed the data; Frank Blaauw developed the Web application. All authors have participated in writing the manuscript.

Conflicts of Interest: The authors declare no conflict of interest.

References

1. WHO. *Global Action Plan for the Prevention and Control of Noncommunicable Diseases 2013–2020*; World Health Organization: Genève, Switzerland, 2013; p. 102.
2. Min-Lee, I.; Shiroma, E.J.; Lobelo, F.; Puska, P.; Blair, S.N.; Katzmarzyk, P.T.; Alkandari, J.R.; Andersen, L.B.; Bauman, A.E.; Brownson, R.C.; et al. Effect of physical inactivity on major non-communicable diseases worldwide: An analysis of burden of disease and life expectancy. *Lancet* **2012**, *380*, 219–229.
3. Ekelund, U.; Steene-Johannessen, J.; Brown, W.J.; Fagerland, M.W.; Owen, N.; Powell, K.E.; Bauman, A.; Lee, I.M. Does physical activity attenuate, or even eliminate, the detrimental association of sitting time with mortality? A harmonised meta-analysis of data from more than 1 million men and women. *Lancet* **2016**, *388*, 1302–1310. [PubMed]
4. Losina, E.; Yang, H.Y.; Deshpande, B.R.; Katz, J.N.; Collins, J.E. Physical activity and unplanned illness-related work absenteeism: Data from an employee wellness program. *PLoS ONE* **2017**, *12*, e0176872. [CrossRef] [PubMed]
5. Matthews, C.E.; Hebert, J.R.; Freedson, P.S.; Iii, E.J.S.; Merriam, P.A.; Cara, B.; Ockene, I.S. Sources of Variance in Daily Physical Activity Levels in the Seasonal Variation of Blood Cholesterol Study. *Am. J. Epidemiol.* **2001**, *153*, 987–995. [CrossRef] [PubMed]
6. Tudor-Locke, C.; Burkett, L.; Reis, J.P.; Ainsworth, B.E.; Macera, C.A.; Wilson, D.K. How many days of pedometer monitoring predict weekly physical activity in adults. *Prev. Med. (Baltim.)* **2005**, *40*, 293–298. [CrossRef] [PubMed]
7. Gardner, B.; Smith, L.; Lorencatto, F.; Hamer, M.; Biddle, S.J. How to reduce sitting time? A review of behaviour change strategies used in sedentary behaviour reduction interventions among adults. *Health Psychol. Rev.* **2016**, *10*, 89–112. [PubMed]
8. Baker, P.R.A.; Francis, D.P.; Soares, J.; Weightman, A.L.; Foster, C. Community wide interventions for increasing physical activity. *Sao Paulo Med. J.* **2011**, *129*, 436–437. [CrossRef]
9. Conroy, D.E.; Hedeker, D.; McFadden, H.G.; Pellegrini, C.A.; Pfammatter, A.F.; Phillips, S.M.; Siddique, J.; Spring, B. Lifestyle intervention effects on the frequency and duration of daily moderate-vigorous physical activity and leisure screen time. *Heal. Psychol.* **2017**, *36*, 299–308. [CrossRef] [PubMed]
10. Ng, L.W.C.; Mackney, J.; Jenkins, S.; Hill, K. Does exercise training change physical activity in people with COPD? A systematic review and meta-analysis. *Chron. Respir. Dis.* **2012**, *9*, 17–26.
11. Cleland, V.; Squibb, K.; Stephens, L.; Dalby, J.; Timperio, A.; Winzenberg, T.; Ball, K.; Dollman, J. Effectiveness of interventions to promote physical activity and/or decrease sedentary behaviour among rural adults: A systematic review and meta-analysis. *Obes. Rev.* **2017**, *18*, 727–741. [CrossRef] [PubMed]
12. Prince, S.A.; Saunders, T.J.; Gresty, K.; Reid, R.D. A comparison of the effectiveness of physical activity and sedentary behaviour interventions in reducing sedentary time in adults: A systematic review and meta-analysis of controlled trials. *Obes. Rev.* **2014**, *15*, 905–919. [CrossRef] [PubMed]

13. Höchsmann, C.; Schüpbach, M.; Schmidt-Trucksäss, A. Effects of Exergaming on Physical Activity in Overweight Individuals. *Sports Med.* **2016**, *46*, 845–860. [CrossRef] [PubMed]
14. Wu, L.; Sun, S.; He, Y.; Jiang, B. The effect of interventions targeting screen time reduction: A systematic review and meta-analysis. *Medicine (Baltimore).* **2016**, *95*, e4029. [CrossRef] [PubMed]
15. Schoeppe, S.; Alley, S.; van Lippevelde, W.; Bray, N.A.; Williams, S.L.; Duncan, M.J.; Vandelanotte, C. Efficacy of interventions that use apps to improve diet, physical activity and sedentary behaviour: A systematic review. *Int. J. Behav. Nutr. Phys. Act.* **2016**, *13*, 127. [CrossRef] [PubMed]
16. Beishuizen, C.R.L.; Stephan, B.C.M.; van Gool, W.A.; Brayne, C.; Peters, R.J.G.; Andrieu, S.; Kivipelto, M.; Soininen, H.; Busschers, W.B.; van Charante, E.P.M.; et al. Web-Based Interventions Targeting Cardiovascular Risk Factors in Middle-Aged and Older People: A Systematic Review and Meta-Analysis. *J. Med. Internet Res.* **2016**, *18*, e55.
17. Shrestha, N.; Kt, K.; Jh, V.; Ijaz, S.; Hermans, V.; Bhaumik, S. Workplace interventions for reducing sitting at work (Review). *Cochrane Database Syst. Rev.* **2016**, *14*, 105.
18. Commissaris, D.A.; Huysmans, M.A.; Mathiassen, S.E.; Srinivasan, D.; Koppes, L.L.; Hendriksen, I.J. Interventions to reduce sedentary behavior and increase physical activity during productive work: A systematic review. *Scand. J. Work. Environ. Health* **2016**, *42*, 181–191. [CrossRef] [PubMed]
19. Mercer, K.; Li, M.; Giangregorio, L.; Burns, C.; Grindrod, K. Behavior Change Techniques Present in Wearable Activity Trackers: A Critical Analysis. *JMIR mHealth uHealth* **2016**, *4*, e40. [CrossRef] [PubMed]
20. Duncan, M.; Murawski, B.; Short, C.E.; Rebar, A.L.; Schoeppe, S.; Alley, S.; Vandelanotte, C.; Kirwan, M. Activity Trackers Implement Different Behavior Change Techniques for Activity, Sleep, and Sedentary Behaviors. *Interact. J. Med. Res.* **2017**, *6*, e13. [CrossRef] [PubMed]
21. Qiu, S.; Cai, X.; Ju, C.; Sun, Z.; Yin, H.; Zügel, M.; Otto, S.; Steinacker, J.M.; Schumann, U. Step Counter Use and Sedentary Time in Adults: A Meta-Analysis. *Medicine (Baltimore)* **2015**, *94*, e1412. [CrossRef] [PubMed]
22. Stephenson, A.; McDonough, S.M.; Murphy, M.H.; Nugent, C.D.; Mair, J.L. Using computer, mobile and wearable technology enhanced interventions to reduce sedentary behaviour: A systematic review and meta-analysis. *Int. J. Behav. Nutr. Phys. Act.* **2017**, *14*, 105. [CrossRef] [PubMed]
23. de Vries, H.J.; Kooiman, T.J.M.; van Ittersum, M.W.; van Brussel, M.; de Groot, M. Do activity monitors increase physical activity in adults with overweight or obesity? A systematic review and meta-analysis. *Obesity* **2016**, *24*, 2078–2091. [PubMed]
24. Li, L.C.; Sayre, E.C.; Xie, H.; Clayton, C.; Feehan, L.M. A Community-Based Physical Activity Counselling Program for People With Knee Osteoarthritis: Feasibility and Preliminary Efficacy of the Track-OA Study. *JMIR mHealth uHealth* **2017**, *5*, e86. [CrossRef] [PubMed]
25. Miyauchi, M.; Toyoda, M.; Kaneyama, N.; Miyatake, H.; Tanaka, E.; Kimura, M.; Umezono, T.; Fukagawa, M. Exercise Therapy for Management of Type 2 Diabetes Mellitus: Superior Efficacy of Activity Monitors over Pedometers. *J. Diabetes Res.* **2016**, *2016*, 1–7. [CrossRef] [PubMed]
26. Cadmus-Bertram, L.A.; Marcus, B.H.; Patterson, R.E.; Parker, B.A.; Morey, B.L. Randomized Trial of a Fitbit-Based Physical Activity Intervention for Women. *Am. J. Prev. Med.* **2015**, *49*, 414–418. [CrossRef] [PubMed]
27. Mansi, S.; Milosavljevic, S.; Tumilty, S.; Hendrick, P.; Higgs, C.; Baxter, D.G. Investigating the effect of a 3-month workplace-based pedometer-driven walking programme on health-related quality of life in meat processing workers: a feasibility study within a randomized controlled trial. *BMC Public Health* **2015**, *15*, 410. [CrossRef] [PubMed]
28. Lewis, Z.H.; Lyons, E.J.; Jarvis, J.M.; Baillargeon, J. Using an electronic activity monitor system as an intervention modality: A systematic review. *BMC Public Health* **2015**, *15*, 585. [CrossRef] [PubMed]
29. Freak-poli, R.; Cumpston, M.; Peeters, A.; Clemes, S. Workplace pedometer interventions for increasing physical activity (Review). *Cochrane Database Syst. Rev.* **2013**, *4*, CD009209.
30. Compernolle, S.; Vandelanotte, C.; Cardon, G.; de Bourdeaudhuij, I.; de Cocker, K. Effectiveness of a web-based, computer-tailored, pedometer-based physical activity intervention for adults: a cluster randomized controlled trial. *J. Med. Internet Res.* **2015**, *17*, e38. [CrossRef] [PubMed]
31. Slootmaker, S.M.; Chinapaw, M.J.M.; Schuit, A.J.; Seidell, J.C.; van Mechelen, W. Feasibility and Effectiveness of Online Physical Activity Advice Based on a Personal Activity Monitor: Randomized Controlled Trial. *J. Med. Internet Res.* **2009**, *11*, e27. [CrossRef] [PubMed]
32. Poirier, J.; Bennett, W.L.; Jerome, G.J.; Shah, N.G.; Lazo, M.; Yeh, H.-C.; Clark, J.M.; Cobb, N.K. Effectiveness of an Activity Tracker- and Internet-Based Adaptive Walking Program for Adults: A Randomized Controlled Trial. *J. Med. Internet Res.* **2016**, *18*, e34.

33. Finkelstein, E.A.; Haaland, B.A.; Bilger, M.; Sahasranaman, A.; Sloan, R.A.; Nang, E.E.K.; Evenson, K.R. Effectiveness of activity trackers with and without incentives to increase physical activity (TRIPPA): A randomised controlled trial. *Lancet Diabetes Endocrinol.* **2016**, *4*, 983–995. [CrossRef]
34. Mamykina, L.; Lindtner, S.; Lin, J.J.; Mamykina, L.; Lindtner, S.; Delajoux, G.; Strub, H.B. Fish'n'Steps: Encouraging Physical Activity with an Interactive Computer Game. In *Ubicomp 2006: Ubiquitous Computing*; Springer-Verlag: Berlin/Heidelberg, Germany, 2006; Volume 4206.
35. Toscos, T.; Faber, A.; Connelly, K.; Upoma, A.M. Encouraging physical activity in teens. Can technology help reduce barriers to physical activity in adolescent girls? In *Pervasive Computing Technologies for Healthcare, 2008*; IEEE: Tampere, Finland, 2008; Volume 3, pp. 218–221.
36. Wang, J.; Chen, R.; Sun, X.; She, M.F.H.; Wu, Y. Recognizing human daily activities from accelerometer signal. *Procedia Eng.* **2011**, *15*, 1780–1786. [CrossRef]
37. Li, X.; Dunn, J.; Salins, D.; Zhou, G.; Zhou, W.; Rose, S.M.S.; Perelman, D.; Colbert, E.; Runge, R.; Rego, S.; et al. Digital Health: Tracking Physiomes and Activity Using Wearable Biosensors Reveals Useful Health-Related Information. *PLoS Biol.* **2017**, *15*, e2001402. [CrossRef] [PubMed]
38. Catal, C.; Tufekci, S.; Pirmit, E.; Kocabag, G. On the use of ensemble of classifiers for accelerometer-based activity recognition. *Appl. Soft Comput. J.* **2015**, *37*, 1018–1022. [CrossRef]
39. Maman, Z.S.; Yazdi, M.A.A.; Cavuoto, L.A.; Megahed, F.M. A data-driven approach to modeling physical fatigue in the workplace using wearable sensors. *Appl. Ergon.* **2017**, *65*, 515–529. [CrossRef] [PubMed]
40. Mollee, J.S.; Middelweerd, A.; te Velde, S.J.; Klein, M.C.A. Evaluation of a personalized coaching system for physical activity: User appreciation and adherence. In Proceedings of ACM 11th EAI International Conference on Pervasive Computing Technologies for Healthcare, Barcelona, Spain, 23–26 May 2017.
41. Gerdes, M.; Martinez, S.; Tjondronegoro, D. Conceptualization of a Personalized eCoach for Wellness Promotion. In Proceedings of ACM 11th EAI International Conference on Pervasive Computing, Barcelona, Spain, 23–26 May 2017.
42. den Akker, H.O.; Jones, V.M.; Hermens, H.J. Tailoring real-time physical activity coaching systems: A literature survey and model. *User Model. User-Adapt. Interact.* **2014**, *24*, 351–392. [CrossRef]
43. van, M.W.; Ittersum, H.K.E.O.; de Groot, M. Self-Tracking-Supported Health Promotion: A Randomized Trial among Dutch Employees. *Eur. J. Public Heal.* **2017**, in press.
44. Wolpert, D.H. The Lack of A Priori Distinctions Between Learning Algorithms. *Neural Comput.* **1996**, *8*, 1341–1390. [CrossRef]
45. Raschka, S.; Mirjalili, V. *Python Machine Learning*; Packt Publishing Ltd.: Birmingham, UK, 2015.
46. Scikit Learn, Choosing the Right Estimator. Available online: http://scikit-learn.org/stable/tutorial/machine_learning_map/index.html (accessed on 15 February 2018).
47. Machine Learning Algorithm Cheat Sheet for Microsoft Azure Machine Learning Studio. Available online: https://docs.microsoft.com/en-us/azure/machine-learning/studio/algorithm-cheat-sheet (accessed on 15 February 2018).
48. scikit-learn v0.18. Available online: http://scikit-learn.org/0.18/documentation.html (accessed on 15 February 2018).
49. Anaconda. Available online: www.anaconda.com (accessed on 15 February 2018).
50. Jupyter Notebooks. Available online: https://jupyter.org (accessed on 15 February 2018).
51. Oracle Express Edition 11g2. Available online: http://www.oracle.com/technetwork/database/database-technologies/express-edition/overview/index.html (accessed on 15 February 2018).
52. Flask. Available online: http://flask.pocoo.org/ (accessed on 15 February 2018).
53. Chan, C.B.; Ryan, D.A.; Tudor-Locke, C. Relationship between objective measures of physical activity and weather: a longitudinal study. *Int. J. Behav. Nutr. Phys. Act.* **2006**, *3*, 21. [CrossRef] [PubMed]
54. Fogg, B. A behavior model for persuasive design. In Proceedings of the 4th International Conference on Persuasive Technology (Persuasive '09), Claremont, CA, USA, 26–29 April 2009; p. 1.
55. Blok, J.; Dol, A.; Dijkhuis, T. Toward a Generic Personalized Virtual Coach for Self-management: A Proposal for an Architecture. In Proceedings of eTELEMED 2017, the Ninth International Conference on eHealth, Telemedicine, and Social Medicine, Nice, France, 19–23 March 2017.

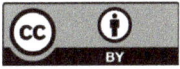

© 2018 by the authors. Licensee MDPI, Basel, Switzerland. This article is an open access article distributed under the terms and conditions of the Creative Commons Attribution (CC BY) license (http://creativecommons.org/licenses/by/4.0/).

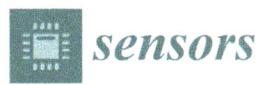

Article

Active2Gether: A Personalized m-Health Intervention to Encourage Physical Activity

Michel C. A. Klein, Adnan Manzoor and Julia S. Mollee *

Department of Computer Science, Vrije Universiteit Amsterdam, De Boelelaan 1081, 1081 HV Amsterdam, The Netherlands; m.c.a.klein@vu.nl (M.C.A.K.); a.manzoor@vu.nl (A.M.)
* Correspondence: j.s.mollee@vu.nl; Tel.: +31-20-598-7743

Received: 5 May 2017; Accepted: 13 June 2017; Published: 19 June 2017

Abstract: Lack of physical activity is an increasingly important health risk. Modern mobile technology, such as smartphones and digital measurement devices, provides new opportunities to tackle physical inactivity. This paper describes the design of a system that aims to encourage young adults to be more physically active. The system monitors the user's behavior, uses social comparison and provides tailored and personalized feedback based on intelligent reasoning mechanisms. As the name suggests, social processes play an important role in the Active2Gether system. The design choices and functioning of the system are described in detail. Based on the experiences with the development and deployment of the system, a number of lessons learnt are provided and suggestions are proposed for improvements in future developments.

Keywords: e-coaching; m-health intervention; personalization; healthy lifestyle; physical activity

1. Introduction

Physical inactivity is an increasingly serious health problem: the World Health Organization (WHO) has identified that it is the fourth leading risk factor for global mortality [1]. The organization estimates that a lack of physical activity leads to 3.2 million deaths per year globally. Physical inactivity has all to do with modern sedentary lifestyles, which are led by 60% to 85% of people worldwide, according to the WHO. One aspect of a sedentary lifestyle is that people are more inclined to passive modes of transportation. Active travelling modes such as biking and walking can contribute to a healthy level of physical activity [2]. Another aspect of a sedentary lifestyle is related to the work environment, where much work is done by people seated in chairs in front of computers. Research suggests that having desk jobs increases health risks up to 50%. Integrating small activities in work routines can help to increase physical activity and lower health risks [3].

At the same time, modern mobile technology, such as smartphones and digital measurement devices, provides new opportunities to tackle physical inactivity. In 2015, 43% of the adults worldwide owned a smartphone, with percentages up to 70% for developed countries [4]. Smartphones allow for continuous and real-time monitoring of activity behavior via built-in sensors such as accelerometers, and provide possibilities for giving contextualized and personalized feedback. This makes the smartphone a potentially powerful device for real-time coaching of people towards a more active lifestyle. To use smartphones and sensors for this aim, they should be integrated into a behavior change support system, which is defined as an information system designed to form, alter, or reinforce attitudes or behaviors [5].

In this paper, we describe the design of such a system in detail, together with lessons learnt and suggestions for future developments. The system is developed in context of an interdisciplinary research project and is called Active2Gether. The goal of the project is to combine domain knowledge from experts in physical activity interventions with modern mobile technology to design an intervention that encourages physical activity among healthy young adults. One of the innovative aspects of the system is that it exploits model-based reasoning techniques for tailoring the coaching to the needs of the user. Up to now, this has hardly been applied within existing interventions [6].

As the name suggests, social processes play an important role in the Active2Gether system. This is reflected in different ways, such as the implementation of social comparison mechanisms on both an individual and a group level. In addition, the system addresses psychological constructs as social norms and social aspects of outcome expectations in its coaching messages.

The aim of the Active2Gether system is to increase or maintain levels of physical activity among young adults in the age group of 18 to 30 years. The system is being evaluated in a trial (see [7] for a detailed description) in which over 100 participants, aged between 18 and 30 years old, used either a variant of the Active2Gether system or the standard website that belongs to a commercial activity tracker for approximately three months. The user evaluation of the system by the participants is described in [8]; in this paper, we focus on the architecture and functionality of the system.

2. System Description

To the user, the Active2Gether system presents itself as an Android-based mobile phone app that continuously monitors the context of a person. One of the distinct features of the system is that it implements evidence-based behavior change techniques, unlike most apps that are currently available in the app stores [9]. The most promising behavior change techniques are employed in the app, including self-monitoring, performance feedback, goal setting and social comparison.

The app performs four main functions: it communicates with the user about his/her objectives regarding physical activity for the next week, provides timely and personalized feedback, facilitates self-monitoring based on several collected data sources, and supports social comparison with the help of Facebook friendship relations. The system focuses on three types of physical activity: leisure time sports activities, active transport and stair walking. Users can choose to be coached on at most one of these three domains at the same time.

In the following sections, we describe the design of the system in detail. We first describe the data that are collected by the system. We then provide an overview of the architecture of the system and describe the layout choices. After that, we explain the working of the reasoning engine and the selection and filtering of coaching messages. Finally, we describe the implementation of the social comparison functionality.

2.1. Data Collection

The system uses several mechanisms to collect information from and about the users. Below, we describe how questionnaires as well as sensor measurements are used to understand the user behavior.

2.1.1. Intake Questionnaires

The user starts with filling in an online intake questionnaire. Besides demographic information, this questionnaire asks about their significant locations (such as home, work, study, etc.), their travel options between these locations, and psychological factors underlying their physical activity behavior (e.g., skills, barriers, goals, and outcome expectations). The answers to these questions are used for tailoring the messages to the user's personal situation and are used in the model-based reasoning about the effect of specific coaching strategies on a specific user (see Section 2.4).

2.1.2. Activity Tracker

The commercial Fitbit One is used as activity tracker that registers the daily number of steps and the number of stairs climbed [10]. Users receive an account on the Fitbit website. The Fitbit device uses Bluetooth LE to automatically synchronize activity data with the Fitbit servers, either via the Fitbit mobile phone app, or via a Bluetooth LE dongle and a pc. After the first login to the Active2Gether system, the user is asked to connect to his/her Fitbit account with the Active2Gether system. A connection is established through an open authentication mechanism. Once the connection is made, Fitbit provides an authentication key for the user. This key is stored in the database, so the Active2Gether system can directly access the Fitbit web service to receive activity data for a user and store it into the Active2Gether database. A script runs every hour to update the database with the most recent activity data. Another script periodically checks whether the battery level is low or whether the last synchronization is more than three days ago, and, in that case, a reminder is sent.

2.1.3. GPS Location

The Active2Gether app uses the built-in GPS sensor for recording the GPS coordinates (latitude and longitude). As soon as a user logs in, he is asked to authorize the use of location tracking. It is possible for a user to turn off the location detection option, but this will disable certain features. In a separate experiment, we compared different time intervals for collecting GPS data [11]. It turned out that a frequency of five minutes provides a good balance between battery consumption and precision. Every 15 min, the data on the mobile phone are synchronized with the server. In the database, latitude, longitude, speed, accuracy and time stamp are stored for each observation.

A script runs every night to see whether a user has visited one of his important locations by comparing the GPS trace with the coordinates of the important locations. Since the user locations are provided in descriptive form, geocoding is used to transform them into latitude and longitude numbers. The system stores the number of minutes at each of the locations. If the duration at a location is larger than 0 min, we can conclude that the user visited that location.

2.1.4. Daily Questions

Every day, a number of questions is posed to the user via the app. Information about the visited locations is used to prompt the user about the travel options that he used to go there. As the users had to list two options (active and inactive) in the intake questionnaire, they are asked to choose between these two options. Since the system is aware of the activity level of the different options for each user, it can derive the types of transport used and the amount of active travel minutes.

In addition, the user is prompted about the sports activities during the day before. When a user regularly answers that he did not participate in sports activities, the frequency of asking about sports is decreased to once per week.

2.2. Architecture

The system is comprised of five main components: (1) an app on a mobile phone; (2) a commercial activity tracker; (3) a database with user (activity) data and persuasive messages; (4) a model-based reasoning engine to interpret the data and predict the effect of different coaching strategies; and (5) a communication engine that selects and sends questions and messages to the app. Figure 1 shows those main components.

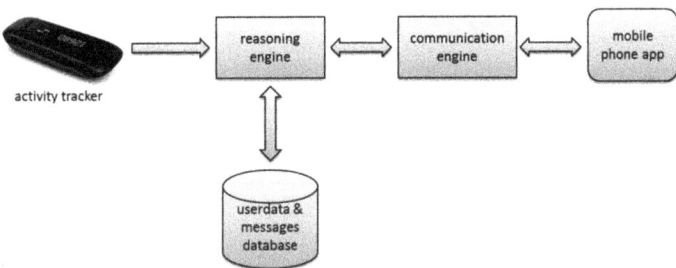

Figure 1. Overall architecture of the Active2Gether system.

Figure 2 provides an overview of the most important data flows in the system. The details are provided in the following sections.

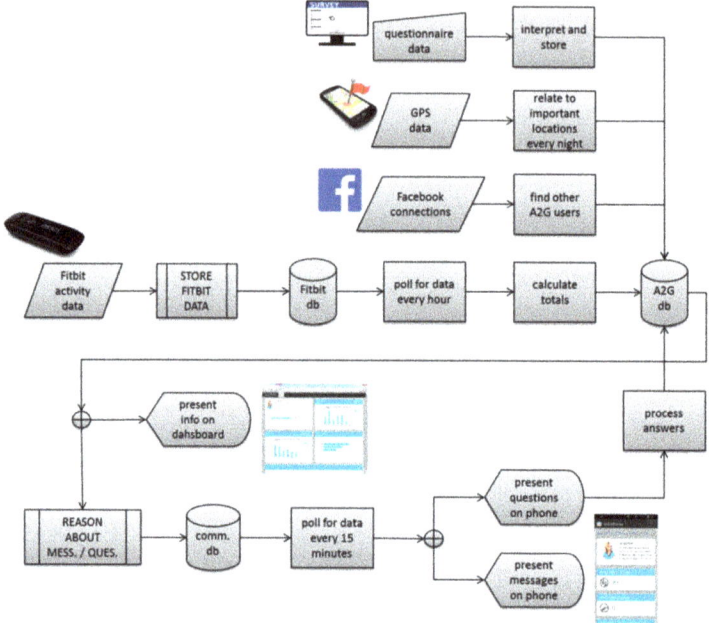

Figure 2. Overall data flow in the Active2Gether system.

Structure of the App

In order to provide users the possibility to also view their information via a website, the main dashboard of the system is developed as a web page. Within the app, the main component is a GUI element (i.e., a WebView component) that renders this web-based dashboard. Since a responsive web design approach is followed, the website automatically adapts to smaller screen sizes. Although the dashboard is actually a website, users do not notice this. The app behaves like a native app and users do not need to login separately via the WebView: once a user has registered his/her account for the Active2Gether system in the Android system, the app uses those credentials to automatically log in the user and to show the appropriate page inside the WebView component as if it is a screen in the app itself.

The other functions of the mobile phone app are to facilitate the communication with the user and to monitor the user's location. The latter is done with the help of Google location services. Using the built-in Android synchronization system, the app connects every 15 min via a web service to the communication engine of the system. Messages or questions that are prepared for the user by the reasoning engine are collected and answers and read notifications are sent back. Whenever a new message or question is sent to a user, it appears in the status bar and when the user clicks on the message, it is shown as an overlay on the main screen.

2.3. Layout and Visual Design

In order to show a consistent look and feel to the user, a professional designer was hired to design and recommend different aspects of the user interface. The designer helped in suggesting layout, fonts and a coloring scheme for the website and consequently the dashboard of the app. There are eight panels (small rectangular windows) on the website, which show different kinds of information to the user depending on the chosen coaching domain for the current week. The first panel shows a picture of the coach and a welcome message corresponding to the current coaching domain. For example, if the current coaching domain is active transportation, the message is: *"Hi Adnan! You have chosen to focus on active transportation this week. Your goal is to spend this week at least 36 minutes of active transportation. I will support your efforts."* The activity data are presented in many different views. Two small panels show the most recent steps and floors count for the present day. Whenever a user visits the website or opens the app, a dynamic script runs to show a summary of the most recent data in the Active2Gether database.

A panel with the caption "Progress to weekly step goal" shows a progress bar towards a weekly goal of 70,000 steps. There is another panel that shows the performance of other users (see Section 2.6 about social comparison below). Another panel shows the type of physical activity based on the chosen domain for the current week (active transport, stair walking or sports activities). In the first week, when no domain has been chosen yet, this panel shows the number of active minutes based on the reported sports activities and active travel choices. A similar panel shows the user's activity in terms of the number of steps. The latter two panels provide an option to the user to view historical data per week, per month or from the beginning. This option is useful for those users who want to see their own past performances. They also provide the user an opportunity to compare his/her performance with the average values of all users. The final panel is dedicated to show the most recent messages. Figure 3 gives an example of the dashboard.

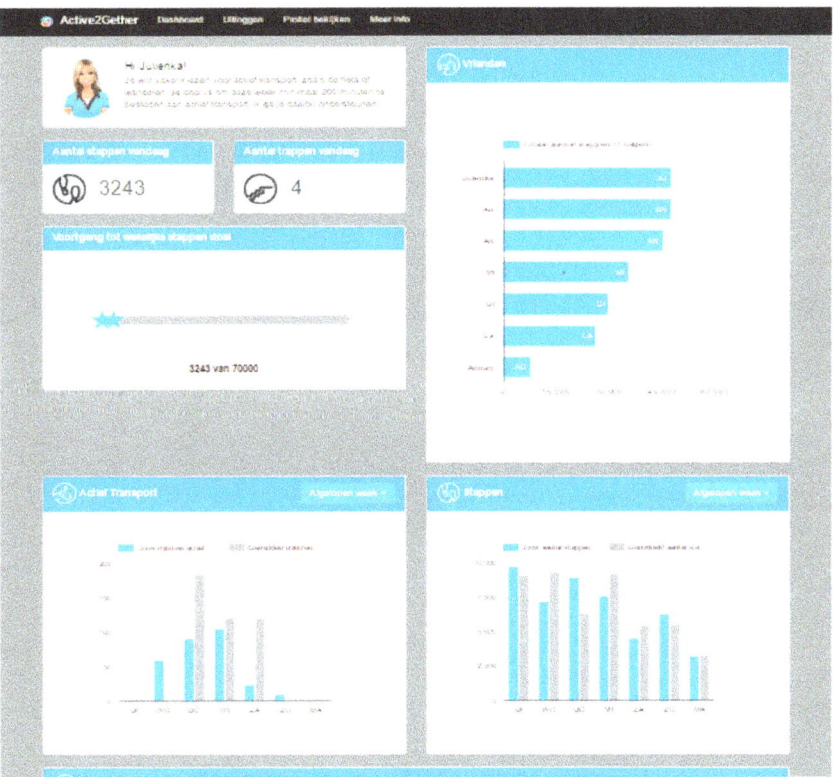

Figure 3. Screenshot of an Active2Gether dashboard.

2.4. Model-Based Reasoning

One of the fundamental components of the Active2Gether system is the so-called reasoning engine, which analyzes and interprets the user's data and determines what type of support the user should receive. A core component of this reasoning engine is a computational model, which is discussed below. The reasoning process can be split up into three parts: assessing the user's activity and awareness level, suggesting a coaching domain based on hypothesized room for improvement, and predicting the most promising coaching determinants. Figure 4 shows a flow chart of the processes taking place in the reasoning engine.

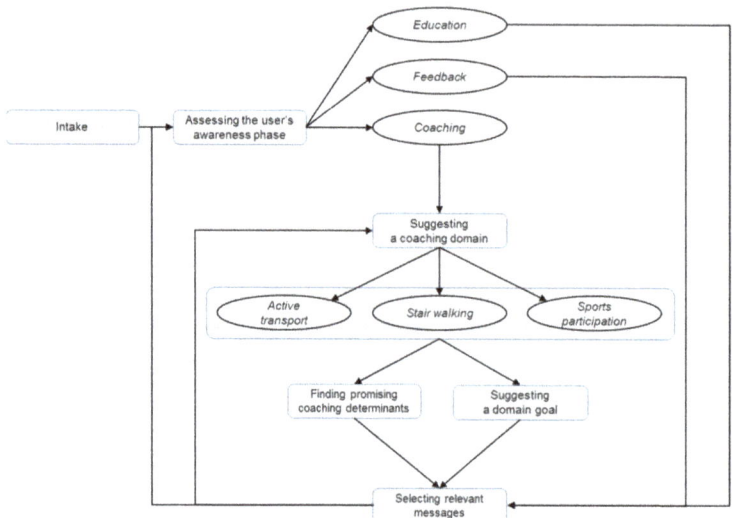

Figure 4. Process flow chart of reasoning engine.

2.4.1. Assessing the User's Awareness Phase

In the first step of the reasoning engine, the user's current activity level and awareness phase are assessed to determine what type of support they need. The assessment is based on two evaluations of the user's physical activity level, namely an objective evaluation (i.e., whether the user meets the norm) and a subjective evaluation (i.e., whether the user thinks he/she is sufficiently physically active). Using that information, the user is assigned to one of four categories, each representing an awareness state regarding their physical activity. The resulting categories are summarized in Table 1. Category 1, in which users believe that they are sufficiently active but objectively do not meet the norm, is more or less comparable with the *precontemplation* phase in Prochaska's Transtheoretical Model of behavior change [12]. In this phase, people are uninformed or under informed about the consequences of their behavior and education about the consequences is needed. Category 4 is similar to the *maintenance* phase, while Categories 2 and 3 are comparable to the *action* phase in Prochaska's model. Because our system can objectively measure whether people meet the norm, we can determine an awareness phase in a simpler and more accurate way than with the questions that are often used for determining the stage according to the transtheoretical model, and without the strong assumption that people always go through all phases.

Table 1. User categories based on objective/subjective evaluation.

No.	Objective	Subjective	User Category
1	Insufficient	Sufficient	The user is unaware that he/she is insufficiently physically active, and will be *educated* to increase this awareness.
2	Insufficient	Insufficient	The user is aware that he/she is insufficiently physically active, and will be *coached* to increase his/her physical activity level.
3	Sufficient	Insufficient	The user is sufficiently physically active, but still wants to be *coached* to increase his/her physical activity level.
4	Sufficient	Sufficient	The user is sufficiently physically active, and wants to maintain his/her physical activity level. This user will not be coached to increase his/her physical activity level, but only receive *feedback*.

Based on the categorization of the awareness of users, the system determines which type of support (i.e., *education*, *coaching* or *feedback*) the user needs. This assessment is reflected in the type of motivational messages that the user receives from the app (see also Section 2.5). In addition, for users who receive coaching, the system guides them to choose a coaching domain, prompts them to set a specific goal, and predicts the most promising coaching determinants, as further explained below. This evaluation is repeated every three weeks, in order to continuously tailor the system to the user's current state. Thus, instead of treating all users the same, their specific needs and wishes are taken into account. This should lead to improved user acceptance and adherence, and consequently to increased effectiveness of the intervention [13].

2.4.2. Suggesting a Coaching Domain and Goal

Users that are assigned to the coaching category are guided by the Active2Gether system to focus their behavior change efforts, by advising on the choice of a specific coaching domain and a goal. This cycle is repeated on a weekly basis. The coaching domains are parts of the user's daily life: (1) stair use at significant locations (e.g., home, work, and university); (2) active transport to significant locations; and (3) leisure-time sports activities.

First, detailed information about the user's context and behavior is used to identify in which domains the user could be more physically active. The user's physical activity in each of the three domains is estimated based on a combination of activity data collected through the activity monitor (number of stairs climbed) and daily user input through the app (selected transport options to visited locations, time spent on sports activities). These physical activity values are then evaluated by comparing them to estimated "maximum" or "ideal" values, which are based on information about the user's context and visits to their important locations. This context information is collected through an intake questionnaire, and includes information about the addresses of their significant locations, (active and non-active) travel options between these locations, relevant floor numbers on these locations, and the availability of stairs. For example, if a user works on the third floor and on average climbs another three floors during the day, a total number of six floors during a work day would be reasonable. For a user that works on the second floor, but on average climbs another eight floors during a work day, a total number of six floors is comparatively low. In addition, the more often the user has gone to work, the higher the expected number of stairs becomes. Similar evaluations are developed for the physical activity level in active transport and sports activities. Using these evaluations, the domain with the largest potential for improvement can be detected, as the evaluation score for that domain will be lowest. This domain is then suggested to the user as focus for the coaching in the upcoming week. However, the user is allowed to overrule this suggestion and opt for another domain.

After selection of a coaching domain, the user is asked to set a specific goal for this coaching domain, i.e., weekly time spent on active transport, weekly time spent on sports or daily number of stairs climbed. If users did meet the previous goal in this coaching domain, the system suggests increasing their goal by 10%. If users did not meet the goal last time, the system advises to keep the goal at the same level. Again, to ensure the user's autonomy, the final decision on the goal is up to the user.

This relative evaluation of the user's behavior and the recommendation of a certain coaching domain respect the individuality of the users more than general physical activity guidelines. It prevents the system from imposing the same expectations on all users, even though their personal situations may be completely different.

2.4.3. Finding the Most Promising Coaching Determinants

Once the coaching domain is selected, the system investigates on which personal determinants the coaching messages should focus to yield the most promising effect on the desired behavior. These behavioral determinants are personal psychological concepts that govern the engagement in healthy behavior. The system contains a large collection of coaching messages, with subsets that each target one of the personal determinants. The messages are based on established behavior change techniques, such as prompting barrier identification, providing information on consequences, and prompting goal setting [7].

In order to determine what messages are most likely to positively affect the user's behavior, the effects of improving each one of the personal determinants are estimated based on simulations of a dynamic computational model. This model is a formalization of the dynamics between these personal determinants and the behavior, where each of the concepts is represented by a numerical value in range [0, 1]. The model is mainly based on the social cognitive theory, that describes the reasons why people fail or succeed to exhibit some desired (health) behavior from both social and cognitive determinants [14,15]. Other theories (e.g., self-regulation theory and health action process approach) and literature were consulted to extend the model to incorporate more relevant aspects. The model that was implemented in the Active2Gether system is an adaptation of the computational model presented in [16]. Revisions between the two versions of the model were motivated by a decrease in conceptual detail and computational complexity of the model, and by suggestions of experts in the domain of behavior change. The resulting model contains determinants such as intentions, self-efficacy and outcome expectations. The values of all parameters in the model can be adjusted by the modeler. In the current implementation, the parameters were chosen based on correlations between the concepts found in literature [17–19]. We performed simulations to find values that keep the ratio between the parameters in accordance with empirical findings [20]. A more detailed description and a preliminary validation of this model on empirical data, which showed promising results, can be found in [21]. Figure 5 shows a graphical representation of the computational model.

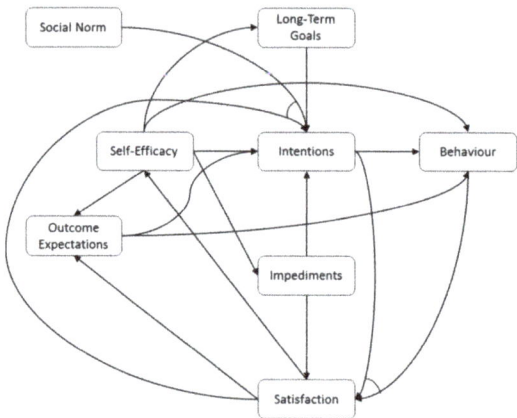

Figure 5. Graphical representation of the computational model.

The simulation process starts with estimating the current states of the personal determinants by means of short questions via the app. The resulting values are used as input for the computational model. To simulate the effect of targeting one of the determinants, one of the values obtained from the app questionnaire is increased according to the hypothesized effect of sending coaching messages about this determinant. Then, the computational model simulates the dynamics between the determinants and estimates the effect on the behavior. By running simulations for each possible targeted determinant, a list of determinants is constructed, ordered by the most promising effect on the behavior variable. This order is taken into account when selecting coaching messages to the user. As with the selection of a coaching domain and goal, the simulation cycle is repeated weekly, in order to tailor to the user's strongest psychological needs at all times.

In contrast to the relative evaluation of the user's behavior for suggesting a coaching domain, this part of the reasoning engine does not tailor the intervention based on information about the user's environment, but rather on information about his/her motivational state of mind. This way, the users will receive support on the aspects that are relevant to their motivation and behavior.

2.5. Selection and Tailoring of Coaching Messages

Once the order of the most promising coaching strategies is established (as described in Section 2.4.3), all necessary elements to send the coaching messages are in place. As explained before, each coaching strategy represents a set of messages targeting one of the concepts from the computational model. The messages are based on established behavior change techniques (e.g., prompting specific goal setting, time management; see [22] for a complete taxonomy), while also taking into account user preferences [23]. They were written to be motivational, personally relevant and trustworthy, and were annotated with restrictions for the circumstances under which they are relevant (e.g., day and time, the user's awareness phase and coaching domain, the user's perceptions reported in the intake questionnaire). A detailed description of the techniques that are applied in the messages and the related determinants is provided in [7]. The messages are sent up to three times a day. In order to send a message, it has to be selected from the set of available messages and (if applicable) tailored to the user.

At given moments in time, the communication engine of the system checks for messages that are relevant to send to the user. Selecting a message is based on elimination: starting from the set of all messages, the selection is narrowed down by filtering inapt or irrelevant messages. As explained in Section 2.4, the user is already assigned an awareness phase and has chosen a coaching domain. In addition, a coaching determinant is picked from the ordered list, with a probability relative to its position in the list. This probability is introduced to increase diversity in the messages during the week. Then, all messages that are aimed at other awareness phases, coaching domains or targeted coaching determinants are filtered out. The system checks for other aspects of the message's relevance as well, such as the day and time, the user's occupational status, answers to questions in the intake questionnaire, whether the user is on track to reach their goal and the current weather.

Once a message is selected, if there are open fields, they have to be filled in to tailor the message to the user and context. In order to increase relatedness, most messages address the user with their first name. Additionally, some messages are completed by filling out the user's current daily number of steps or stairs, their accumulated weekly time spent on sports or active transport, their weekly goal, the percentage of their weekly goal they have reached so far, the maximum number of stairs they would consider to walk, or the current weather score.

The coaching strategies are only relevant if the user is in the coaching phase (see Section 2.4), as only then certain determinants from the computational model are targeted. However, also when users are in the education phase or in the feedback phase, they receive messages on a regular basis. In the education phase, users receive messages that put their (insufficient) performance into perspective, as well as messages that emphasize the need for and benefits of physical activity. In the feedback phase, users receive positive feedback on their satisfactory behavior. In addition, users in all awareness

2.6. Social Comparison

The Active2Gether system uses social comparison, as one of the core ideas behind the system is that a healthy lifestyle can be maintained and achieved in the presence of social support network. Social comparison is implemented in two ways in the Active2Gether system, namely on a group level and on an individual level. On the group level, social comparison is implemented by showing group averages adjacent to the user's physical activity data in the graphs on the dashboard. This allows the user to compare his/her daily performance to other Active2Gether users anonymously.

On the individual level, social comparison is implemented as a ranking of the user's performance within a list of other users, which is shown in one of the panels in the app/website. The ranking automatically updates every time a user visits the website or opens the app. Overall physical activity is used as basis for the comparison, which is determined by the number of steps taken by an individual in the last seven days, but implementations based on activity data for one of the coaching domains are also conceivable.

In order to increase the relevance of the comparative data, the system tries to show actual friends of the user in the ranking. To do so, it extracts friendship relations from Facebook. Facebook is an obvious choice, since it is one of the most popular social media websites globally and also very popular among Dutch young adults. A connection to the Facebook Graph API is established through an open authentication mechanism. As a new user logs in for the first time on the system, it asks the user whether he/she wants to grant access to Active2Gether to check for friendships with other Active2Gether users. If permission is granted and a match is found, the friendship connection is also registered in the Active2Gether system. It is not mandatory for users to grant access, but individuals who do not opt for such explicit social comparison can only observe the activities of other users anonymously, which will probably make the social comparison less effective.

Social comparison can be either *upward* or *downward*, depending on whether an individual compares to targets that perform better or worse. Both variants address different underlying motivational processes. Upward comparison can be beneficial if individuals use the target as a role model and motivation to self-improve, but it can have a discouraging effect if the target's performance seems unattainable [24,25]. Downward comparison can boost an individual's self-esteem and thereby lay the groundwork for self-improvement [26]. However, downward comparison could also have an adverse effect, since it leads to relatively low goals and since it does not challenge an individual to minimize the discrepancy with a better performing individual. An experiment testing the effects of presenting people with their preferred or opposite direction of social comparison in the domain of physical activity showed that it is important to take personal preferences into account [27]. Participants who were shown the type of social comparison opposite to their preference showed a decrease in overall physical activity. Showing the preferred direction of social comparison typically resulted in an upward trend, which was not statistically significant however. Even though the preferences were based on a simple question (whether the participants prefer to compare themselves to individuals who perform better or worse) and the sample size was small, the results demonstrated that these preferences matter: if not to enhance the motivational effects of social comparison, then at least to avoid the potential adverse effects of social comparison [27].

When creating the ranking, the Active2Gether system takes the social comparison preference (upward or downward) of the users into account. The comparison preference of users was determined in the intake questionnaire with the same question as in the experiment described above [27]. The system first tries to find up to six friends whose activity level is in line with the preferred comparison direction. If there are more than six friends that match the preferred direction, the six friends that are closest to the current user in terms of step total of the last seven days are selected. If there are less than six friends in the preferred direction, the system selects other users in the preferred direction. If not sufficient people are found to create the ranking, then the system searches for users in the opposite direction, since it is not appropriate to show an empty ranking list to the user. This could happen, for example, if an individual's preference for social comparison is upward, but his performance is among the best of the users. The data of befriended users are shown with their first name, but data of other users are shown with their initials only, to maintain a level of anonymity. Figure 6 shows the step-by-step process of selecting the friends or other users to show in the ranking.

```
Goal: show up to 7 users in total: the actual user plus maximum 6 other users

// select up to 6 friends most suited for the comparison
IF preference = downward:
    • select up to 6 friends with a lower total step count than the user ordered from high to
      low
ELSE IF preference = upward:
    • select up to 6 friends with a higher total step count than the user ordered from low to
      high
RESULTING_#FRIENDS = number of selected friends

IF RESULTING_#FRIENDS < 6 users:
    // add other users until there are 6 other users shown in total
    IF preference = downward:
        • select all users with a lower step total than the user, and then select the top
          (6 - RESULTING_#FRIENDS) of that list
    ELSE IF preference = upward:
        • select all users with a higher step total than the user, and then select the bottom
          (6 - RESULTING_#FRIENDS) of that list
Merge resulting list with list of friends
RESULTING_#USERS = number of user in list

IF RESULTING_#USERS < 6 users:
    IF preference = downward:
        • select all users with a higher step total than the user, and then select the
          bottom (6 - RESULTING_#USERS) of that list
    ELSE IF preference = upward:
        • select all users with a lower step total than the user, and then select the top
          (6 - RESULTING_#USERS) of that list

Order the resulting list from highest to lowest step count
Show the full name of the friends
Show the other users anonymized (only initials)
```

Figure 6. Algorithm for selecting users for the social comparison.

3. Discussion

In this section, we offer suggestions for improvements based on our experiences with the development and use of the current Active2Gether system.

3.1. Data Collection

Advances in (mobile) technology open up ways to improve the location and travel monitoring in the Active2Gether system.

First, for determining modes of transportation, we currently use daily questions in combination with location data (i.e., prompted user input). At the time of the design, this was a reasonable choice, considering the state-of-the-art and the consequences on battery consumption during full-time use of accelerometers in the mobile phone. Nowadays, the Google Activity Recognition API and the iOS CM Motion Activity class would be logical candidates, as they are the de-facto standards for providing location information [28,29]. Power consumption remains an important issue, however.

Second, we used a complicated questionnaire for reporting significant locations and their characteristics (such as relevant floors). It is difficult and cumbersome to answer, and also difficult to update during the intervention. Therefore, we recommend to automatically detect significant locations [11], which can also be done via Google location services. A remaining drawback, however, is that the users are required to provide this privacy-sensitive information.

3.2. Architecture

The decision to use a combination of a web-based approach and a native app, which requires more-or-less permanent Internet connection, turned out well. Most users in the Netherlands apparently have good Internet connections on their phones. A drawback of our current choice was that integration with third-party APIs (i.e., Fitbit and Facebook authentication) was difficult, since Fitbit does not allow using their authentication API through the WebView. This can be solved with the newer Chrome tabs approach.

We decided to copy the data from Fitbit servers to our own database: a Cron job runs periodically to fetch the data through a web service. The advantage is that we could do our analyses more easily (e.g., summarizing the data for different time periods every hour) and have a good performance when we query the data. A disadvantage is that the information sometimes lags behind. If the performance is sufficient, we would recommend to dynamically invoke a web service at runtime. Another possible solution is the use of the use of more advanced services, such as the Fitbit subscription API, which allows sending notification to our system when new data are available.

Related to the point above, we let participants use the Fitbit app to synchronize their data with the activity tracker. This was necessary because it is not possible to read out the Fitbit device directly. As a consequence, the Fitbit app or a computer was needed in addition to our own system. It also required an additional step in the initialization, as users had to create an account on the Fitbit website. For future applications, direct communication between the coaching system and activity trackers is preferred; however, this is likely not easy with commercially available trackers.

We have decided to partly develop a native app for Android. A native app was necessary for implementing the location detection. New developments in standardization of location detection APIs and more advanced techniques for platform-independent development might result in a different choice, which could enlarge the potential user base. Another option would be to use the Google Fit API for getting information about the activity of users. Since its introduction, many systems and wearables directly integrate with this service.

3.3. Layout and Visual Design

Although the user interface of the app was designed in collaboration with a graphic designer, we put only minimal effort in its design. We did not receive any signs that this hampered the use of the app, but we imagine that following the design guidelines of the respective platform (Android and iOS) would improve the users' perception.

3.4. Model-Based Reasoning

Some of the design choices in the personalization process described in Section 2.4 seem successful, but we identified opportunities for improvement in others. Our findings on these elements of the Active2Gether system are described below.

Based on anecdotic feedback, we conclude that determining the user's awareness phase by comparing their actual behavior to their perception works well. Acknowledging the users' awareness of the need to change is a useful way of tailoring the coaching messages.

In contrast, the suggestion of a coaching domain could be improved. The current approach is not very flexible, as the scores for active transport and stair walking are based on the characteristics of the significant locations that were identified via the intake questionnaire. Any physical activity related to these domains on other locations is ignored during the evaluation of the user's behavior.

Since that activity is not taken into account for either the actual behavior or the "ideal" behavior, this simplification should not distort the behavior scores. However, it is recommended to also take behavior on (or during transit to) other locations into account, to get a more complete picture of the user's behavior. This could be achieved by using more adaptive behavior evaluation algorithms, which learn the user's potential or ideal from past behavior, possibly in combination with other (web) sources.

Part of the selection of coaching messages is based on the simulations of a computational model. Although a preliminary validation of the model showed very promising results [21], the added value of the model in predicting the most effective coaching determinants still has to be evaluated. In theory, an adaptive approach can be used to learn the effect of specific (sets of) messages on a person's behavior, which might lead to better suggestions for coaching determinants. The outcome of evaluating the model could for example lead to the decision to use personal and adaptive parameters in the computational model, or to take an entirely different approach (e.g., machine learning techniques).

3.5. Selection and Tailoring of Coaching Messages

The messages that people receive are very diverse, but sometimes still give the impression that they are redundant or not on topic. For a more detailed investigation of the user experience of the messages, see [8]. We have a number of suggestions for improvement.

First, the personal relevance of the messages could be improved. For example, the messages are only sent at specific times during the day, but the users' physical location could be used to trigger messages as well. Furthermore, the selection of messages to be sent could be based on more complex combinations of information. For instance, combining the current location with the relevant floors on that location and the availability of stairs and the maximum number of stairs that a user is willing to walk. Incorporating these ideas would increase the context-awareness of the system. In addition, the messages should contain less trivial content in order to better fit the expectations of the target group.

Next, we implemented the selection of the message to be sent in such a way that the system sends the message that has been sent the longest time ago. However, if only a few messages are relevant, the users will still receive the same messages in a short time period. Therefore, it is important to adhere to a minimum amount of time between resending the same message. In addition, the interdependence or similarity between messages should be taken into account: if messages are different formulations of the same content, the system should be aware of that. If such improvements imply that a user does not receive any coaching messages for some period of time, the system could observe this and send a warning to the developers to make sure that this lack of relevant messages is noticed and possibly remedied.

Finally, the coaching messages could be improved by implementing a feedback mechanism. Instead of only being able to click "OK" to close a message, the user could rate the message, and this feedback could be used to further tailor the system.

3.6. Social Comparison

As explained in Section 2.6, the position of users in the ranking is based on their indicated preference. If people prefer upward comparison, they are shown users who perform better, and vice versa. This implies that users are always at the top or bottom position in the overview, irrespective of their performance. Although a study has shown that it matters to take the preferred direction of social comparison into account [27], the specific implementation might still allow room for improvement. A negative consequence of the current design decision is that users may become demotivated if they do not see any acknowledgment of their efforts. Therefore, a less strict selection of other users to show in the ranking might work better to motivate users through social comparison.

In addition, social comparison is more effective if you know the people you are comparing with. If users only have a few Facebook connections that are also using the system, it is likely that they mostly see anonymized other users that they do not know. Therefore, it might be better to allow adding connections via the system directly, or to invite friends to start using the system as well. Another option could be to select similar users (in terms of occupational status, home town, gender, age, etc.) to show in the ranking, and to show and emphasize these similarities in the design, in order to strengthen the perceived closeness to the other users.

Related to this is the issue that social comparison might not be equally beneficial for all types of people. For example, it is expected that patients and individuals managing chronic conditions are not so much interested in social comparison, but could benefit from social support. Although our system targets healthy individuals, in general it is important to take such personal characteristics into account when reasoning about the specific behavior change techniques that are applied by the system to the users.

A final consideration is of ethical nature. In the current implementation, it is easily possible that user A is shown the data of user B, but not vice versa. This means that individual reciprocity of information sharing is not ensured, which could cause objections from potential users. In that case, a more sophisticated selection mechanism should be developed, in which such reciprocity is maintained.

4. Conclusions and Future Work

In this paper, we have described the design of the Active2Gether coaching system in detail. The coaching system aims to encourage physical activity among young adults by combining evidence-based behavior change techniques with elements from modern (mobile) technology, such as location monitoring and model-based reasoning.

The effectiveness of the system is currently being evaluated in a three-month trial with more than 100 participants between 18 and 30 years old. To determine the added value of the tailored messaging, a three-armed design has been chosen. One group uses the full version of the Active2Gether system, a second group uses the Active2Gether system but does not receive tailored messages, and the third group uses the standard website and app that belong to the Fitbit tracker. The participants start with an intake questionnaire that contains questions about their personal situation, their current exercise behavior and perceptions about physical activity. After three months, a similar questionnaire is sent out. The participants are also asked to wear a validated activity monitor in the first week of the intervention and after three months. This allows us to conclude whether using the system leads to a significant increase in physical activity. However, because several behavior change techniques have been employed in the system, it is difficult to identify *which* technique actually influences behavior. In the case a positive overall effect is found, we will further analyze which messages were sent to users to identify the contribution of specific techniques (focusing on specific determinants) on the behavior change. In addition, future research is needed with variants of the system in which only specific components (i.e., social comparison, self-monitoring and goal setting) are functional.

In the current paper, we have discussed the architecture and the implementation of the Active2Gether system. In addition, we have shared lessons learnt during the design, implementation and evaluation of the system, as well as recommendations for further development and improvement. We believe that these insights and the detailed description of the technological choices will prove helpful to designers and developers of healthy lifestyle interventions to produce effective and appealing coaching systems.

Acknowledgments: This research is supported by Philips and Technology Foundation STW, Nationaal Initiatief Hersenen en Cognitie NIHC under the partnership program Healthy Lifestyle Solutions (grant no. 12014). The authors would like to thank Anouk Middelweerd, Saskia J. te Velde and Aart van Halteren for their contribution to the conceptual design of the Active2Gether system.

Author Contributions: M.C.A.K., A.M. and J.S.M. conceived, designed and implemented the described system. M.C.A.K., A.M. and J.S.M. wrote the paper. All three authors contributed equally to this article, and are therefore in alphabetical order.

Conflicts of Interest: The authors declare no conflict of interest.

References

1. WHO. Physical Activity. Available online: http://www.who.int/topics/physical_activity/en/ (accessed on 13 June 2017).
2. Sahlqvist, S.; Song, Y.; Ogilvie, D. Is active travel associated with greater physical activity? The contribution of commuting and non-commuting active travel to total physical activity in adults. *Prev. Med.* **2012**, *55*, 206–211. [CrossRef] [PubMed]
3. Levine, J. Killer Chairs: How Desk Jobs Ruin Your Health. *Sci. Am.* **2014**, *311*, 34–35. [CrossRef] [PubMed]
4. Poushter, J. Smartphone Ownership and Internet Usage Continues to Climb in Emerging Economies. Available online: http://www.pewglobal.org/2016/02/22/smartphone-ownership-and-internet-usage-continues-to-climb-in-emerging-economies/ (accessed on 13 June 2017).
5. Oinas-Kukkonen, H. Behavior change support systems: A research model and agenda. In Proceedings of the International Conference on Persuasive Technology, Copenhagen, Denmark, 7–10 June 2010; pp. 4–14.
6. Mollee, J.S.; Middelweerd, A.; Kurvers, R.L. What technological features are used in smartphone apps that promote physical activity? A review and content analysis. *Pers. Ubiquitous Comput.* **2017**, in press.
7. Middelweerd, A.; te Velde, S.J.; Mollee, J.S.; Klein, M.C.A.; Brug, J. Development of Active2Gether: An app-based intervention combining evidence-based behavior change techniques with a model-based reasoning system to promote physical activity among young adults. *J. Med. Internet Res.* **2017**, in press.
8. Mollee, J.S.; Middelweerd, A.; te Velde, S.J.; Klein, M.C.A. Evaluation of a personalized coaching system for physical activity: User appreciation and adherence. In *Health-i-Coach, Intelligent Technologies for Coaching in Health, Proceedings of ACM 11th EAI International Conference on Pervasive Computing Technologies for Healthcare, Barcelona, Spain, 23–26 May 2017*; ACM Digital Library: New York, NY, USA, 2017.
9. Middelweerd, A.; Mollee, J.S.; van der Wal, C.N.; Brug, J.; te Velde, S.J. Apps to promote physical activity among adults: A review and content analysis. *Int. J. Behav. Nutr. Phys. Act.* **2014**, *11*, 97. [CrossRef] [PubMed]
10. Fitbit One. Available online: https://www.fitbit.com/one (accessed on 13 June 2017).
11. Manzoor, A.; Mollee, J.S.; van Halteren, A.T.; Klein, M.C.A. Real-life validation of methods for detecting locations, transition periods and travel modes using phone-based GPS and activity tracker data. In Proceedings of the 9th International Conference on Computational Collective Intelligence, Nicosia, Cyprus, 27–29 September 2017. in press.
12. Prochaska, J.O.; DiClemente, C.C. Transtheoretical therapy: Toward a more integrative model of change. *Psychother.: Theory Res. Pract.* **1982**, *19*, 276–288. [CrossRef]
13. Kroeze, W.; Werkman, A.; Brug, J. A systematic review of randomized trials on the effectiveness of computer-tailored education on physical activity and dietary behaviors. *Ann. Behav. Med.* **2006**, *31*, 205–223. [CrossRef] [PubMed]
14. Bandura, A. Health promotion from the perspective of social cognitive theory. *Psychol. Health* **1998**, *13*, 623–649. [CrossRef]
15. Bandura, A. Health promotion by social cognitive means. *Health Educ. Behav.* **2004**, *31*, 143–164. [CrossRef] [PubMed]
16. Mollee, J.S.; van der Wal, C.N. A computational agent model of influences on physical activity based on the social cognitive theory. In Proceedings of the PRIMA 2013: Principles and Practice of Multi-Agent Systems, Dunedin, New Zealand, 1–6 December 2013; pp. 478–485.
17. Rovniak, L.S.; Anderson, E.S.; Winett, R.A.; Stephens, R.S. Social cognitive determinants of physical activity in young adults: A prospective structural equation analysis. *Ann. Behav. Med.* **2002**, *24*, 149–156. [CrossRef] [PubMed]
18. Plotnikoff, R.C.; Lippke, S.; Courneya, K.S.; Birkett, N.; Sigal, R.J. Physical activity and social cognitive theory: A test in a population sample of adults with type 1 or type 2 diabetes. *Appl. Psychol.* **2008**, *57*, 628–643. [CrossRef]
19. Plotnikoff, R.C.; Costigan, S.A.; Karunamuni, N.; Lubans, D.R. Social cognitive theories used to explain physical activity behavior in adolescents: A systematic review and meta-analysis. *Prev. Med.* **2013**, *56*, 245–253. [CrossRef] [PubMed]
20. Mollee, J.S.; Araújo, E.F.M.; Klein, M.C.A. Exploring parameter tuning for analysis and optimization of a computational model. In Proceedings of the 30th International Conference on Industrial, Engineering, Other Applications of Applied Intelligent Systems, Arras, France, 27–30 June 2017. in press.

21. Mollee, J.S.; Klein, M.C.A. Empirical validation of a computational model of influences on physical activity behavior. In Proceedings of the 30th International Conference on Industrial, Engineering, Other Applications of Applied Intelligent Systems, Arras, France, 27–30 June 2017. in press.
22. Abraham, C.; Michie, S. A taxonomy of behavior change techniques used in interventions. *Health Psychol.* **2008**, *27*, 379. [CrossRef] [PubMed]
23. Middelweerd, A.; van der Laan, D.M.; van Stralen, M.M.; Mollee, J.S.; Stuij, M.; te Velde, S.J.; Brug, J. What features do dutch university students prefer in a smartphone application for promotion of physical activity? A qualitative approach. *Int. J. Behav. Nutr. Phys. Act.* **2015**, *12*, 31. [CrossRef] [PubMed]
24. Lockwood, P.; Kunda, Z. Superstars and me: Predicting the impact of role models on the self. *J. Pers. Soc. Psychol.* **1997**, *73*, 91. [CrossRef]
25. Maddux, J.E. Self-efficacy theory. *Self-Effic. Adapt. Adjust.* **1995**, 3–33.
26. Wills, T.A. Downward comparison principles in social psychology. *Psychol. Bull.* **1981**, *90*, 245. [CrossRef]
27. Mollee, J.S.; Klein, M.C.A. The effectiveness of upward and downward social comparison of physical activity in an online intervention. In Proceedings of the International Conference on Ubiquitous Computing and Communications and 2016 International Symposium on Cyberspace and Security (IUCC-CSS), Granada, Spain, 14–16 December 2016; pp. 109–115.
28. Google APIs for Android. Available online: https://developers.google.com/android/reference/com/google/android/gms/location/package-summary (accessed on 13 June 2017).
29. Core Motion. Available online: https://developer.apple.com/reference/coremotion (accessed on 13 June 2017).

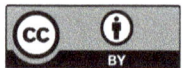

© 2017 by the authors. Licensee MDPI, Basel, Switzerland. This article is an open access article distributed under the terms and conditions of the Creative Commons Attribution (CC BY) license (http://creativecommons.org/licenses/by/4.0/).

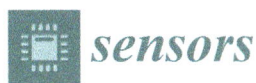

Article

The Feasibility and Usability of RunningCoach: A Remote Coaching System for Long-Distance Runners [†]

Daniel Aranki * [ID], Gao Xian Peh [ID], Gregorij Kurillo [ID] and Ruzena Bajcsy

Department of Electrical Engineering and Computer Sciences, UC Berkeley, Berkeley, CA 94720, USA; pehgaoxian@berkeley.edu (G.X.P.); gregorij@eecs.berkeley.edu (G.K.); bajcsy@eecs.berkeley.edu (R.B.)
* Correspondence: daranki@cs.berkeley.edu
† The paper extends on the work reported in Aranki, D.; Balakrishnan, U.; Sarver, H.; Serven, L.; Asuncion, C.; Du, K.; Gruis, C.; Peh, G.X.; Xiao, Y.; Bajcsy, R. RunningCoach—Cadence Training System for Long-Distance Runners. In Proceedings of 2017 Health-i-Coach—Intelligent Technologies for Coaching in Health, Barcelona, Spain, 23–26 May 2017.

Received: 1 November 2017; Accepted: 23 December 2017; Published: 10 January 2018

Abstract: Studies have shown that about half of the injuries sustained during long-distance running involve the knee. Cadence (steps per minute) has been identified as a factor that is strongly associated with these running-related injuries, making it a worthwhile candidate for further study. As such, it is critical for long-distance runners to minimize their risk of injury by running at an appropriate running cadence. In this paper, we present the results of a study on the feasibility and usability of RunningCoach, a mobile health (mHealth) system that remotely monitors running cadence levels of runners in a continuous fashion, among other variables, and provides immediate feedback to runners in an effort to help them optimize their running cadence.

Keywords: remote coaching; telemonitoring; telehealth; cadence; marathon; elevation change analysis

---

1. Introduction

Researchers have found that up to 79% of long-distance runners are expected to sustain a running-related injury in the lower extremities [1]. Such injuries could potentially be avoided if the long-distance runner runs within the boundaries of the recommended cadence throughout the entire run. Findings have shown that optimal control over one's cadence can aid the runner in reducing the impact forces on joints [2], reducing muscle soreness and fatigue [3] and increasing efficiency of oxygen use [4]; all of which reduce the possibility of injuries to the runner. Given the numerous advantages of maintaining an optimal cadence throughout a run for long-distance runners, we are interested in examining a mobile health (mHealth) solution to monitoring and coaching cadence for long-distance runners, aimed at minimizing their risk of injury.

There are many commercial apps that are widely used by runners, including MapMyFitness, Runtastic, Adidas miCoach, Nike+, RunKeeper and Endomondo [5–10]. The primary function of most of these apps is to monitor the runner's performance and to provide an interface for the runner to view statistics related to her or his runs. Some of these apps allow the runner to import workout plans that are aimed at motivating the runner and improving her or his performance. These apps, however, do not address minimizing the risk of injury, which creates a gap in the technology that we attempt to fill in this work.

To close this gap, we have designed an Android smartphone app, RunningCoach, to coach long-distance runners. In this work, we define "long-distance runners" as individuals who every week: (i) run for at least five kilometers (or three miles) in distance; or (ii) run at least one session that is one hour or longer in duration; which is the definition of the Association of Athletics Federations (IAAF). RunningCoach is designed to monitor the runner's cadence, among other parameters, and to coach her or him based on the collected data. In this paper, we discuss the design and findings of a pilot study that aimed to explore the feasibility and usability of this app. This is the first of a series of studies that aim to refine the system and validate its efficacy regarding the reduction of injuries.

This paper extends on previous published work in [11]. Our previous paper was focused on the design and implementation details of the system. In this paper, we describe a feasibility and usability study for RunningCoach and report the findings of this study. Distinctly from the previously published paper, the contributions of this paper are (i) presenting evidence for the feasibility and usability of a coaching system based on remote monitoring for long-distance running; and (ii) reporting on lessons learned that developers can rely on to build robust mobile coaching solutions for fitness and health applications.

Concretely, we aim to understand the following factors related to the use of RunningCoach. First, we study the battery consumption incurred by the app as a usability factor. Second, this work examines general usability-related scenarios that are related to the robustness of the system, such as its ability to recover from faults (e.g., server is down, lost internet connection, etc.). Third, we examine the accuracy of the system in estimating the runner's cadence, speed, and other variables, as perceived by the runner. Fourth, we examine the privacy-related aspects of using this app and study the acceptability of the users to this technology through a post-study questionnaire. Finally, we explore a possible analysis relating cadence, speed and the gradient of elevation (in the path of the run) as a potential way to assess injury-related performance, which is a gateway to future directions of this research effort.

The rest of the paper is organized as follows. In Section 2, we survey the literature on related research. Subsequently in Section 3, we describe the study objectives and the study protocol. In Section 4, we give a brief summary of the architecture and implementation of RunningCoach before presenting and discussing the results of the study in Section 5. We finally close the paper in Section 6 by reflecting on our conclusions and directions of future research.

2. Related Work

Injuries stemming from long-distance running are studied extensively in the literature. In addition, there are many commercial products available in the market that aim to assist runners to avoid injuries and to provide motivational support to lead a healthier lifestyle. These commercial products include variety of smartphone apps, often paired with wearables or insoles, that measure fitness markers such as energy expenditure, speed, distance, heart rate, and cadence (see the review of related fitness trackers in [12] and apps in [11,13,14]).

In this section, we focus on reviewing scientific literature on (i) studies that utilize remote monitoring systems for runners, (ii) studies that link running cadence to running-related injuries and (iii) studies that explore the usability and feasibility of mHealth systems in the context of running.

2.1. Monitoring Systems for Runners

Researchers have studied the effectiveness of various features present in remote monitoring systems for runners. Boratto et al. studied the effectiveness of u4fit, a human-in-the-loop remote monitoring system linking runners with professional fitness coaches to enhance runner safety and engagement [15]. Similarly, Vos et al. describe the design process and evaluation of Inspirun, a smartphone application for recreational runners [16]. Both papers emphasize the importance of personalized running experience and coaching. Both u4fit and Inspirun track heart rate, running speed, and GPS coordinates to keep track of the runs and to determined the intensity of the training. Given an intensity profile and training results, u4fit relies on a human fitness coach to provide feedback on compliance with the personalized training regimen. On the other hand, Inspirun relies on the smartphone application itself to provide coaching feedback. u4fit is aimed at improving and sustaining runner motivation, while Inspirun is designed to help recreational runners set new performance-related goals. The authors, however, do not report on any quantitative results in their publications. Unlike u4fit or Inspirun, our efforts are focused on minimizing injuries in a specific subpopulation of runners, i.e., long-distance runners. Moreover, in RunningCoach, the training regimen is focused on cadence, which has been reported as one of the factors associated with injury and performance.

Our long-term goal, which we aim to achieve after a series of further studies, is to develop a recommendation algorithm that outputs an optimal cadence level for an individual runner, based on her or his physical parameters (e.g., age, gender, height and weight), data from previous runs (e.g., performance, heart rate, etc.) and other factors related to injuries.

2.2. Taxonomy of Running Cadence

Up to 79% of long-distance runners are expected to sustain a running-related injury within a six month period, most commonly located at the knee [1,17]. Patellofemoral pain syndrome (PFPS) was observed as the most frequent issue encountered in running injuries out of the 26 most common running injuries [18]. PFPS is a condition that causes severe to mild knee pain, which often starts due to a dramatic change in the training regimen [19]. In addition to this reason, numerous biomechanical risk factors can contribute to causing PFPS. These factors include kinematic abnormalities, patellar maltracking, overuse, and excessive compressive stresses on the patellofemoral joint cartilage [20–24]. Running as an activity generates much larger cartilage stress at the patellofemoral joint as compared to other everyday activities [25,26]. A clear way forward to mitigate PFPS would be to find a method to reduce the magnitude of the patellofemoral joint force during running. By running at 5% to 10% above one's preferred cadence has been shown to be beneficial in reducing pain, increasing training ability in runners with PFPS and minimizing the risk of injury to the patellofemoral joint. For instance, Lenhart et al. report a decrease of 14% in peak patellofemoral joint force as a result of a 10% increase in cadence relative to the preferred cadence level [27]. Heiderscheit et al. report a significant decrease in the absorbed mechanical energy at the knee as a result of 5% to 10% increase in cadence relative to the runner's preferred cadence level [2]. These reductions in peak patellofemoral joint force and absorbed mechanical energy may reduce the risk of running-related knee injuries [2,27].

The importance of optimizing one's cadence as a long-distance runner is twofold. First, subtly increasing and optimizing cadence during a run assists runners with preventing common running-related injuries [2]. From an injury-prevention standpoint, this enables both professional and hobbyist long-distance runners to continue running. Second, optimizing and maintaining a consistent cadence throughout a run enables long-distance runners to conserve energy and as such enhance performance [28,29]. Unlike novice long-distance runners, advanced long-distance runners avoid deviations from their optimal cadence when they are in a fatigued state as such deviations lead to an increased energy cost [30–32].

Given the numerous benefits of optimizing cadence for long-distance runners, many mHealth technologies were created to meet this need. In order to provide effective feedback on running cadence, many have studied the relationship between music and setting the running cadence through auditory-motor synchronization [33,34]. These studies provide evidence of the ability of music to affect the running cadence and ultimately improve performance [33] and reduce injuries [2,34].

2.3. Feasibility and Usability of mHealth Systems

In spite of findings that show that a lack of focus on usability and feasibility issues for mHealth systems would lead to an increase in overall costs and delays in successful implementation, few mHealth interventions have explained the attributes that contribute to their success and the aspects that have led to failed implementations [35–37]. A 2013 systematic review of mHealth literature by Fiordelli et al. identified that only 14% of the studies reported on user assessment of the technology [38].

Through post-study questionnaires in the first user study, Vos et al. managed to surface issues with Inspirun on the accuracy of speed measurements which were later addressed in the third release of Inspirun [16].

In mHealth, understanding the privacy preferences of users and their acceptability of the technology is a determining factor in its success and adoption due to the amount of sensitive data typically collected by the apps. Very few studies, however, report on the privacy-related aspects of the mHealth systems they adopt [13,39].

3. Materials and Methods

3.1. Study Objectives

The short-term objective of the study is to assess the feasibility and usability of RunningCoach, a mobile health (mHealth) remote coaching system for long-distance runners which aims to optimize their running cadence. We are particularly interested in understanding (i) how long-distance runners interact with RunningCoach; (ii) how long-distance runners perceive the accuracy of the data collected by RunningCoach; and (iii) what running-related analyses can be performed with the collected data to provide further insights into the system and runner's performance. These immediate objectives are set for the purpose of guiding the future iterations of the study. Understanding the interactions of the user with the system, and investigating any potential usability issues with the system allow us to address those issues in the future. Moreover, exploring potential running-related analyses helps us devise hypotheses, that can be validated in future studies.

The long-term objective of our research is to achieve personalized coaching for an individual runner that will be integrated in the proposed telemonitoring system. We envision this coaching system to include the ability to take advantage of the anthropometric parameters of each individual, the individual's previous performance, and other factors related to injuries in order to devise a training regimen that is tailored to that individual. Ultimately, this personalized training regimen shall provide recommendations to the runner regarding cadence and speed, depending on the specific consecutive day of training and the previously-collected running data.

In order to achieve these objectives, we have designed a series of user studies, which are approved by the Institutional Review Board at University of California, Berkeley. In this paper, we describe the design and findings of the first study in this series, which is concerned with the feasibility and acceptability of such telemonitoring technology.

3.2. Training Regimen

In order to guide the runners to improve their running cadence, the system has to provide a training regimen tailored to each subject. Before establishing the plan for improving the runner's cadence, the system has to establish the runner's baseline cadence. Note that the different runners may have different levels of experience and different body types. As such, a single and fixed training regimen may not be generalizable to all runners. Therefore, RunningCoach collects two types of information from the runner in order to set her or his personalized training regimen. First, RunningCoach collects information about the runner's physical parameters. The collected physical parameters in the app include age, gender, height, weight, and leg length as measured from the hip joint to the ground (Figure 1a). Second, RunningCoach sets the desired cadence improvement curve, by collecting information about the runner's baseline, target cadence and the length of the proposed training regimen. In the current version of RunningCoach, all of the aforementioned parameters are manually set by the runner.

In future iterations of the app, a recommended training regimen will be determined by collecting data over a small set of consecutive runs and comparing runner's own baseline with similar runners. Similar runners will be identified using the provided physical parameters and their baseline data.

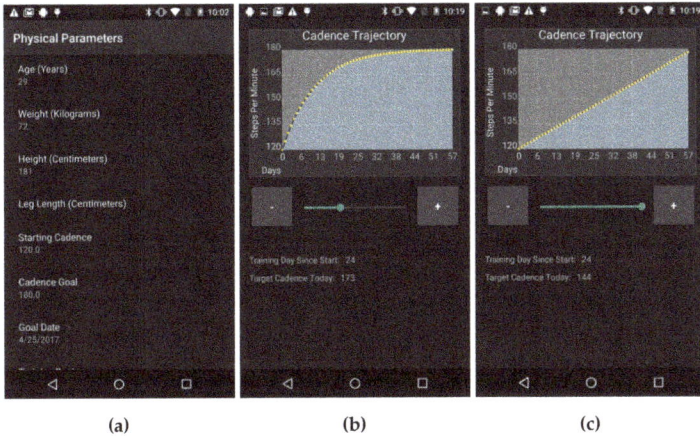

Figure 1. (a) A screenshot depicting the physique profile screen; (b) a screenshot depicting an exponential cadence training regimen; and (c) a screenshot depicting a linear training regimen [11].

After the runner provides her or his physical parameters, a default training regimen is suggested. This training regimen consists of a starting cadence level (baseline), a target cadence level, the length of the training regimen, and the steepness of the cadence improvement curve. The default length of the training regimen is 90 days, which can be altered by the subject. The reason for selecting 90 days as a default value was to maintain the length of the training regimen with the length of the study. The family of parametric cadence training regimens adopted by RunningCoach follows an exponential improvement curve, as follows.

$$C(d) = \frac{C_N \cdot e^{\alpha N} - C_0}{e^{\alpha N} - 1} - \frac{C_0 - C_N}{e^{-\alpha N} - 1} \cdot e^{-\alpha d}, \tag{1}$$

In Equation (1), $C(d)$ denotes the suggested cadence on day d. C_0 denotes the baseline cadence of the runner, where C_N denotes the target cadence. The parameter α controls the steepness of the personalized training regimen (larger values imply steeper improvements) and N denotes the length of the training regimen in days. By setting values for C_0, N, C_N and α, a training regimen is established that guides the runner to achieve the target cadence level C_N within N days.

The family of training regimens described in Equation (1) is the solution of the function $C(d) = A + B \cdot e^{-\alpha d}$ with initial conditions $C(0) = C_0$ and $C(N) = C_N$. Moreover, as α approaches 0, the training regimen described in Equation (1) approaches a training regimen with a linear improvement curve. Concretely, $\lim_{\alpha \to 0} C(d) = C_0 + \frac{C_N - C_0}{N} \cdot d$. This claim is formally shown in [40]. The reasoning behind devising training regimens with gradual improvements in cadence is to minimize the risk of injury due to sudden changes in the runner's training routine. In addition, the exponential training regimen allows for larger increases around the baseline and then levels off towards the higher target cadence to prevent over-training.

Examples of the training regimens are depicted in Figure 1b,c, where Figure 1b shows a training regimen with exponential improvements in cadence ($\alpha > 0$) and Figure 1c shows a training regimen with a linear improvement curve of cadence ($\alpha \to 0$).

As stated earlier, in the current version of RunningCoach, the cadence training regimen settings are manually set by the runner. Eventually, we aim to develop an algorithm that would recommend, to each runner, her or his ideal cadence level (C_N), and a personalized improvement steepness curve (α), that are based on her or his physique profile depicted in Figure 1a as well as data from her or his previous runs. In addition, we aim to use heart rate data to dynamically alter the training regimen for the runner in a way that is sensitive to the runner's physical ability. In order to achieve this goal, we aim to use the data collected in this study (and the future iterations of this study) to train a recommendation algorithm in a way that mimics the true improvement trajectories of the runners. Further studies are needed to validate the efficacy of such a recommendation algorithm. More details about the adopted training regimen can be found in [11,40].

3.3. Study Protocol

3.3.1. Screening and Recruitment

Members of the University of California Berkeley community were sought for participation in this study. Potential participants were screened according to two criteria. First, participation was only allowed to those who are current long-distance runners. This requirement was placed in an effort to not subject the study participants to the risks of running, if they do not regularly run (e.g., injury). By limiting participation in the study to those who regularly run long distances, we are taking measures to minimize the risks of participation in the study. For screening purposes, we use the definition of "long-distance runner" that is used by the International Association of Athletics Federations (IAAF), which states the following:

> A long-distance runner is someone who every week (i) runs for at least 5 km (or 3 miles) in distance; or (ii) runs at least one session that is 1 h or longer in duration.

The second screening criterion limited participation to subjects who owned an Android smartphone running Android 4.3 (Jelly Bean MR2) or newer. This requirement allowed us to better assess acceptability and usability qualities of the proposed system, by requesting that participants use their own smartphones for the purposes of the study. In turn, any feasibility or usability issues arising from using an unfamiliar smartphone, if it were to be provided by the study, are thus eliminated.

After the screening of each candidate subject, the researcher administering the process obtained her or his consent for participation in the study. After the consent process, the researcher conducted the initial set up procedure for the subject. This procedure entailed providing the subject with a Jarv Run heart rate chest strap monitor [41]. Afterwards, the RunningCoach app was installed on the subject's smartphone and paired with the heart rate monitor. Subsequently, the subjects were instructed on the proper way of using the system by providing instructions specific to pre-, during, and post-running use (e.g., how to wear the heart rate chest strap, where to secure the phone during the run, etc.). Finally, the researcher demonstrated the use of the RunningCoach app and its features to the subject. The subjects were encouraged to ask any questions related to the system or the protocol.

In total, six subjects were recruited for the study. The study spanned from February 2017 to July 2017. The subject demographics and physical parameters are summarized in Table 1.

Table 1. The demographics of the recruited subjects.

Subject Identifier	Gender	Age (years)	Weight (kg)	Height (cm)
s28ikk	Male	23	67	183
i989kje	Female	24	60	168
w32jbl	Female	24	70	178
b01k1o	Female	25	55	165
p542ok	Male	25	72.5	177
j83bbl	Male	26	72.5	185

3.3.2. Study Procedures

During the main part of the study, the subjects were asked to secure the phone on their body in a comfortable area (e.g., on the shoulder or on the hip) during their routine runs with the RunningCoach app. In addition, the subjects were asked to wear the heart rate chest strap that was provided to them, which connects to the app via Bluetooth and sends the data in real time. The subjects were not specifically asked to use the app during each run but rather to use it on their own terms. The reason subjects were not instructed to use the app during each run is that some recruited subjects are competitive runners who preferred to use a smartphone only during a part of their weekly training routine.

During each run, the app collects information about the runners' estimated energy expenditure, cadence, speed, heart rate from the chest strap, and total distance covered. In addition to these estimates, the app collects the following two variables: (i) whether or not the screen light is on; and (ii) the battery level. Before and after each run, the app collects single estimates of the heart rate using two different vision algorithms, one from a video of the subject's face and another from a video of the subject's index finger [11]. These algorithms were previously only validated under controlled conditions. Since an external heart monitor was used in the study, we used this opportunity to get an insight on the usability of the implemented heart rate measurement algorithms in the field. Note that this was not a controlled validation and should therefore be treated as exploratory only. Table 2 summarizes the types of data collected before, during and after the run.

Table 2. The data types collected about every run.

Data Type	Source of Estimation	Collection Frequency
Energy expenditure	Accelerometer.	Every 60 s.
Cadence	Accelerometer.	Every 15 s.
Speed	GPS.	Every 5 s.
Heart rate	External sensor (chest strap).	Every 1 s.
Heart rate	Video of the runner's face.	Once before the run and once after the run.
Heart rate	Video of the runner's index finger.	Once before the run and once after the run.
Distance covered	GPS.	Every 5 s.
Screen light	Android API.	Every 30 s.
Battery consumption	Android API.	Every 60 s.

After each run, subjects were asked to fill a post-run survey inquiring about the run. The questions asked in the post-run survey were: (i) "How tired were you on a scale of 1-5 where 3 is your typical level of fatigue after long runs prior to using the app, 5 is very tired and 1 is least tired?" (ii) "After viewing your run data, were any of the measurements inaccurate to the best of your assessment? (Choose all that apply from Speed, Cadence, Heart Rate, Energy Expenditure, Distance);" (iii) "If you selected any of the choices in the previous question, please explain;" and (iv) "Please provide any other comments regarding your experience using the app." Figure 2a depicts an example screen showing some of the run statistics after the run, and Figure 2b depicts an example of a question from the post-run survey as displayed in the app. The post-run survey provides information about (i) the perceived accuracy of the system; (ii) the usability of the system; and (iii) how hard the training regimen is pushing the runners in terms of performance. The post-run questions about the perceived accuracy of the app's collected data are shown to the subject after the run statistics are presented (e.g., Figure 2a).

In the process of designing the post-run survey, the 1 to 5 scale of fatigue was selected for the following reasons. The adopted scale is a reduced version of rating-of-fatigue (ROF), which is a 10-point scale designed to measure level of fatigue [42]. Other seemingly relevant measures have been studied in the sports literature, including Borg's perceived exertion scale [43]. Borg's scale is not a good fit for our purposes because it is designed to capture subjective exertion. Some researchers argue that perceived exertion, the subjective experience of how hard a physical task feels, is different from perceived fatigue and should not be used to measure perceived fatigue levels [42]. Moreover, Borg's scale is designed to follow the heart rate of the subject by multiplying it by 10. Since we are collecting heart rate data, Borg's score would not provide additional information, and therefore, a reduced fatigue scale that is similar to ROF was selected for our purposes.

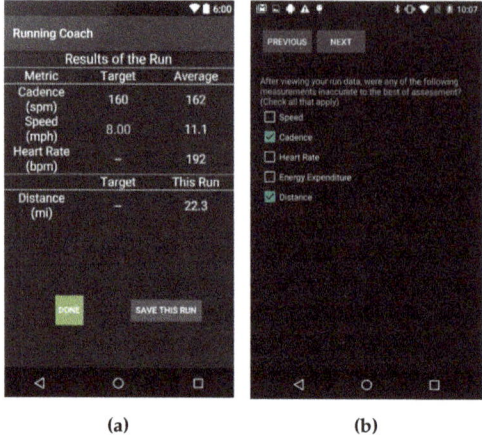

Figure 2. (**a**) A screen showing some of the run-statistics after a run; and (**b**) an example of a question in the post-run survey [11].

Subjects were asked to perform the aforementioned procedure for a period of 3 months. By the end of that period, the subjects answered an exit acceptability and privacy survey about the system and the study.

4. System Design

The architecture and implementation of the system, which are based on the Berkeley Telemonitoring framework [44], are described in [11]. For completeness, we briefly discuss them in this section; for more details, we refer the reader to [11,39,44].

4.1. RunningCoach App

The purpose of the RunningCoach app is to serve as the remote monitoring node. As such, it collects data about each run, including energy expenditure, cadence, speed, heart rate, and distance covered. In addition, the app administers the surveys after each run. Figure 3 depicts various screens from the RunningCoach app. Concretely, Figure 3a depicts the home screen of the app, listing previous runs; Figure 3b,c depict two screens shown during the run, presenting the runner's cadence and speed, respectively.

Finally, the app delivers the real-time feedback to the runners regarding their cadence and/or speed levels (depending on the settings). If the cadence or speed are outside of a preset range around the target values of the day, according to the training regimen, the phone provides haptic feedback (vibration) and auditory cues (beeping) to the runner. The vibration and beeping patterns depend on whether the runner is higher than the target value or lower than it, allowing the runner to adjust accordingly. This preset range can be set by the subject in the app, with a default value of 10% (around the target cadence or speed).

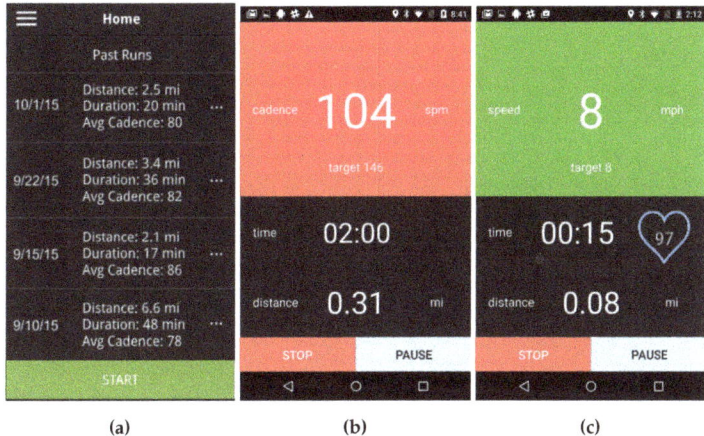

Figure 3. (**a**) A screenshot of the home screen of RunningCoach, summarizing the past runs; (**b**) a screenshot from the app during a run showing the cadence significantly lower than its target value (outside the 10% range of the target cadence); and (**c**) a screenshot from the app during the run showing the speed within acceptable range of its target value (within 10% of the target speed) [11].

4.2. Backend

The RunningCoach server backend is written in Java and uses the Berkeley Telemonitoring framework as well. To communicate with the client nodes, the backend uses the Tele-Interfacing (TI) protocol with Transport Layer Security (TLS), as described in [44]. The backend receives the data from the client nodes in the form of data jobs, unpacks the jobs back into encapsulators using job handlers (conforming to the Berkeley Telemonitoring framework) and stores the data in a MySQL database. Each data job is attached to a subject identifier that is uniquely set to each runner in the app. The identifiers are used to identify the source of the data (Table 1). The subject identifier is stored in the database along with the corresponding data.

4.3. Dashboard

In addition to the backend, we designed a dashboard that provides a way to visualize the data about the runs. The dashboard can be accessed on the web using a browser. Figure 4 depicts an example plot of cadence data for three different runs by three different subjects. In the runs reported in Figure 4, runner s28ikk reported holding the phone in his hand during run 11, contrary to the instructions given to the subjects to place the smartphone around the hip or on the shoulder during the run. In all of the runs in the figure, we observe that the runners stopped momentarily, which is corroborated by the other data variables (e.g., speed, GPS, etc.). This explains the seemingly low cadence readings in these figures. These issues will be discussed further in Section 5.

The paths of the runs can also be visualized with a colored overlay, representing the recorded values from various data sources, such as cadence, speed, or heart-rate. For example, the dashboard can provide a plot of the path of the run with the color from green to red indicating the value of cadence (range: zero to 200), as depicted in Figure 5.

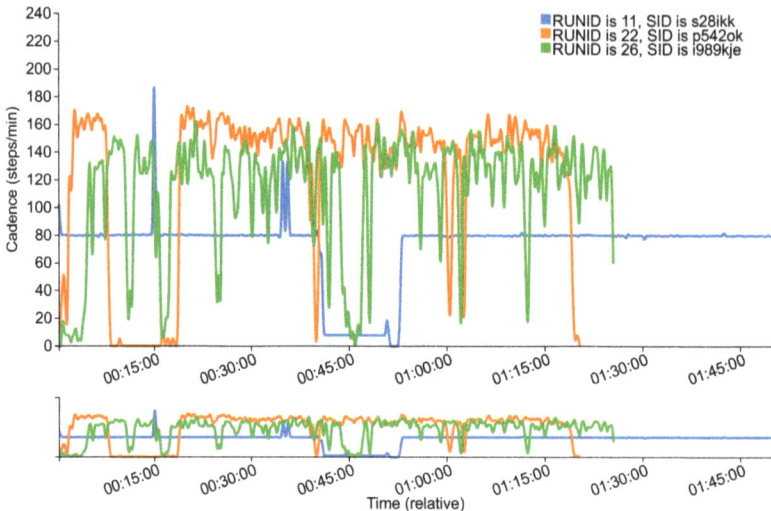

Figure 4. An example plot from the dashboard, depicting the estimated cadence during runs 11, 22 and 26 by subjects s28ikk, p542ok and i989kje, respectively [11].

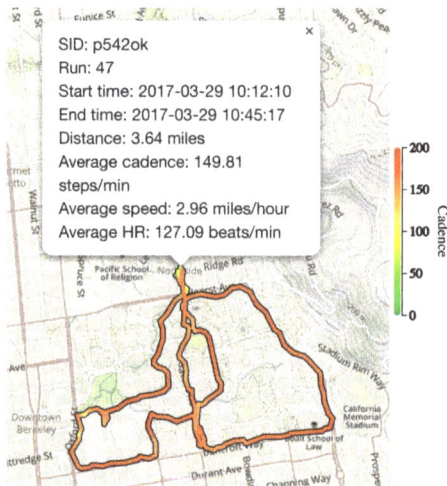

Figure 5. An example plot of the path of run 47 by subject p542ok.

5. Results and Discussion

5.1. General Statistics

The six subject enrolled in this study used the app to collect data of a total of 22 runs amounting to more than 22.5 h of data. In Figure 6a, we present the durations of the runs for the different subjects. In addition, Figure 6b depicts the total distances traveled during each run for the different subjects. Finally, Figure 7a presents the deviation of the runner from his or her target cadence for the run in question. Note that in some runs, the subjects elected to disable GPS data collection, and those runs were omitted from Figure 6b, which is why the number of runs per runner is different in the different plots.

We note that for the majority of runs, runners were running at a cadence lower than the recommended cadence for the run, signaling the need for more personalized training regimens as stated in our long-term goals. Moreover, we note that the auditory and haptic feedback is provided whenever the cadence is more than 10% off the target value for the run, for a period of 30 s or longer. Therefore, runs that had a deviation in cadence within a 10% window of the target cadence level should be considered as ones that met the target cadence. Moreover, runner s28ikk reported running with the phone in his hand. As will be detailed in Section 5.3.2, this violates the design assumptions of the cadence estimation algorithm, which explains the large deviation from the target cadence for that runner.

In order to provide contextual perspective, we present the self-reported levels of fatigue after each run by the different subjects in Figure 7b.

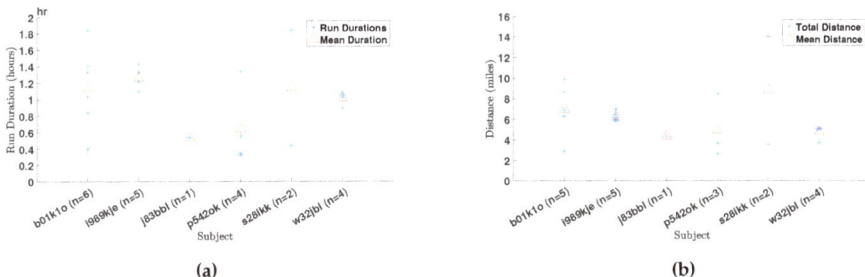

Figure 6. (a) The durations of the different runs as observed in each subject ($N = 22$); and (b) the total distances of the different runs as observed in each subject ($N = 20$).

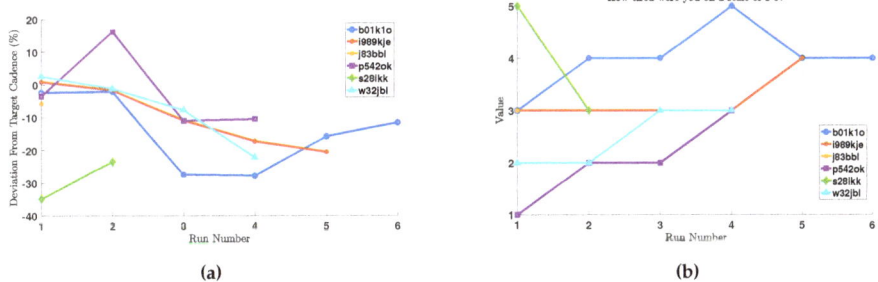

Figure 7. (a) The deviation of the average cadence from the target cadence for each run, expressed in percentage points ($N = 22$); and (b) subject-reported level of fatigue after each run. A value of three represents the level of fatigue reported after an average run; a value of one is least fatigued; and value five is most fatigued after an average run ($N = 22$).

5.2. Usability

5.2.1. Battery

Optimizing battery consumption is key to adoption of smartphone-based telemonitoring applications [39,45]. In this study, the subjects did not report any usability issues regarding battery consumption. However, as described earlier, battery levels were collected during every run (once a minute). From these data, we calculate the amount of battery that is consumed during each run. Note that the battery consumption captures the total battery consumption of the smartphone, not just of our app. Since the different runs are different in duration, we normalize this consumption by time, in order to get a measure of "battery percentage consumed per hour". These results are depicted in Figure 8a.

We note that different subjects have different battery consumption profiles, which may be caused by one or a combination of the following factors. First, different phones have different battery consumption profiles; and the phones used in this study were not provided by us and therefore are heterogeneous. Second, battery consumption depends on factors that are external to RunningCoach, such as listening to music and whether the music is streamed or played locally. Third, battery consumption profiles depend on the carrier and the strength of cellular coverage [46]. However, the data provide evidence that RunningCoach alone is not very burdensome on battery and can consume as low as 5% battery/h. This is even true for subject b01k1o, who manifests high battery consumption patterns in general. In one run, RunningCoach consumed less than 5% battery/h, which can be explained by the factors listed above.

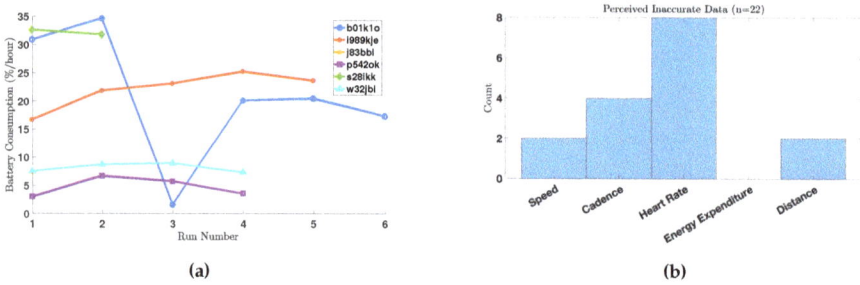

Figure 8. (**a**) The amount of battery consumption (in %) per hour during the different runs by the different subjects ($N = 22$); and (**b**) the perceived accuracy of the collected data by the runners ($N = 22$).

5.2.2. General Usability

We now turn to general usability issues as reported by the subjects. First, there were two instances where extreme fault-tolerance was tested during the study. In one instance, a subject reported that the phone's operating system malfunctioned in the middle of a run; but when the phone was restarted after the run, the app resumed its operation from the previous state. In this instance, the data before the crash were not lost, even though they were not submitted to the server prior to the crash.

In another instance, the server was down for a prolonged period of time, during which several runs were taken by the different subjects. Because of the built-in fault-tolerance mechanisms in the Berkeley Telemonitoring framework, no data were lost during the server downtime. The app was able to recover all the data and send them to the server once the server was back online. It is worth reporting that one subject uninstalled the app manually before the server was restarted; which caused the data not yet sent to the server to be lost. These incidents validate the fault-tolerance implementation described in [44].

Besides the aforementioned issues, we further summarize general usability reports made by the study subjects in Table 3.

Table 3. Summary of usability reports by the subjects.

Usability Issue	Description
Equipment	Subject b01k1o complained that the heart rate chest strap caused skin irritation. The subject was asked to stop using the strap immediately in order to limit the risk of harm. The strap itself was later tested and no fault in it was found.
Screen light	Data from the screen light sensor shows that subject i989kje regularly checked the app's interface to view his or her running parameters such as cadence, speed, distance, time and heart rate throughout the run (the screen was turned on more than 80% of the time during subject i989kje's runs). All other runners ran generally with the screen turned off, only using the haptic vibration and auditory cues as the primary means of feedback (the screen was turned off more than 80% of the time during their runs).
User Experience	Subject i989kje provided a usability feedback in the app regarding the speed and cadence estimates, stating "I stopped a few times during the run and the app did not take it into account". The data corroborate the feedback by the subject, which seems to have stopped on multiple occasions as can be seen from Figure 4 (run 26). It is worth noting that the app provides an option to pause the current run, which the subject did not use in this instance. Moreover, multiple subjects suggested that speed should be presented in units of mins/mile rather than miles/h

5.3. Perceived Accuracy

As part of the routine post-run surveys, we inquired about the perceived levels of accuracy of the collected data. Concretely, we asked the subjects: "After viewing your run data, were any of the measurements inaccurate to the best of your assessment? (Choose all that apply from Speed, Cadence, Heart Rate, Energy Expenditure, Distance)". The responses to this question are presented in Figure 8b. As follow-up to this question, the subjects were also asked to provide additional information when they thought any measurements were inaccurate.

Energy expenditure was not perceived as inaccurate by the runners. A possible explanation to this is that it is difficult for people to gauge their own energy expenditure during physical activity. For distance, one subject reported: "if you're counting total miles traveled, then it should be closer to 5, but if you're just counting miles run, that's maybe accurate." The measured distance (from GPS data) during this particular run was 3.72 miles, which reflects the total miles traveled. After carefully reviewing the data, it seems that the run monitoring was not started until the runner was in the middle of the run. We concluded this because the runner always took the same route, except in this run where the monitoring started from a middle point in that route (which accounts for the difference in mileage). In the following sections, we discuss in more detail the perceived accuracy for the heart rate and cadence measurements.

5.3.1. Heart Rate

We note that the heart-rate measurements were deemed to be the least accurate in our system. According to the responses of the follow-up questions in the post-run survey, the subjects found the pre- and post-run single heart-rate measurements using the computer vision algorithms to be inaccurate. This discontent can be explained by the fact that these algorithms were mainly tested in a controlled lab environment, and failed to perform at the same level when taken in uncontrolled settings. For example, on different occasions, subject p542ok responded to the follow-up questions with "I am not at 70 bpm immediately after a run [(referring to the vision-based estimates)]", "face and finger[-based estimates] are way off as usual", (they were lower than 55 bpm) "finger[-based estimates] is still way too low after the run" and "finger heart rate after run was 45". In the first instance reported above, the heart-rate chest strap did indeed record 70 bpm at the end of the run. In all other instances when the subject complained about the accuracy of the vision-based heart-rate estimates, the heart-rate chest strap recorded values that were significantly higher than the vision-based ones. No feedback was given regarding the accuracy of the chest heart-rate strap.

On one occasion, the same subject took video-based heart rate estimates without actually running. The subject did not report any perceived inaccuracy in the estimates, which were 61 bpm and 62 bpm for the finger-video-based and face-video-based estimates, respectively. Other subjects did not provide textual feedback regarding the accuracy of the heart-rate measurements.

5.3.2. Cadence

The subjects' responses to the follow-up question provided valuable insight as to why they perceived certain cadence measurements as inaccurate. These reasons are sometimes explained by improper use of the system. For example, as a follow-up to choosing "cadence" as inaccurate in the survey, one subject responded: "Cadence too low; possibly because I held phone in hand". The cadence algorithm was designed to work around the hip area or on the shoulder, which explains why during this run the average cadence of the runner was as low as 72 steps/min.

In another example, a subject reported that "My measured cadence was also lower than expected—I was mostly running on beat to songs that had 150+ bpm". The measured cadence of the run is depicted in Figure 9b. The average cadence of the run was 111 steps/min, which includes the segments in the beginning of the run as well as some segments when the runner slowed down (or perhaps momentarily stopped running). After excluding these data points, the average increased to 124 steps/min, which is still lower than the subject's self-reported cadence of 150 steps/min. For reference, Figure 9a depicts the speed during the same run, which shows that the runner would slow down in many instances. One potential reason for those momentary slow-downs is the urban path that the runner selected, which is corroborated by the run's GPS data (the path passed through many street intersections).

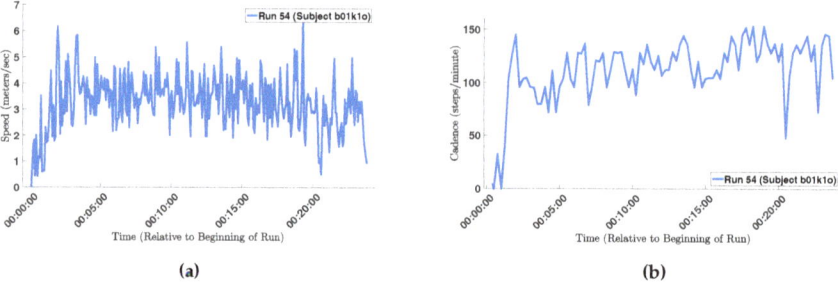

Figure 9. (a) The estimated speed (m/s) during run 54 by subject b01k1o; and (b) the estimated cadence (steps/min) during run 54 by subject b01k1o.

5.4. *Acceptability*

In Figure 10 we present the results of the acceptability portion of the post-study questionnaire. It is worth noting that the study subjects' acceptability of this technology is lower than the acceptability reported in other telemonitoring applications such as in congestive heart failure (CHF) [46,47]. This can be attributed to multiple factors. First, some subjects voiced preference for using a monitoring device with a smaller form factor than a smartphone for this application. For example, one subject stated: "I'm a big fan of using running watches instead of phone apps because the form factor is much more comfortable. That's the main reason I was so negative about using a phone-based athletic trainer". In that regard, we note that the Berkeley Telemonitoring framework supports general Android devices, not only Android smartphones. Therefore, an Android smart watch application can be implemented using the same framework, averting the form factor challenge. Second, people may be more likely to tolerate certain drawbacks in a technology if they perceive a higher utility and value in it. As such, the higher levels of acceptability in CHF telemonitoring and intervention (e.g., [46]) may be attributed to the potentially higher perceived utility and value of the technology to the subjects in that application [47].

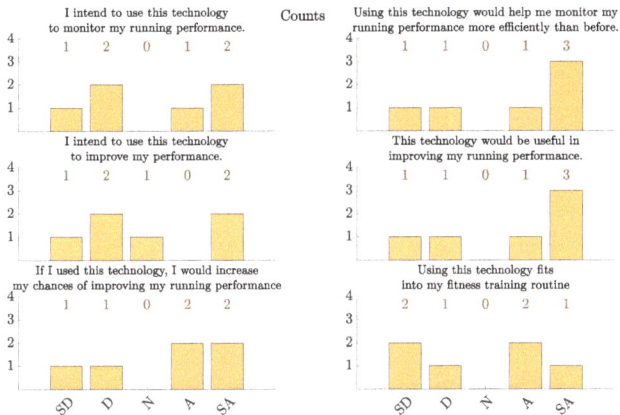

Figure 10. The results from the acceptability portion of the post-study questionnaire ($N = 6$). SD = "strongly disagree", D = "disagree", N = "neutral", A = "agree" and SA ="strongly agree" [47].

Another aspect of the post-study questionnaire focused on the privacy aspects of the technology, as perceived by the subjects. In that portion of the questionnaire, the subjects were asked the following set of questions. "Sometimes the smartphone might automatically record, or ask you to report, specific kinds of information about your health or behavior, such as your weight, your mood, or your blood pressure. The following questions will help us understand how comfortable you are with the idea of other people knowing these things about you". In Figure 11 we present the subjects' responses indicating their levels of comfort in sharing data about their (i) weight; (ii) level of physical activity; (iii) exact physical location at any point in time; (iv) heart-beat rate; (v) types of physical activity they do; and (vi) mood at any point in time, with: (i) doctors and nurses who provide them healthcare; (ii) researchers who study athletic training technology; (iii) public health professionals who study the effects of exercise and athleticism; (iv) insurance companies that set their health insurance prices; and (v) close family members who care about their health [47].

In particular, the data provide an indication that the subjects' level of comfort in sharing data about their fitness, GPS, health and mood with technology researchers is comparable to sharing those variables with their family and physicians [47]. In contrast, the subjects were noticeably less comfortable sharing these variables with their health insurance companies, suggesting that they are not privacy indifferent. These two observations combined suggest that the provided technology is at an acceptable level from a privacy point of view. In addition to the ethical reasons for designing privacy-aware data-collection systems, these findings are of great significance because they have direct implications on the adoption of these systems [39].

We note that the privacy acceptability levels are similarly high to those reported in the other applications such as CHF [46,47].

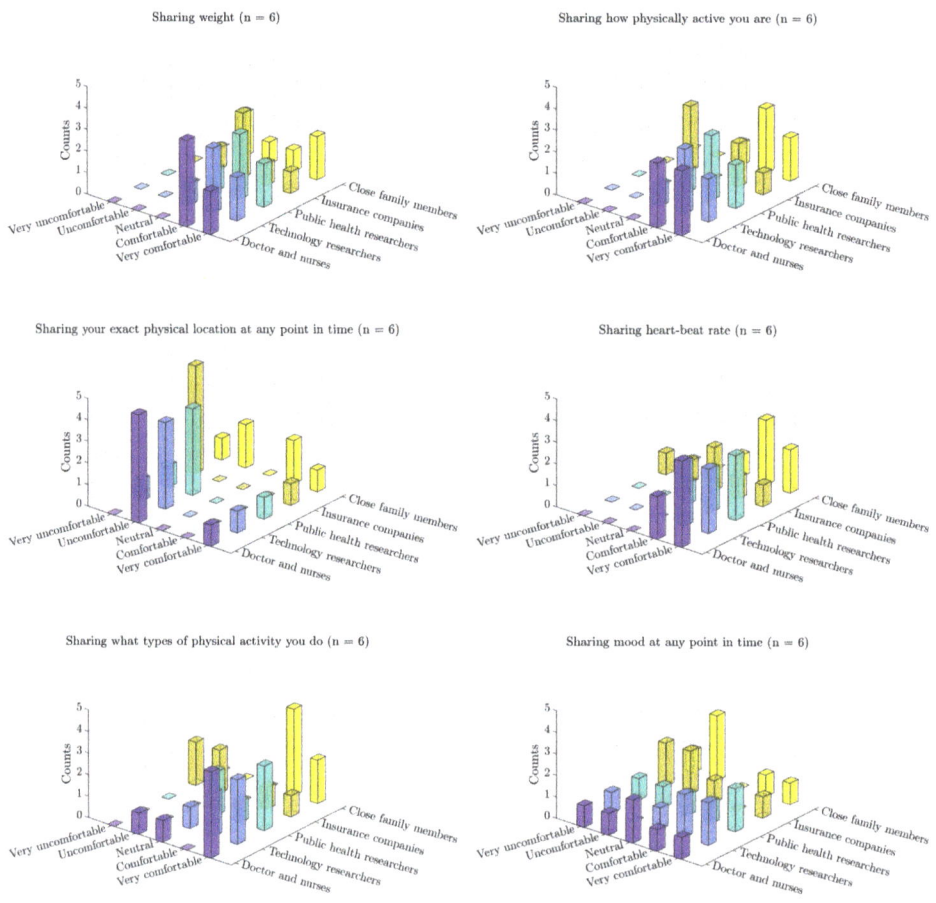

Figure 11. The responses to the privacy portion of the post-study questionnaire about the subjects' comfort levels sharing different data variables with different parties ($N = 6$) [47].

5.5. Elevation, Cadence and Speed

It is interesting to understand whether runner's speed or cadence change as a result in elevation changes during the run. That is, we ask whether cadence or speed drop as a result of running uphill and whether they increase as a result of running downhill, relative to the cadence and speed during running on a flat surface. This type of analysis can be beneficial in analyzing the performance of each runner for each run. In order to perform this analysis, we split each run into segments of one minute each. Each segment was defined as "running uphill" if the net change in elevation is at least $+2$ m. Each segment was defined as "running downhill" if the net change in elevation is at most -2 m. All other segments were marked as running on flat surface. In order to estimate elevation for each data point, we used the Digital Terrain Elevation Data (DTED) maps from the United States Geological Survey (USGS) [48] to estimate the elevation of each GPS data point during the run.

During each run and for each surface type (uphill, flat and downhill), we explored the distribution of cadence and speed. It is ideal if the speed and cadence remained unaffected due to terrain elevation changes. The data indicate that, for most runners, cadence is less affected by terrain elevation changes than speed. Figure 12 displays this analysis for two runs by two different runners. In run 50, there seems to be a noticeable change in speed due to terrain elevation changes; however, cadence is less affected. In run 52, there is a smaller effect of terrain elevation changes on both speed and cadence, indicating a more consistent pace during the run (which is desired). This type of running performance analysis is possible with the type of data collected by RunningCoach. One can envision this analysis as a source of intervention to help the runner minimize injuries, although further longitudinal studies are necessary to validate this claim.

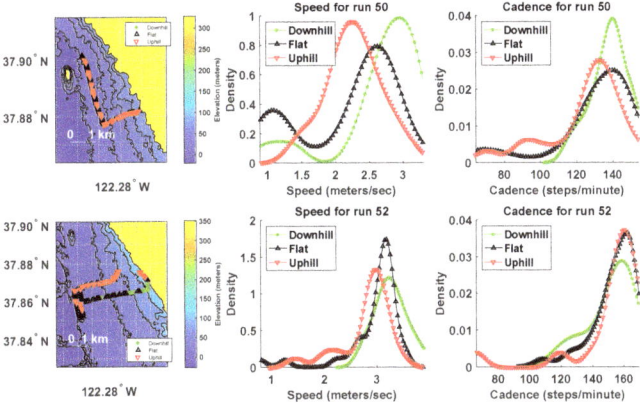

Figure 12. The relationship between elevation changes (ascending/descending), cadence and speed for runs 50 and 52 by subjects i989kje and b01k1o, respectively.

5.6. Limitations of the Study

The presented study has several limitations. First, the number of subjects in the study (sample size) is small. While all recruited subjects are considered long-distance runners per definition, their training regimens in total distances traveled per run were quite diverse. Some subjects were in general not users of smartphone apps for running, therefore their expectations and responses may have been different than of the subjects who are users of such applications on a more regular basis. Since the goal of this study was to assess the feasibility and the usability of the developed telemonitoring framework, less emphasis was given on the rigid study protocol that would perhaps result in larger number of collected runs during the three months. The study instead aimed to investigate how often the runners would use RunningCoach app during their runs and what type of information can be extracted from the collected data. A sample of the results was presented in this paper. To evaluate in more detail the running performance of individual runners and their changes over time, given the feedback on the cadence, the subjects in future studies will be required to perform certain number of runs per week. Such data collection across larger pool of subjects would provide the data needed to achieve the long-term goal of this research, i.e., to tune the training models to individual runner's physique and to evaluate the efficacy and potential benefits of such training for prevention of injuries.

Furthermore, feedback from the users indicated that the large form factor of the smartphone may not be as convenient for long-distance runners due to the mounting inconvenience and additional weight. The use of a smartphone for casual monitoring of daily activities may be preferred over wearable devices as people tend to carry their smartphone throughout the day. On the other hand, to measure the athletic performance, wearable sensors may be more convenient. As the Berkeley Telemonitoring framework is compatible with any Android device, the future iterations of this system may include the use of a smart watch or other wearable technology.

6. Conclusion

Studies suggest that optimizing cadence is an important factor in reducing the risk of sustaining a running-related injury and in improving overall running performance. In this work, we presented a feasibility study utilizing an mHealth solution to long-distance running cadence-based coaching, called RunningCoach. Future versions of the system will include a music player that selects music with beats that are on the desired cadence for the day. The feedback from the subjects in this study will also be incorporated in the next version of the system.

Based on the findings of the study, there are early signs of satisfaction from a usability and perceived accuracy point of view, with one exception. The video-based heart rate estimates were perceived as inaccurate in this study. As such, the study findings indicate that there is a need for tools that systematically assess the accuracy of sensory estimates and guide the estimation algorithms accordingly. For example, the algorithms for estimating cadence would be different when the phone is secured on the hip versus when the phone is held by the runner in her or his hand. In these cases, it is the responsibility of the system to employ the correct estimation algorithm by detecting the conditions under which the system is being used. More generally, the study findings suggest that audit mechanisms need to be developed and employed for each estimation algorithm, in order to ensure, verify and quantify the accuracy of its outputs.

One important usability issue to be studied in the future is the motivation of runners to use this and similar mHealth technologies for tracking their runs. There is clearly an interest of (novice) runners to improve cadence for performance gains as is evident from a number of apps that provide feedback through music or otherwise [5–10]. However, the evidence for the motivation of using apps for injury prevention is to the best of our knowledge limited. There are several behavioral factors, specific to runners [49], that influence their attitudes towards the level of training and higher risk of injuries. As noted by [50], injury-preventive actions that require behavior modification need to take into account that runners' perceived susceptibility to sport has multiple predictors, including previous experiences, neuroticism and obsessive passion. Mobile applications for runners thus provide an opportunity to address injury prevention through individualized feedback and various motivational mechanisms, which were out of the scope of this pilot study.

Acknowledgments: We would like to thank David M. Liebovitz, MD for suggesting long-distance running as an application to the Berkeley Telemonitoring Project and advising on the design of the app. Eugene Song, Uma Balakrishnan, Hannah Sarver, Lucas Serven and Carlos Asuncion contributed to the design of the study protocol, and to the design and implementation of the RunningCoach system. Kaidi Du, Caitlin Gruis, Yu Xiao contributed to the implementation of the RunningCoach system that was used in this study. We would like to thank everyone involved in the Berkeley Telemonitoring Project at UC Berkeley for their hard work that made this work possible. We would also like to thank the anonymous reviewers and the editors for their invaluable suggestions and assistance. This work was supported in part by the Center for Long-Term Cybersecurity (CLTC) at UC Berkeley, including the fees to publish in open access. The views expressed in this paper are those of the authors and do not necessarily represent the official views of the CLTC.

Author Contributions: D.A. and R.B. contributed to the design of the study protocol and conducted the study. D.A. and G.X.P. contributed to the design and implementation of the RunningCoach system used in this study. D.A., G.X.P. and G.K. analyzed the data. All authors contributed to the writing of the paper.

Conflicts of Interest: The authors declare no conflict of interest. The funding sponsors had no role in the design of the study; in the collection, analyses or interpretation of data; in the writing of the manuscript; nor in the decision to publish the results.

References

1. Van Gent, B.R.; Siem, D.D.; van Middelkoop, M.; van Os, T.A.; Bierma-Zeinstra, S.S.; Koes, B.B. Incidence and determinants of lower extremity running injuries in long distance runners: A systematic review. *Br. J. Sports Med.* **2007**, *41*, 469–480.
2. Heiderscheit, B.C.; Chumanov, E.S.; Michalski, M.P.; Wille, C.M.; Ryan, M.B. Effects of step rate manipulation on joint mechanics during running. *Med. Sci. Sports Exerc.* **2011**, *43*, 296–302.

3. Rowlands, A.V.; Eston, R.G.; Tilzey, C. Effect of stride length manipulation on symptoms of exercise-induced muscle damage and the repeated bout effect. *J. Sports Sci.* **2001**, *19*, 333–340.
4. Hamill, J.; Derrick, T.R.; Holt, K.G. Shock attenuation and stride frequency during running. *Hum. Mov. Sci.* **1995**, *14*, 45–60.
5. Mapmyfitness. Available online: www.mapmyfitness.com (accessed on 1 December 2017).
6. Runtastic. Available online: www.runtastic.com (accessed on 1 December 2017).
7. micoach. Available online: www.Adidas.com/fi/micoach (accessed on 1 December 2017).
8. Nike+gps. Available online: nikerunning.nike.com (accessed on 1 December 2017).
9. Runkeeper. Available online: www.runkeeper.com (accessed on 1 December 2017).
10. Endomondo. Available online: www.endomondo.com (accessed on 1 December 2017).
11. Aranki, D.; Balakrishnan, U.; Sarver, H.; Serven, L.; Asuncion, C.; Du, K.; Gruis, C.; Peh, G.X.; Xiao, Y.; Bajcsy, R. RunningCoach—Cadence Training System for Long-Distance Runners. In Proceedings of the 2017 Health-i-Coach—Intelligent Technologies for Coaching in Health, Barcelona, Spain, 23–26 May 2017.
12. Kaewkannate, K.; Kim, S. A comparison of wearable fitness devices. *BMC Public Health* **2016**, *16*, 433.
13. Hussain, M.; Al-Haiqi, A.; Zaidan, A.; Zaidan, B.; Kiah, M.L.M.; Anuar, N.B.; Abdulnabi, M. The landscape of research on smartphone medical apps: Coherent taxonomy, motivations, open challenges and recommendations. *Comput. Methods Programs Biomed.* **2015**, *122*, 393–408.
14. Higgins, J.P. Smartphone applications for patients' health and fitness. *Am. J. Med.* **2016**, *129*, 11–19.
15. Boratto, L.; Carta, S.; Mulas, F.; Pilloni, P. An e-coaching ecosystem: Design and effectiveness analysis of the engagement of remote coaching on athletes. *Pers. Ubiquitous Comput.* **2017**, *21*, 689–704.
16. Vos, S.; Janssen, M.; Goudsmit, J.; Lauwerijssen, C.; Brombacher, A. From problem to solution: Developing a personalized smartphone application for recreational runners following a three-step design approach. *Procedia Eng.* **2016**, *147*, 799–805.
17. Lun, V.; Meeuwisse, W.; Stergiou, P.; Stefanyshyn, D. Relation between running injury and static lower limb alignment in recreational runners. *Br. J. Sports Med.* **2004**, *38*, 576–580.
18. Taunton, J.E.; Ryan, M.B.; Clement, D.; McKenzie, D.C.; Lloyd-Smith, D.; Zumbo, B. A retrospective case-control analysis of 2002 running injuries. *Br. J. Sports Med.* **2002**, *36*, 95–101.
19. Dixit, S.; Difiori, J.P.; Burton, M.; Mines, B. Management of patellofemoral pain syndrome. *Am. Fam. Physician* **2007**, *75*, 194–202.
20. Farrokhi, S.; Keyak, J.; Powers, C. Individuals with patellofemoral pain exhibit greater patellofemoral joint stress: A finite element analysis study. *Osteoarthr. Cartil.* **2011**, *19*, 287–294.
21. Fredericson, M.; Powers, C.M. Practical management of patellofemoral pain. *Clin. J. Sport Med.* **2002**, *12*, 36–38.
22. Juhn, M.S. Patellofemoral pain syndrome: A review and guidelines for treatment. *Am. Fam. Physician* **1999**, *60*, 2012–2022.
23. Pal, S.; Besier, T.F.; Beaupre, G.S.; Fredericson, M.; Delp, S.L.; Gold, G.E. Patellar maltracking is prevalent among patellofemoral pain subjects with patella alta: An upright, weightbearing MRI study. *J. Orthop. Res.* **2013**, *31*, 448–457.
24. Pal, S.; Draper, C.E.; Fredericson, M.; Gold, G.E.; Delp, S.L.; Beaupre, G.S.; Besier, T.F. Patellar maltracking correlates with vastus medialis activation delay in patellofemoral pain patients. *Am. J. Sports Med.* **2011**, *39*, 590–598.
25. Chen, Y.J.; Scher, I.; Powers, C.M. Quantification of patellofemoral joint reaction forces during functional activities using a subject-specific three-dimensional model. *J. Appl. Biomech.* **2010**, *26*, 415–423.
26. Reilly, D.T.; Martens, M. Experimental analysis of the quadriceps muscle force and patello-femoral joint reaction force for various activities. *Acta Orthop. Scand.* **1972**, *43*, 126–137.
27. Lenhart, R.L.; Thelen, D.G.; Wille, C.M.; Chumanov, E.S.; Heiderscheit, B.C. Increasing running step rate reduces patellofemoral joint forces. *Med. Sci. Sports Exerc.* **2014**, *46*, 557.
28. Cavagna, G.; Mantovani, M.; Willems, P.; Musch, G. The resonant step frequency in human running. *Pflügers Arch.* **1997**, *434*, 678–684.
29. Williams, K.R.; Cavanagh, P.R. Relationship between distance running mechanics, running economy, and performance. *J. Appl. Physiol.* **1987**, *63*, 1236–1245.
30. Cavanagh, P.R.; Williams, K.R. The effect of stride length variation on oxygen uptake during distance running. *Med. Sci. Sports Exerc.* **1982**, *14*, 30–35.

31. Verbitsky, O.; Mizrahi, J.; Voloshin, A.; Treiger, J.; Isakov, E. Shock transmission and fatigue in human running. *J. Appl. Biomech.* **1998**, *14*, 300–311.
32. Candau, R.; Belli, A.; Millet, G.; Georges, D.; Barbier, B.; Rouillon, J. Energy cost and running mechanics during a treadmill run to voluntary exhaustion in humans. *Eur. J. Appl. Physiol. Occup. Physiol.* **1998**, *77*, 479–485.
33. Bood, R.J.; Nijssen, M.; Van Der Kamp, J.; Roerdink, M. The power of auditory-motor synchronization in sports: Enhancing running performance by coupling cadence with the right beats. *PLoS ONE* **2013**, *8*, e70758.
34. Van Dyck, E.; Moens, B.; Buhmann, J.; Demey, M.; Coorevits, E.; Dalla Bella, S.; Leman, M. Spontaneous entrainment of running cadence to music tempo. *Sports Med.-Open* **2015**, *1*, 15.
35. Johnson, C.M.; Johnson, T.R.; Zhang, J. A user-centered framework for redesigning health care interfaces. *J. Biomed. Inform.* **2005**, *38*, 75–87.
36. Abbott, P.A.; Foster, J.; de Fatima Marin, H.; Dykes, P.C. Complexity and the science of implementation in health IT—Knowledge gaps and future visions. *Int. J. Med. Inform.* **2014**, *83*, e12–e22.
37. Vedanthan, R.; Blank, E.; Tuikong, N.; Kamano, J.; Misoi, L.; Tulienge, D.; Hutchinson, C.; Ascheim, D.D.; Kimaiyo, S.; Fuster, V.; et al. Usability and feasibility of a tablet-based Decision-Support and Integrated Record-keeping (DESIRE) tool in the nurse management of hypertension in rural western Kenya. *Int. J. Med. Inform.* **2015**, *84*, 207–219.
38. Fiordelli, M.; Diviani, N.; Schulz, P.J. Mapping mHealth research: A decade of evolution. *J. Med. Internet Res.* **2013**, *15*, e95.
39. Aranki, D.; Kurillo, G.; Bajcsy, R. Smartphone Based Real-Time Health Monitoring and Intervention. In *Handbook of Large-Scale Distributed Computing in Smart Healthcare*; Springer: Berlin, Germany, 2017; pp. 473–514.
40. Song, E.; Asuncion, C.; Balakrishnan, U.; Sarver, H.; Serven, L. A Telemonitoring Solution to Long-Distance Running Coaching. Master's thesis, EECS Department, University of California, Berkeley, CA, USA, 2016. UCB/EECS-2016-99. Available online: http://www2.eecs.berkeley.edu/Pubs/TechRpts/2016/EECS-2016-99.html (accessed on 9 January 2018).
41. Jarv. Jarv Run BT Premium Bluetooth Heart Rate Monitor for Android Devices. Available online: http://www.jarvmobile.com/productdetail.asp?productid=33499 (accessed on 1 December 2017).
42. Micklewright, D.; Gibson, A.S.C.; Gladwell, V.; Al Salman, A. Development and Validity of the Rating-of-Fatigue Scale. *Sports Med.* **2017**, *47*, 2375–2393.
43. Borg, G.A. *Physical Performance and Perceived Exertion*; CWK Gleerup: Lund, Sweden, 1962.
44. Aranki, D.; Kurillo, G.; Mani, A.; Azar, P.; van Gaalen, J.; Peng, Q.; Nigam, P.; Reddy, M.P.; Sankavaram, S.; Wu, Q.; et al. A Telemonitoring Framework for Android Devices. In Proceedings of the 2016 IEEE First International Conference on Connected Health: Applications, Systems and Engineering Technologies (CHASE), Washington, DC, USA, 27–29 June 2016; pp. 282–291.
45. Alshurafa, N.; Eastwood, J.A.; Nyamathi, S.; Liu, J.J.; Xu, W.; Ghasemzadeh, H.; Pourhomayoun, M.; Sarrafzadeh, M. Improving compliance in remote healthcare systems through smartphone battery optimization. *IEEE J. Biomed. Health Inform.* **2015**, *19*, 57 63.
46. Aranki, D.; Kurillo, G.; Yan, P.; Liebovitz, D.M.; Bajcsy, R. Real-Time Tele-Monitoring of Patients with Chronic Heart-Failure Using a Smartphone: Lessons Learned. *IEEE Trans. Affect. Comput.* **2016**, *7*, 206–219.
47. Aranki, D. Towards Predictive Medicine – On Remote Monitoring, Privacy and Scientific Bias. PhD thesis, EECS Department, University of California, Berkeley, CA, USA, 2017. UCB/EECS-2017-145. Available online: https://www2.eecs.berkeley.edu/Pubs/TechRpts/2017/EECS-2017-145.html (accessed on 9 January 2018).
48. United States Geological Survey (USGS). EarthExplorer. Available online: https://earthexplorer.usgs.gov/ (accessed on 1 December 2017).
49. Johnson, R. Exercise dependence: When runners don't know when to quit. *Sports Med. Arthrosc. Rev.* **1995**, *3*, 267–273.
50. Stephan, Y.; Deroche, T.; Brewer, B.W.; Caudroit, J.; Le Scanff, C. Predictors of perceived susceptibility to sport-related injury among competitive runners: The role of previous experience, neuroticism, and passion for running. *Appl. Psychol.* **2009**, *58*, 672–687.

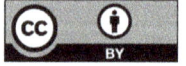

© 2018 by the authors. Licensee MDPI, Basel, Switzerland. This article is an open access article distributed under the terms and conditions of the Creative Commons Attribution (CC BY) license (http://creativecommons.org/licenses/by/4.0/).

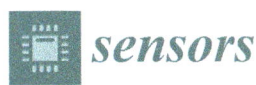

Article

Real-Time Monitoring in Home-Based Cardiac Rehabilitation Using Wrist-Worn Heart Rate Devices

Javier Medina Quero [1,*], María Rosa Fernández Olmo [2], María Dolores Peláez Aguilera [3] and Macarena Espinilla Estévez [1]

1. Department of Computer Science, University of Jaen, Campus Las Lagunillas, 23071 Jaén, Spain; mestevez@ujaen.es
2. Heart Rehabilitation Unit of the Hospital Complex of Jaén, Av. del Ejército Español 10, 23007 Jaén, Spain; mr.fernandez.olmo.sspa@juntadeandalucia.es
3. Council of Health for the Andalucian Health Service, Av. de la Constitucion 18, 41071 Sevilla, Spain; mdolores.pelaez.sspa@juntadeandalucia.es
* Correspondence: jmquero@ujaen.es; Tel.: +34-953-21-28-97

Received: 31 October 2017; Accepted: 5 December 2017; Published: 12 December 2017

Abstract: Cardiac rehabilitation is a key program which significantly reduces the mortality in at-risk patients with ischemic heart disease; however, there is a lack of accessibility to these programs in health centers. To resolve this issue, home-based programs for cardiac rehabilitation have arisen as a potential solution. In this work, we present an approach based on a new generation of wrist-worn devices which have improved the quality of heart rate sensors and applications. Real-time monitoring of rehabilitation sessions based on high-quality clinical guidelines is embedded in a wearable application. For this, a fuzzy temporal linguistic approach models the clinical protocol. An evaluation based on cases is developed by a cardiac rehabilitation team.

Keywords: wrist-worn heart rate devices; cardiac rehabilitation; real-time wearable monitoring; fuzzy logic; fuzzy linguistic approach; m-health

1. Introduction

Home-based e-health programs are being increasingly used due to the proliferation of wearable devices and portable medical sensors which are seamlessly integrated into the daily lives of users to monitor vital signs and physical activity [1]. In this way, wearable devices, together with connectivity and ubiquitous computing in mobile applications [2], have provided a solution for monitoring a greater number of patients under prevention and rehabilitation programs in a personalized manner [3].

Moreover, wearable devices have been demonstrated to favor strategies for changes to healthy habits and the promotion of healthy physical activity [4]. To achieve this, a key aspect is to adapt high-quality clinical guidelines and protocols from health centers to home-based solutions [5] in order to provide real-time activity monitoring by means of wearable devices [6].

Motivated by these recent advances, in this work a cardiac rehabilitation program is embedded in a wrist-worn device with a heart rate sensor, which provides real-time monitoring of physical activity during sessions in a safe and effective way. For this, a linguistic approach based on fuzzy logic [7] is proposed in order to model the cardiac rehabilitation protocol and the expert knowledge from the cardiac rehabilitation team. Fuzzy logic has provided successful results in developing intelligent systems from sensor data streams [8–12], and more specifically, it has been described as an effective modeling tool in cardiac rehabilitation [13].

The remainder of the paper is structured as follows: in Section 1.1, the principles and motivation of cardiac rehabilitation together with previous related works are presented; in Section 2, we detail a standardized protocol for cardiac rehabilitation, and based on it, a fuzzy model is proposed for real-time monitoring the heart rate of patients. In Section 3, the developed architecture based on wrist-worn wearable and mobile applications for patients and a cloud web application for the cardiac rehabilitation team is presented; in Section 4, an evaluation of fuzzy modifiers and temporal windows from heart rate sessions is provided by the cardiac rehabilitation team in order to adjust the real-time monitoring of the fuzzy model in practice; and finally, in Section 5, conclusions and suggestions for future works are presented.

1.1. Home-Based Cardiac Rehabilitation

Cardiovascular diseases represent a major health problem in developed countries according to the World Health Organization (WHO) [14]. Around 17 million people die annually from cardiovascular pathologies [15]. Fortunately, its prognosis has been improved by primary prevention, drug treatment, secondary prevention, and cardiac rehabilitation, the latter of which has been shown to be the most effective tool [16]. In this way, cardiac rehabilitation has been revealed by multiple studies as effective for reducing morbidity and mortality by around 20–30% in acute myocardial infarctions [17]. *Cardiac rehabilitation* (CR) is defined as the sum of the activities required to favorably influence the underlying cause of heart disease, as well as ensuring the best physical, social and mental conditions, thus enabling patients to occupy by their own means a normal place in society [18]. For these reasons, in recent years, secondary prevention programs and cardiac rehabilitation units (CRUs) have been developed in several countries [17,19,20]. However, there is a lack of accessibility due to several factors, such as lack of time, comorbidities, geographical area, and access to health services [18,20,21]. Minimizing these limitations by means of home-based programs and wearable devices is the motivation of this work, which is underway with respect to the development of CR at the primary and home-care level in order to increase the number of patients who benefit from these programs. These are fundamentally low-risk patients [16].

1.2. Related Works

In the literature, we highlighted recent works and reviews where the effectiveness of smart health monitoring systems is described and summarized [15,22,23]. In recent years, some works have been carried out in which information and communication technologies and/or wearable device have enabled the telemonitoring of these patients. These are the most representative of the following works.

In [24], a home-based CR with telemonitoring guidance is evaluated. It includes *individual coaching by telephone weekly* after uploading training data. In [25], a home-based walking training program is presented. The approach includes a health device with four electrodes. At the end of the sessions, the data are transmitted using a mobile device to a monitoring center, which provides indicators of adherence and evaluation. In [26], a combination of e-textiles, wireless sensor networks, and a transmission board provide monitoring of several physiological parameters, such as the electrocardiogram (ECG), heart rate, and body temperature for *future healthcare environments*. In [13], the cardiac and aortic data are collected by wearable t-shirts with embedded electrodes. Then, they are processed by a mobile device to acquire biosignals. In addition, fuzzy logic is presented as an effective modeling tool with monitoring of the vital signs by means of fuzzy rules. In [27], a mobile application uploads the sessions from a wearable device to enable the coaching of health personnel. The wearable device is presented as a data collector without providing a real-time feedback of sessions. In [28], Fitbit wearable sensor devices, and personalized coaching with SMS are proposed. In the same way, an ad hoc application was not embedded in the wearable device. Finally, in [29], the heart rate was measured by the index finger on a built-in camera for one minute at each exercise stage in order to evaluate the quality of the session.

In this way, previous works have foregrounded the relevance and efficacy of integrating cardiac rehabilitation programs (CRPs) into home-based solutions, but with the limitations of non-programmable heart rate sensors or burdensome devices in the early stages of implantation. However recently, a new generation of smart-watches and wrist-worn devices has improved the quality of measures in heart rate (HR), achieving a median error below 5% in laboratory-based activities [30]. Moreover, smart-watches and wrist-worn devices are expected to *be a boon to mHealth technologies* in physical activity sensing thanks to the recent tools and operating systems which enable application development [31].

Based on this context, in this work, we describe real-time monitoring and evaluation of cardiac rehabilitation sessions (CRSs) at home using wearable wrist-worn devices with heart rate sensors. The highlights of this approach are:

- *Wear and play* devices. Wrist-worn devices are noninvasive because of the heart rate sensor is embedded. In addition, they do not require placement of electrodes on the body prior to physical activity. Moreover, they are worn as a watch in an everyday manner.
- *Modeling a theoretical high-quality CRP*. A standardized CRP, which was developed by the CRU of Hospital Complex of Jaen (Spain) was introduced in the home-base approach for each patient's care in a personalized way. A linguistic approach based on fuzzy logic [7] is included to model the CRP and the expert knowledge from the cardiac rehabilitation team.
- *Real-time smart monitoring* is embedded in the wrist-worn device in order to: (1) show patients the adherence to CRP during physical activity; and (2) prevent unsuitable and inadequate HR ranges.
- *Practical methods* are described for applying the theoretical model to wearable computing.

2. Methodology

In Section 2, we detail the standardized protocol for the CRP where this work is focused for proposing a fuzzy model for real-time monitoring of the heart rate of patients by means of wrist-worn wearable devices.

2.1. Setting a Cardiac Rehabilitation Program

In this section, we describe a standardized CRP for patients with ischemic heart disease, a disease where patients suffer from a kind of restriction in the blood supply to the tissues. In the literature, several models for handling CRPs have been proposed and analyzed in many countries [32]. In this work, we proposed the use of a general model for cardiac rehabilitation [33] based on the heart rate, which is focused on determining the values of the heart rate training zones in the CRS. This model was developed at the CRU of the Hospital Complex of Jaen, Spain, where this work is centered.

As a previous step before starting the CRP, a first evaluation for each new patient of CR is required in health centers. In this initial evaluation, the patients are connected to an ECG and undergo a controlled cardiac stress test, which is evaluated by a cardiologist in terms of symptoms and blood pressure response for diagnosing patients. From this test, a cardiologist determines the next thresholds for each patient [34]:

- The maximal or peak heart rate (HR_{max}), that is, the number of contractions of the heart per minute (bpm) when it is working at its maximum capacity without severe problems.
- The basal or resting heart rate (HR_{rest}), that is, the bpm when the patient is awake, relaxed, and has not recently exercised.
- The first ventilatory threshold (VT_1), that is, the bpm which represents a level of intensity when blood lactate accumulates faster than it can be cleared, this being related to the aerobic threshold.
- The second ventilatory threshold (VT_2), that is, the bpm which represents the point where lactate is rapidly increasing with an intensity that generates hyperventilation; this being related to the anaerobic threshold.

Once patient thresholds are defined in the health center, a set of sessions are designed for configuring CRP by the cardiac rehabilitation team defining the:

- Duration range. The exercise duration of sessions, which is increased from initial sessions in an interval of (15–20) min to an interval of (30–40) min for trained patients [35].

- The optimal heart rate training zones (OHRTZs). These are defined by the clinical protocol in each session, as percentage ranges $[p_+^*, p_-^*]$ from HR_{max} and HR_{rest}. The methodology of Marvonen [33] allows translating the percentage range to absolute bpm $[r_+^*, r_-^*]$ that is defined by $r^* = HR_{rest} + p^*(HR_{max} - HR_{rest})$.

  The middle point between $[r_+^*, r_-^*]$ is known as *target heart rate* HR_{tar}, which is related to the ideal heart rate to maintain in the session.

- Duration of the progressive stage (d_w). The progression of HR within from basal state needs for a lineal increase, which starts from the resting point until reaching the OHRTZ. The duration of this progressive stage is defined in minutes.

2.2. A Fuzzy Model for Real-Time Monitoring and Evaluation of Cardiac Rehabilitation Sessions

In this section, we describe a fuzzy model for real-time monitoring and evaluation of the heart rate of patients in accordance with the cardiac rehabilitation program described in Section 2.1.

This fuzzy model is proposed to describe, in real-time, the heart rate stream, which is composed of the measured values and the time-stamps when they are collected by the heart rate sensor. In Section 2.2.1, we focus on fuzzification of the measures from heart rate sensor. In the Section 2.2.3, we describe a fuzzy aggregation of the terms using temporal windows. Moreover, in order to model the progressive stage, a fuzzy transformation from progressive to maintenance stage is detailed in Section 2.2.2. Finally, in Section 2.2.4, we detail an interpretable evaluation based on the previous steps to describe the further heart rate stream at the end of the rehabilitation session.

2.2.1. Fuzzification of Heart Rate Measures by Optimal Heart Rate Training Zones

In this section, we describe a linguistic approach based on fuzzy logic for the OHRTZ. In fuzzy logic methodology, a variable can be defined by means of terms, which are described by means fuzzy sets. Each fuzzy set is defined in terms of a membership function which is a mapping from the universal set to a membership degree between 0 and 1.

Based on the fuzzy logic methodology, we proceed to describe the HR under a linguistic representation defined by the parameters from the CRP, detailed in Section 2.1. Specifically, we propose three intuitive terms *{low, adequate and high}*, which are defined by fuzzy sets, for describing the variable *heart rate*, which is measured by a 2-tuple value $\bar{hr}_i = hr_i, t_i$. hr_i represents a given value in the heart rate stream and t_i its time-stamp. Hence, the heart rate stream is composed of a set of measured values $S_{\bar{hr}} = \{\bar{hr}_0, \ldots, \bar{hr}_i, \ldots, \bar{hr}_n\}$ which are collected by the heart rate sensor.

In this section, we focus on the fuzzification of a heart rate measure individually, $\bar{hr}_i$. On one hand, because of prior definitions in cardiac rehabilitation, which are, (1) the OHRTZs as values of HR between the ranges $[r_+, r_-]$; and (2) the ventilatory thresholds $[VT_1, VT_2]$ as the efficient and safe ranges of aerobic physical activity, we define the term as *adequate*. This term is described by a fuzzy set characterized by a membership function whose shape corresponds to a trapezoidal function. The well-known trapezoidal membership functions are defined by a lower limit l_1, an upper limit l_4, a lower support limit l_2, and an upper support limit l_3 (See Equation (1)):

$$TS(x)[l_1, l_2, l_3, l_4] = \begin{cases} 0 & x \leq 0 \\ (x - l_1)/(l_2 - l_1) & l_1 \leq x \leq l_2 \\ 1 & l_2 \leq x \leq l_3 \\ (l_4 - x)/(l_4 - l_3) & l_3 \leq x \leq l_4 \\ 0 & l_4 \leq x \end{cases} \quad (1)$$

For the term *adequate*, the fuzzy set is characterized by the trapezoidal membership function that is defined by Equation (2):

$$\mu_{adequate}(hr_i) = TS(hr_i)[VT_1, r_-^*, r_+^*, VT_2], VT_1 < r_-^* < r_+^* < VT_2 \quad (2)$$

On the other hand, with VT_2 being the threshold from aerobic to anaerobic activity, and r_+^* the upper limit range for OHRTZs, we define the term *high*, which is described by a fuzzy set characterized by the trapezoidal membership function that is defined by Equation (3):

$$\mu_{high}(hr_i) = TS(hr_i)[r_+^*, VT_2, VT_2, VT_2], VT_2 > r_+^* \quad (3)$$

In a similar way, with VT_1 being the lower threshold of the aerobic activity and r_- the lower limit range for OHRTZs, we define the term *low*, which is described by a fuzzy set characterized by the trapezoidal membership function that is defined by Equation (4):

$$\mu_{low}(hr_i) = TS(hr_i)[VT_1, VT_1, VT_1, r_-^*], VT_1 < r_-^* \quad (4)$$

The relation between the thresholds from cardiac rehabilitation program and the membership functions is shown in Figure 1. Moreover, thanks to the use of linguistic modifiers, in fuzzy logic, we can model different semantics over the membership functions for describing the linguistic terms [36]. To represent the impact of a linguistic modifier m over a linguistic term v, such as *great* or *fair*, a straightforward power operation of the membership function is proposed [37] and defined by $\mu_{m,v}(x) = \mu_v(x)^{\alpha_m}$.

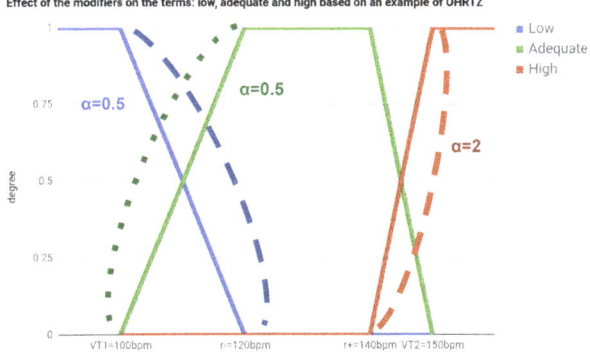

Figure 1. Example of membership functions for the terms low, normal, and high. In the example, the optimal heart rate training zones (OHRTZs) of the sessions are for trained patients, which are closer to VT_2 than to VT_1. In the example of modifiers, the impacts of the weak modifier in short-dashed lines and the strong modifier in long-dashed lines are shown.

If $\alpha_m < 0$, we obtain a weak modifier, such as *fair*; and a strong modifier with $\alpha_m > 0$, such as *great*. In Figure 1, we describe the impact of the linguistic modifiers, and in Section 4, we describe the comparative results of provided by the cardiac rehabilitation team.

At this point, based on the current value of the heart rate hr_i and the thresholds for the session $[VT_1, VT_2]$ and $[r_+^*, r_-^*]$, we are able to calculate the degree of the fuzzy terms {*low, adequate, and high*} in order to advise the patient in real-time with respect to the adequacy of the sessions.

The degrees of membership of the HR to the fuzzy sets {*low, adequate, and high*} can provide an intuitive evaluation for the real-time monitoring of sessions in wrist-worn wearable devices. For example, in this work, gradually changing colors in the evaluation of the HR are used to paint the screen of the wearable device and to evaluate the session using a 4-star scale, as described in Section 3.

However, in practice, it is necessary to handle additional issues in order to provide real-time monitoring during the rehabilitation sessions: the monitoring in the progressive stage and the temporal evaluation of heart rate streams.

2.2.2. Fuzzy Transformation from the Progressive to Maintenance Stage

In the literature there is a lack of proposals for modeling of the progressive stage in cardiac rehabilitation. This is related to the fact that it does not contain critical HRs. To resolve this issue, we propose a straightforward method to translate the model of OHRTZs from the aerobic state to define the initial basal state. In this way, the basal state is described by the following parameters:

- Basal ranges $[r_+^0, r_-^0]$ in bmp, where the HRs of patient are adequate in order to start the session.
- Lower basal threshold in bmp VT_1^0. This represents a minimal value of HR not recommended before starting the session.
- Upper basal threshold in bmp VT_2^0. This represents a maximal value of HR not recommended before starting the session.

Next, for calculating the time evolution in real-time within the progressive stage, we define a weight progression $w = \Delta t_0 / d_w, w \in [0, 1]$, where Δt_0 is the duration of session in the current time t_0 and d_w is the total duration of the progressive stage defined by the cardiac rehabilitation team.

Based on the temporal evolution of the weight progression as well as the initial and final values of each threshold, we can define the threshold in the progressive stage for each current time frame using a linear progression as shown in Equation (5).

$$
\begin{aligned}
r_-(w) &= r_-^0 + (r_-^* - r_-^0) \cdot w, w = \Delta t_0 / d_w \\
r_+(w) &= r_+^0 + (r_+^* - r_+^0) \cdot w, w = \Delta t_0 / d_w \\
VT_1(w) &= VT_1^0 + (VT_1 - VT_1^0) \cdot w, w = \Delta t_0 / d_w \\
VT_2(w) &= VT_2^0 + (VT_2 - VT_2^0) \cdot w, w = \Delta t_0 / d_w
\end{aligned} \quad (5)
$$

In Figure 2, we show an example of a CRS, where the linear progression of thresholds from progressive to maintenance stages is plotted.

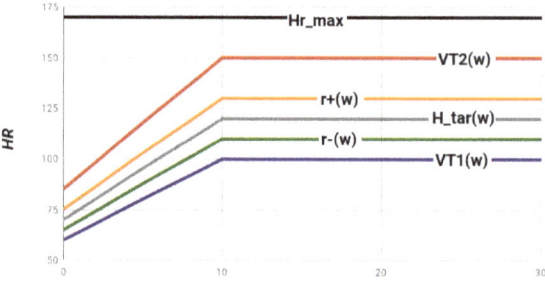

Figure 2. Evolution of the values of parameters from progressive to maintenance stages for a rehabilitation session: duration range (30 min), duration of progressive stage (10 m), OHRTZ $r_{+,-}^* = [130 \text{ bpm}, 110 \text{ bpm}]$, $HR_{max} = 170$ bpm, and $VT_{1,2} = [100 \text{ bpm}, 150 \text{ bpm}]$. This includes the basal ranges $[r_+^0, r_-^0] = [65 \text{ bpm}, 75 \text{ bpm}]$, and the lower and upper basal threshold $VT_{1,2}^0 = [60 \text{ bpm}, 85 \text{ bpm}]$ for the patient. HR: heart rate; bpm: number of contractions of the heart per minute.

2.2.3. Fuzzy Temporal Aggregation of the Heart Rate Stream

In the practice of developing based-sensor systems, the temporal component in the data streams is a critical aspect to analyze [38]. For example, in a given current time when we evaluate the heart rate sensor stream, we can take into account the last single sample of HR or calculate an average within a sliding window.

In this work, we propose fuzzy temporal aggregation [8], which provides a model to: (1) weight linguistic terms based on temporal membership functions; (2) define progressive and interpretable temporal linguistic terms; and (3) give flexibility in the presence of eventual signal loss or variance in the sample rate.

Based on previous works [8,39], we have integrated a fuzzy aggregation of the terms in the heart rate sensor stream using fuzzy temporal windows, which are straightforwardly described in function of the distance from each sample time-stamp $ts = \{t_0, \ldots, t_n\}$ to the current time $\Delta t_i = t_i - t_0$.

First, the degrees of a fuzzy term, in our case $V = \{low, adequate, high\}$, are weighted by the degree of their time-stamps evaluated by a fuzzy temporal window T_k defined by Equation (6).

$$V_r \cap T_k(\bar{hr}_i) = V_r(hr_i) \cap T_k(\Delta t_i) \in [0,1] \tag{6}$$

Secondly, the degrees of membership over the fuzzy temporal window are aggregated using the t-conorm operator in order to obtain a single degree of both fuzzy sets $V_r \cap T_k$ by Equation (7).

$$V_r \cup T_k(S_{\bar{hr}}) = \bigcup_{\bar{hr}_i \in S_{\bar{hr}}} V_r \cap T_k(\bar{hr}_i) \in [0,1] \tag{7}$$

We note several fuzzy operators can be applied to implement the aggregation. However in this paper, we propose a fuzzy weighted average [40] as is recommended in the case of high sample rates from wearable sensors [8]. The aggregation process is defined by Equation (8).

$$V_r \cup T_k(S_{\bar{hr}}) = \frac{1}{\sum T_k(\Delta t_i)} \sum V_r(hr_i) \times T_k(\Delta t_i^j) \in [0,1] \tag{8}$$

The definition and adequacy of several temporal windows, which model the evolution of linguistic terms in the heart rate stream, are discussed in Section 4.

2.2.4. Evaluating the Cardiac Rehabilitation Sessions

Previous sections describe real-time monitoring of heart rate stream within a wearable device based on fuzzy logic. Once the rehabilitation session has been finished by the patient, evaluating the further session at the end to provide a feedback is fairly intuitive.

Based on the degree of a fuzzy term V_r and its temporal window T_r, we compute an accumulative degree in the complete data stream $S_{\bar{hr}}$ by Equation (9).

$$\begin{aligned} low(S_{\bar{hr}}) &= \sum low \cup T_{low}(\bar{hr}_i) \\ adequate(S_{\bar{hr}}) &= \sum adequate \cup T_{adequate}(\bar{hr}_i) \\ high(S_{\bar{hr}}) &= \sum high \cup T_{high}(\bar{hr}_i) \end{aligned} \tag{9}$$

Under this approach, the accumulative degrees are calculated as the average degree of the terms in the heart rate stream ahead, providing upright and interpretable analytical data for the session. For example, the accumulative value of the term *adequate* has been used to fill a 4-star scale in the mobile application of this work in order to provide an evaluation of the rehabilitation session for the patient.

3. Development as a Wearable Mobile Cloud Platform

In this section, we describe the technical development of the proposed approach to be deployed in wearable wrist-worn devices, mobile devices, and a cloud web platform. The proposed architecture is inspired by current advances in wearable and mobile development tools [41], which provide real-time monitoring in wearable devices and data synchronization between mobile and web applications.

For the client, we have implemented two applications using Android Platform [42], both in wearable wrist-born and mobile devices. On the server side, we have implemented a web server under Java Tomcat, which web services orchestrate and synchronize the flow data between the cardiac rehabilitation team and patients. In Figure 3, we show the architecture and data flow of components.

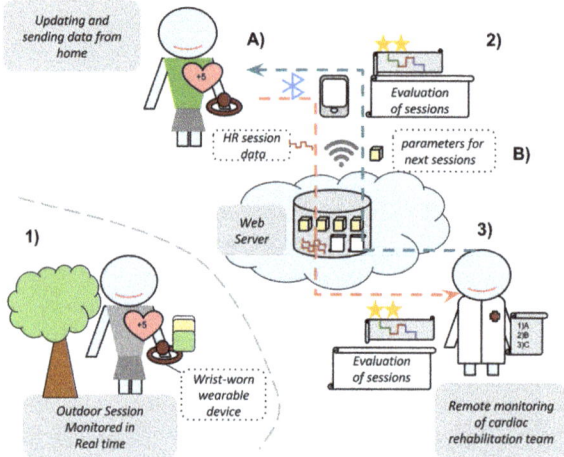

Figure 3. Architecture of components: (**1**) wearable device with real-time monitoring; (**2**) mobile application for evaluating the sessions; and (**3**) a web platform for evaluating the sessions by the cardiac rehabilitation team. The data from the patient and the team are synchronized (**A**) from wearable to mobile by Bluetooth; and (**B**) from mobile to cloud services by 4G/WiFi.

Hence, the approach includes three applications: a wearable application, a mobile application, and a web application, whose use cases are:

- A cloud web application for the cardiac rehabilitation team. Requiring previous authentication through login credentials, this includes the next use cases:

    - Registration and updating of patient data, including the thresholds for CRP: maximal heart rate HR_{max}, ventilatory thresholds $[VT_1, VT_2]$, basal ranges $[r_+^0, r_-^0]$ and basal limits $[VT_1^0, VT_2^0]$.
    - Creation and modification of the parameters of the sessions in the rehabilitation programs. They are: optimal heart rate training zones $[r_+^*, r_-^*]$, duration range $[d_1, d_2]$, and duration of progressive stage d_w.
    - Showing the CRSs from patients. The sessions developed by patients are synchronized from the mobile application to the web server. From them, the cardiac rehabilitation team can observe: (1) the raw data from the HR of the session in a timeline (with an option to zoom and scale); (2) the real-time monitoring provided for the patient using gradual colors: *blue, green, red* based on the degree of the terms $\{low, adequate, high\}$, respectively; and (3) a summarized indicator which evaluates the session using a 4-star scale.

- A mobile application for patients in order to show the sessions and communicate the data between the web server and the wearable devices. It has been developed for Android and included the next use cases:

    - Synchronization of the parameters of the next sessions from the CRP, which are defined by the cardiac rehabilitation team and are collected in the web server, in the mobile device using a web service under wireless network technology (3G/4G or WiFi).

- Synchronization of the session data from the wrist-worn wearable device into the mobile device using an ad-hoc Bluetooth connection.
- Uploading of the session data from the mobile device into the web server using a web service under wireless network technology (3G/4G or WiFi).
- Showing and evaluating the CRSs. In the same way as the cardiac rehabilitation team, patients can observe the following information in their mobile devices for each session: (1) the raw data from the HR of sessions in a timeline; (2) the real-time monitoring provided using gradually changing colors *blue, green, red*; and (3) a summarized indicator of the session using a 4-star scale.

- A wearable application for patient in order to develop the sessions with regard to the CRP. This has been developed for Android to include the next use cases:

  - Updating the the parameters of sessions from the mobile device into the wrist-worn wearable device using an ad-hoc Bluetooth connection.
  - Monitoring the session in the wearable device with regard to the CRP providing a real-time monitoring by means of showing (1) the current HR of the patient; (2) the target HR; (3) a graphical evaluation using gradually changing colors *blue, green, red* based on the degree of the terms $\{low, adequate, high\}$ respectively; and (4) the time of session and the graphical time progression in proportion to the proposed duration.
  - To synchronize the data of sessions, which contains the monitoring and raw HR, from the wrist-worn wearable device into the mobile device using an ad hoc Bluetooth connection.

Images from wearable, mobile, and web applications are shown in Figure 4, where we detail the evaluation and real-time monitoring developed under the methodology described in Section 2 by means of the technological components of the approach.

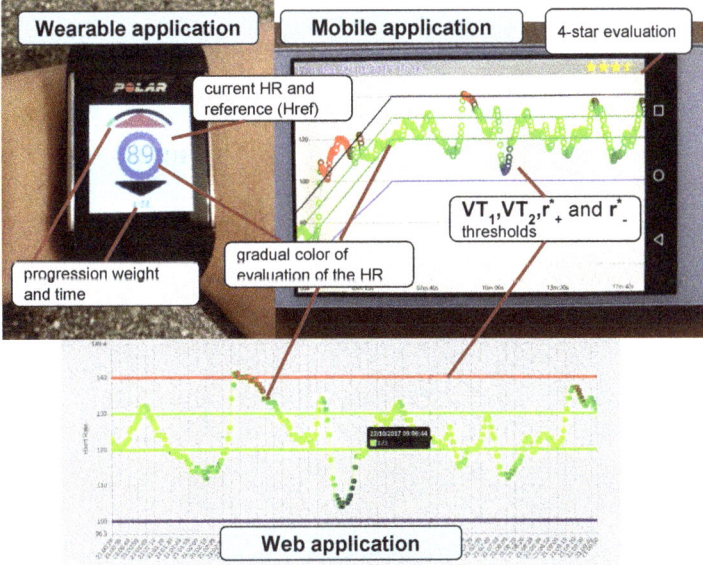

Figure 4. Pictures of the wearable, mobile, and web applications. In the wearable application in Polar M600, we show (1) a gradual color change in the evaluation of the HR; (2) progression and total time; and (3) the current and reference HR. In the mobile application, the VT_1, VT_2, r_+^* and r_-^* thresholds and the 4-star evaluations are described. In the web application, the cardiac rehabilitation team has access to heart streams and VT_1, VT_2, r_+^* and r_-^* thresholds of patients with zoom and scale options.

Polar M600 (https://www.polar.com/us-en/products/sport/M600-GPS-smartwatch) was chosen as an Android Wear device due to the high-quality optical heart rate monitor. The strength specifications of Polar M600 include : (1) optical heart rate measurement with six LEDs; (2) its waterproof nature (IPX8 10 m); (3) low weight (63 g); (4) reduced dimensions (45 × 36 × 13 mm); and (5) long-life battery (500 mAh Li-pol for a 2-day average uptime per charge or 8 h of training).

Based on the further evaluation of [43], Polar M600 is highly accurate. The HR value is ±5 bpm or less from the ECG HR value during periods of steady-state sports (cycling, walking, jogging, and running), which are the focus of cardiac rehabilitation. However, the accuracy was reduced during some intensity change exercises. No statistically significant was found in this sample on the basis of sex, body mass index, VO2max, skin type, or wrist size.

4. Results

In this section, we present an evaluation of the fuzzy model for real-time monitoring of cardiac rehabilitation sessions (CRSs) at home using wearable wrist-worn devices with heart rate sensors. As we discussed previously in Section 2, the theoretical aspects of cardiac rehabilitation are well defined in the literature. However, we can model different semantics over the membership functions for describing the linguistic terms by means of linguistic modifiers and temporal windows. In the next sections, we discuss the impact and adequacy of them based on the expert knowledge of a cardiac rehabilitation team.

4.1. Impact of Modifiers over Linguistic Terms

In this section, we describe an evaluation of the linguistic modifiers for the terms defined in Section 2.2.1. As we detailed previously, the OHRTZs define the ranges where the values of HR are totally *adequate*, VT_1 defines the basal-aerobic threshold from which inferior values of HR are totally *low*, and VT_2 the aerobic-anaerobic threshold from which upper values of HR are totally *high*. However, the values of HR between these optimal zones need to change gradually. This progression between optimal zones has been modeled and evaluated using several modifiers.

In this work, we have evaluated three models using different modifiers to adjust the progression in the trapezoidal membership functions of the terms *low, adequate, and high* with regards to Section 2.2.1.

First, we have evaluated low–adequate values of the heart rate by means of three models: (A) a severe model, where the *low* term is strong and the *adequate* term is weak; (B) a neutral model, where neutral modifiers are applied to both terms; and (C) a yielding model, where the *adequate* term is stronger than the *low* term, which is weaker. The strong, neutral, and weak properties have been defined by the parameters $\alpha = 0.5, \alpha = 1$, and $\alpha = 2.0$ of the modifier, respectively. In Figure 5, we show a representation of the impact of the modifiers on the degree of the linguistic terms in a HR stream.

To evaluate the impact of fuzzy modifiers, we have included a survey of 10 cases with key fragments of low values from the heart rate of a sessions, which were colored with blue and green, based on the degree of the terms low and adequate, respectively. In Figure 5, we show an example of a survey case. In a clinical session, the cardiac rehabilitation team evaluates them using a 5-point Likert scale: *{value -2, value -1, value 0, value +1, value +2}*, for which results are detailed in Table 1.

Second, in a similar way, high–adequate values of heart rate have been evaluated by means of three models: (A) a severe model; (B) a neutral model; and (C) a yielding model. A second survey, which contains 10 cases with key fragments of high values from the heart rate of sessions, was evaluated by the cardiac rehabilitation team using the 5-point Likert scale. Results are detailed in Table 1 and two examples of cases from the surveys are presented in Figure 5.

Table 1. The columns are related in order of: (1) survey; (2) model; (3) modifiers; and then percentages of responses for (4) value −2; (5) value −1; (6) value 0; (7) value +1; and (8) value +2.

Survey	Model	α Modifiers	Value −2	Value −1	Value 0	Value +1	Value +2
High values	severe	$\alpha_{high} = 2, \alpha_{adequate} = 0.5$	0	0.2	0.6	0.2	0
	neutral	$\alpha_{high} = \alpha_{adequate} = 1$	0	0	0.2	0.5	0.3
	yielding	$\alpha_{high} = 0.5, \alpha_{adequate} = 2$	0.3	0.4	0.3	0.0	0
Low values	severe	$\alpha_{low} = 2, \alpha_{adequate} = 0.5$	0	0.3	0.3	0.3	0.1
	neutral	$\alpha_{low} = \alpha_{adequate} = 1$	0	0	0.2	0.4	0.4
	yielding	$\alpha_{low} = 0.5, \alpha_{adequate} = 2$	0	0.4	0.5	0.1	0

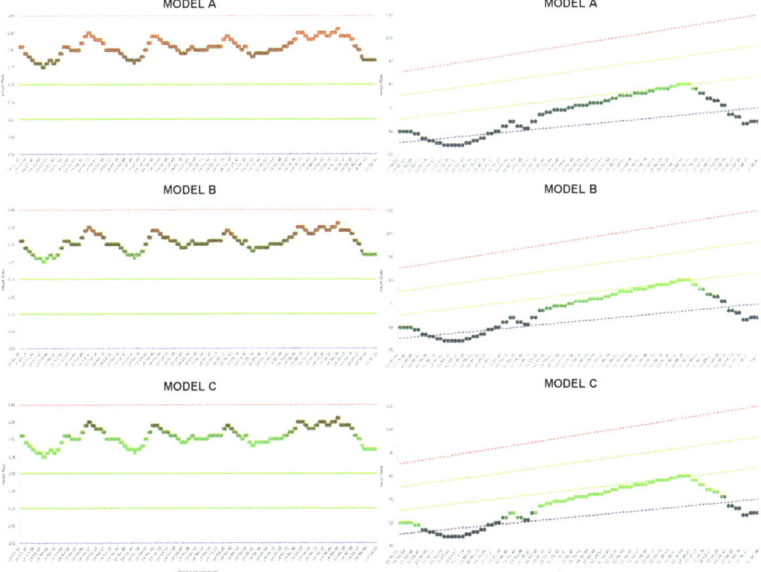

Figure 5. Impact of the fuzzy modifiers on heart rate streams. Heart rate is plotted using gradually changing colors blue, green, red based on the degree of the terms $\{low, adequate, high\}$, respectively. Green dotted lines determine the OHRTZs of patient. Blue and red dotted lines determine aerobic thresholds VT_1, VT_2 of the patient, respectively. The impact of the models A, B and C for a case of high–adequate HRs (**right**); and the impact of the models A, B, and C for a case of low–adequate HRs (**left**).

4.2. Impact of Temporal Window over Linguistic Terms

In this section, we describe an evaluation on the fuzzy temporal windows over linguistic terms which describe the heart rate stream during rehabilitation sessions. As we detailed previously, the theoretical thresholds of the heart range zones from CRP are defined theoretically missing the temporal permanence in OHRTZs. In some critical situations when patients develop the CRP, the evolution of heart rate between OHRTZs is prompt and inconstant. In those cases, the adherence and adequacy could not be just defined by the current value of HR.

In order to analyze the impact of the temporal windows, a survey with 15 key fragments of prompt and inconstant heart rate streams from the CRSs was designed to evaluate three temporal windows. The cardiac rehabilitation team from the Hospital Complex of Jaen (Spain) analyzed the impact of temporal windows for each term $\{low, adequate, high\}$ based on their expert knowledge.

The temporal windows to evaluate are (t_1): the last single sample; (t_2): a 3–5 s window; and (t_3): a 5–10 s window. In the two last cases (t_2 and t_3), we have defined the next fuzzy temporal windows

$\mu_{t2}(\Delta t_i) = TS(3s, 3s, 3s, 5s)$ and $\mu_{t3}(\Delta t_i) = TS(5s, 5s, 5s, 10s)$ based on the temporal fuzzification described in Section 2.2.3. In Figure 6, we detail an example of the semantics and impact of the three temporal windows on a heart rate streams.

In Table 2, we show the results of the evaluation described by a 5-point Likert scale: {value −2, value −1, value 0, value +1, value +2}. We can observe that the short-term temporal window t_1 is more recommendable when evaluating the term *high* because of corresponding critical values of HR, which require an immediate response from the patient to decrease the heart rate, whereas the long-term window t_3 is strongly not recommended. On the other hand, the longer temporal window t_2 is more properly related to the temporal term *adequate* because of the correct adherence the HR stream needs for a temporary stabilization in OHRZs. Finally, the term *low* is more appropriate with the temporal window t_2, and is adequate with other windows too.

Table 2. The columns are related in order of: (1) term; (2) model; and the percentage of responses for: (3) value −2; (4) value −1; (5) value 0; (6) value +1; and (7) value +2.

Term	Model	Value −2	Value −1	Value 0	Value +1	Value +2
High	t_1	0	0	0.3	0.3	0.4
	t_2	0	0	0.3	0.4	0.3
	t_3	0.3	0.4	0.3	0	0
Adequate	t_1	0	0	0.3	0.4	0.3
	t_2	0	0	0.2	0.2	0.6
	t_3	0	0.2	0.4	0.4	0
Low	t_1	0	0	0.3	0.4	3.0
	t_2	0	0	0.3	0.3	0.4
	t_3	0	0	0.3	0.4	3.0

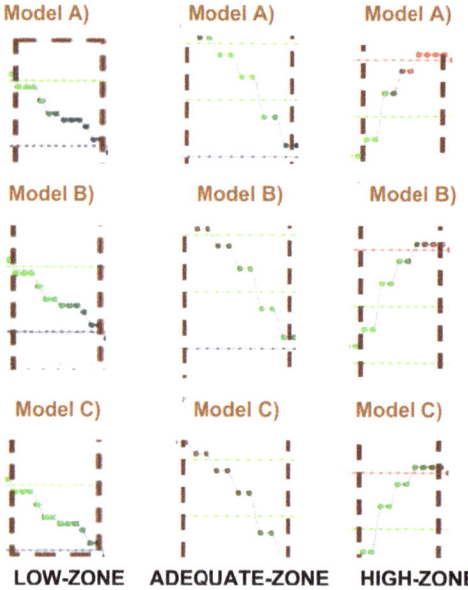

Figure 6. Impact of temporal windows on a case of prompt heart rate streams within the zones described by the linguistic terms {*low, adequate, high*}. Based on expert evaluation: Model A (short-term temporal window) suits in *high* zones detecting immediately critical HRs; Model B (middle-term temporal window) suits in *adequate* zone requiring a minimal permanence within; and Model B suits in the *low* zone without critical differences with regard to other models.

4.3. Discussion

On one first hand, from the results presented in Section 4.1, where the impact of modifiers are evaluated, we observe the preferences for the neutral model, where neutral modifier $\alpha_m = 1.0$ is applied to the linguistic terms. It indicates the non-predominance of a linguistic term over another when defining transition zones between OHRTZs and the aerobic thresholds VT_1, VT_2. We note that in the case of high values of HR, which are more sensitive for patients, the yielding model is strongly not recommended by the experts.

On the other hand, based on expert evaluation presented in Section 4.2 where the impact of temporal windows are evaluated, we note that the short-term temporal window suits in *high* zones detecting immediately critical heart rates. Model B (the middle-term temporal window) suits in the *adequate* zone requiring a minimal permanence within, and also suits in the *low* zone without critical differences with regard to other models.

In this way, we can note the adequacy of the clinical protocol for real-time monitoring the CRSs in wrist-worn devices. In addition, the use of a fuzzy model including modifiers and temporal windows has provided a methodology to obtain more accurate terms. This methodology can be extended to model other health contexts based on data stream processing.

Although previous works have been mainly focused on ECG sensors [13,26], the use of a wrist-worn device with the new generation of heart rate sensors provides high accuracy with respect to ECGs [43] for low-risk patients performing low- and medium-intensity exercise. The proposed approach has been implemented within Polar M6000 with Android Wear. Moreover, this wrist-worn device is noninvasive, light and comfortable, but with powerful computing capacity.

On translating the approach to other devices and health contexts, we advise that the quality and precision of heart rate is critical to ensure patient safety. High-risk patients and those with other pathologies could require more accurate devices such as ECGs. In this way, the proposed wrist-worn device just provides a measurement of HR. ECG devices could provide further signal processing of HR where heart rate variability or QRS could be described by means of the here-proposed linguistic terms and fuzzy temporal windows, due to the expanding importance of short-term beat windows in patient analysis [44].

Finally, we note the light processing to compute our methodology, which is based on fuzzy logic, enabling low-cost wrist-worn devices to incorporate it without a computational burden. Other approaches based on similar devices, such as the Fitbit [28] or Garmin [45], could be extended to develop embedded applications providing real-time monitoring during rehabilitation sessions.

5. Conclusions and Future Work

The main motivation of this work is enabling the high-quality real-time monitoring of CRPs at the homes of patients, designed and supervised remotely by the cardiac rehabilitation team. For this, we have proposed: (1) integrating a high-quality protocol based on clinical guidelines for monitoring the HR of the patient in a personalized way; (2) providing a real-time monitoring during sessions using a wearable wrist-worn device with heart rate sensor; and (3) using a wearable-mobile-cloud platform for collecting and synchronizing data between patients and the cardiac rehabilitation team.

The methodology of this work has been focused on modeling the theoretical approaches for developing an wearable application for real-time monitoring using wrist-worn devices. In order to address this challenge, first, a fuzzy model is proposed to describe under a linguistic approach the heart rate stream by means of three representative terms: *low, adequate, and high*. Fuzzy modifiers and fuzzy temporal windows are included in the methodology. The fuzzy approach provides a flexible evaluation of the HR stream: (1) enabling a intuitive real-time monitoring in wrist-worn wearable devices during sessions; and (2) providing visual and gradual advice, for which intensity is related to the degree of the terms.

On the other hand, an evaluation of fuzzy modifiers and fuzzy temporal windows is included to generate more accurate and flexible terms. In Section 4, the impact of fuzzy modifiers and temporal windows over the linguistic terms is analyzed by means of surveys based on cases. They have been evaluated by the cardiac rehabilitation team from the Hospital Complex of Jaen (Spain), indicating the most appropriated semantics for each linguistic term.

In future works, the approach will be extended to generate linguistic recommendations and summaries of the further sessions for the patients and the cardiac rehabilitation team. In this work, we have introduced the aggregation as a straight indicator in a 4-star scale, but a further analysis of the heart rate stream will provide intelligent and automatic feedback for cardiologists to detect weak points in the sessions of patients.

Acknowledgments: This contribution has been supported by the project PI-0203- 2016 from the Council of Health for the Andalucian Health Service, Spain together the research project TIN2015-66524-P from the Spanish government.

Author Contributions: J.M.Q. designed the methodology and wrote the paper; M.R.F.O. designed the rehabilitation protocol and led the experiments; M.D.P.A. contributed materials and analysis tools; M.E.E. analyzed and improved the methodology and the paper.

Conflicts of Interest: The authors declare no conflict of interest.

Abbreviations

The following abbreviations are used in this manuscript:

CR	Cardiac Rehabilitation
CRU	Cardiac Rehabilitation Units
CRP	Cardiac Rehabilitation Program
CRS	Cardiac Rehabilitation Sessions
ECG	Electrocardiogram
VT1	First Ventilatory Threshold
VT2	Second Ventilatory Threshold
HR	Heart Rate
bpm	Number of contractions of the heart per minute
OHRTZ	Optimal Heart Rate Training Zone

References

1. Butte, N.F.; Ekelund, U.; Westerterp, K.R. Assessing physical activity using wearable monitors: Measures of physical activity. *Med. Sci. Sports Exerc.* **2012**, *44* (Suppl. S1), S5–S12.
2. Espinilla, M.; Liu, J.; Garcia-Chamizo, J.M. Recent Advancements in Ubiquitous Computing. *J. Ambient Intell. Humaniz. Comput.* **2017**, *8*, 467–468.
3. Gouaux, F.; Simon-Chautemps, L.; Fayn, J.; Adami, S.; Arzi, M.; Assanelli, D.; Forlini, M.C.; Malossi, C.; Martinez, A.; Placide, J.; et al. Ambient intelligence and pervasive systems for the monitoring of citizens at cardiac risk: New solutions from the EPI-MEDICS project. In Proceedings of the IEEE Computers in Cardiology, Memphis, TN, USA, 22–25 September 2002; pp. 289–292.
4. Case, M.A.; Burwick, H.A.; Volpp, K.G.; Patel, M.S. Accuracy of smartphone applications and wearable devices for tracking physical activity data. *JAMA* **2015**, *313*, 625–626.
5. Krupinski, E.A.; Bernard, J. Standards and guidelines in telemedicine and telehealth. *Healthcare* **2014**, *2*, 74–93.
6. Chiauzzi, E.; Rodarte, C.; DasMahapatra, P. Patient-centered activity monitoring in the self-management of chronic health conditions. *BMC Med.* **2015**, *13*, 77.
7. Zadeh, L.A. Fuzzy sets. *Inf. Control* **1965**, *8*, 338–353.
8. Medina, J.; Martinez, L.; Espinilla, M. Subscribing to fuzzy temporal aggregation of heterogeneous sensor streams in real—Time distributed environments. *Int. J. Commun. Syst.* **2017**, *30*, doi:10.1002/dac.3238.
9. Medina, J.; Espinilla, M.; Garcia-Fernandez, A.L.; Martinez, L. Intelligent multi-dose medication controller for fever: From wearable devices to remote dispensers. *Comput. Electr. Eng.* **2017**, in press.
10. Espinilla, M.; Medina, J.; Garcia-Fernandez, Á.L.; Campaña, S.; Londoño, J. Fuzzy Intelligent System for Patients with Preeclampsia in Wearable Devices. *Mob. Inf. Syst.* **2017**, *2017*, 7838464.

11. Shewell, C.; Medina, J.; Espinilla, M.; Nugent, C.; Donnelly, M.; Wang, H. Comparison of Fiducial Marker Detection and Object Interaction in Activities of Daily Living Utilising a Wearable Vision Sensor. *Int. J. Commun. Syst.* **2017**, *30*, doi:10.1002/dac.3223.
12. Espinilla, M.; Nugent, C. Computational Intelligence for Smart Environments. *Int. J. Comput. Intell. Syst.* **2017**, *10*, 1250–1251.
13. Oliveira, C.C.; Dias, R.; da Silva, J.M. A Fuzzy Logic Approach for a Wearable Cardiovascular and Aortic Monitoring System. In *ICT Innovations 2015*; Springer: Cham, Switzerland, 2016; pp. 265–274.
14. World Health Organization. *Needs and Action Priorities in Cardiac Rehabilitation and Secondary Prevention in Patients with Coronary Heart Disease*; WHO Regional Office for Europe: Geneva, Switzerland, 1993; Volume 6.
15. Baig, M.M.; Gholamhosseini, H. Smart health monitoring systems: An overview of design and modeling. *J. Med. Syst.* **2013**, *37*, 9898.
16. De la Cuerda, R.C.; Diego, I.M.A.; Martín, J.J.A.; Sánchez, A.M.; Page, J.C.M. Cardiac rehabilitation programs and health-related quality of life. State of the art. *Rev. Esp. Cardiol. (Engl. Ed.)* **2012**, *65*, 72–79.
17. Grima-Serrano, A.; García-Porrero, E.; Luengo-Fernández, E.; León, L.M. Preventive cardiology and cardiac rehabilitation. *Rev. Esp. Cardiol.* **2011**, *64*, 66–72.
18. Balady, G.J.; Ades, P.A.; Bittner, V.A.; Franklin, B.A.; Gordon, N.F.; Thomas, R.J.; Tomaselli, G.F.; Yancy, C.W.; Association Science Advisory and Coordinating Committee. Referral, enrollment, and delivery of cardiac rehabilitation/secondary prevention programs at clinical centers and beyond. *Circulation* **2011**, *124*, 2951–2960.
19. Heran, B.S.; Chen, J.M.; Ebrahim, S.; Moxham, T.; Oldridge, N.; Rees, K.; Thompson, D.R.; Taylor, R.S. Exercise-based cardiac rehabilitation for coronary heart disease. *Cochrane Database Syst. Rev.* **2011**, *7*, CD001800.
20. Yue, C.S.S. Barriers to participation in a phase II cardiac rehabilitation programme. *Hong Kong Med. J.* **2005**, *11*, 472–475.
21. Daly, J.; Sindone, A.P.; Thompson, D.R.; Hancock, K.; Chang, E.; Davidson, P. Barriers to participation in and adherence to cardiac rehabilitation programs: A critical literature review. *Prog. Cardiovasc. Nurs.* **2002**, *17*, 8–17.
22. Taylor, R.S.; Dalal, H.; Jolly, K.; Zawada, A.; Dean, S.G.; Cowie, A.; Norton, R.J. *Home—Based versus Centre—Based Cardiac Rehabilitation*; The Cochrane Library: London, UK, 2015.
23. Taylor, R.S.; Dalal, H.; Jolly, K.; Moxham, T.; Zawada, A. Home-based versus centre-based cardiac rehabilitation. *Cochrane Database Syst. Rev.* **2010**, *1*, CD007130.
24. Kraal, J.J.; Peek, N.; van den Akker-Van, M.E.; Kemps, H.M. Effects and costs of home-based training with telemonitoring guidance in low to moderate risk patients entering cardiac rehabilitation: The FITA Home study. *BMC Cardiovasc. Disord.* **2013**, *13*, 82.
25. Worringham, C.; Rojek, A.; Stewart, I. Development and feasibility of a smartphone, ECG and GPS based system for remotely monitoring exercise in cardiac rehabilitation. *PLoS ONE* **2011**, *6*, e14669.
26. Lopez, G.; Custodio, V.; Moreno, J.I. LOBIN: E-textile and wireless sensor-network-based platform for healthcare monitoring in future hospital environments. *IEEE Trans. Inf. Technol. Biomed.* **2010**, *14*, 1446–1458.
27. Rawstorn, J.C.; Gant, N.; Meads, A.; Warren, I.; Maddison, R. Remotely delivered exercise-based cardiac rehabilitation: Design and content development of a novel mHealth platform. *JMIR mHealth uHealth* **2016**, *4*, e57.
28. Kitsiou, S.; Thomas, M.; Marai, G.E.; Maglaveras, N.; Kondos, G.; Arena, R.; Gerber, B. Development of an innovative mHealth platform for remote physical activity monitoring and health coaching of cardiac rehabilitation patients. In Proceedings of the 2017 IEEE EMBS International Conference on Biomedical & Health Informatics (BHI), Orlando, FL, USA, 16–19 February 2017; pp. 133–136.
29. Lee, E.S.; Lee, J.S.; Joo, M.C.; Kim, J.H.; Noh, S.E. Accuracy of Heart Rate Measurement Using Smartphones During Treadmill Exercise in Male Patients with Ischemic Heart Disease. *Ann. Rehabil. Med.* **2017**, *41*, 129–137.
30. Shcherbina, A.; Mattsson, C.M.; Waggott, D.; Salisbury, H.; Christle, J.W.; Hastie, T.; Wheeler, M.T.; Ashley, E.A. Accuracy in wrist-worn, sensor-based measurements of heart rate and energy expenditure in a diverse cohort. *J. Personalized Med.* **2017**, *7*, 3.
31. Rawassizadeh, R.; Price, B.A.; Petre, M. Wearables: Has the age of smartwatches finally arrived? *Commun. ACM* **2015**, *58*, 45–47.

32. Price, K.J.; Gordon, B.A.; Bird, S.R.; Benson, A.C. A review of guidelines for cardiac rehabilitation exercise programmes: Is there an international consensus? *Eur. J. Prev. Cardiol.* **2016**, *23*, 1715–1733.
33. American College of Sports Medicine. *ACSM's Guidelines for Exercise Testing and Prescription*; Lippincott Williams & Wilkins: Philadelphia, PA, USA, 2013.
34. Binder, R.K.; Wonisch, M.; Corra, U.; Cohen-Solal, A.; Vanhees, L.; Saner, H.; Schmid, J.P. Methodological approach to the first and second lactate threshold in incremental cardiopulmonary exercise testing. *Eur. J. Cardiovasc. Prev. Rehabil.* **2008**, *15*, 726–734.
35. Anari, L.M.; Ghanbari-Firoozabadi, M.; Ansari, Z.; Emami, M.; Nasab, M.V.; Nemaiande, M.; Boostany, F.; Neishaboury, M. Effect of cardiac rehabilitation program on heart rate recovery in coronary heart disease. *J. Tehran Univ. Heart Cent.* **2015**, *10*, 176–181.
36. Holldobler, S.; Khang, T.D.; Storr, H.P. A fuzzy description logic with hedges as concept modifiers. In Proceedings of the Third International Conference on Intelligent Technologies and Third Vietnam-Japan Symposium on Fuzzy Systems and Applications (InTech/VJFuzzy), Hanoi, Vietnam, 3–5 December 2002; pp. 25–34.
37. Kerre, E.E.; De Cock, M. Linguistic modifiers: An overview. *Fuzzy Log. Soft Comput.* **1999**, *9*, 69–85.
38. Baños, O.; Galvez, J.M.; Damas, M.; Pomares, H.; Rojas, I. Window size impact in human activity recognition. *Sensors* **2014**, *14*, 6474–6499.
39. Medina, J.; Espinilla, M.; Nugent, C. Real-time fuzzy linguistic analysis of anomalies from medical monitoring devices on data streams. In Proceedings of the 10th EAI International Conference on Pervasive Computing Technologies for Healthcare, Cancun, Mexico, 16–19 May 2016; ICST (Institute for Computer Sciences, Social-Informatics and Telecommunications Engineering): Brussels, Belgium, 2016; pp. 300–303.
40. Dong, W.M.; Wong, F.S. Fuzzy weighted averages and implementation of the extension principle. *Fuzzy Sets Syst.* **1987**, *21*, 183–199.
41. Paez, D.G.; de Buenaga Rodríguez, M.; Sánz, E.P.; Villalba, M.T.; Gil, R.M. Big data processing using wearable devices for wellbeing and healthy activities promotion. In Proceedings of the International Workshop on Ambient Assisted Living, Puerto Varas, Chile, 1–4 December 2015; Springer: Cham, Switzerland, 2015; pp. 196–205.
42. Meier, R. *Professional Android 4 Application Development*; John Wiley & Sons, Ltd.: Hoboken, NJ, USA, 2012.
43. Horton, J.F.; Stergiou, P.; Fung, T.S.; Katz, L. Comparison of Polar M600 Optical Heart Rate and Ecg Heart Rate during Exercise. *Med. Sci. Sports Exerc.* **2017**, *49*, 2600–2607.
44. Smith, A.L.; Owen, H.; Reynolds, K.J. Heart rate variability indices for very short-term (30 beat) analysis. Part 2: Validation. *J. Clin. Monit. Comput.* **2013**, *27*, 577–585.
45. Avila, A.; Goetschalckx, K.; Vanhees, L.; Cornelissen, V. A randomized controlled study comparing home-based training with telemonitoring guidance versus center-based training in patients with coronary heart disease: Rationale and design of the tele-rehabilitation in coronary heart disease (TRiCH) Study. *J. Clin. Trials* **2014**, *4*, 1–5.

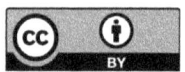

© 2017 by the authors. Licensee MDPI, Basel, Switzerland. This article is an open access article distributed under the terms and conditions of the Creative Commons Attribution (CC BY) license (http://creativecommons.org/licenses/by/4.0/).

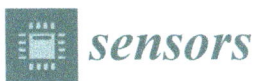

Article

Modular Bayesian Networks with Low-Power Wearable Sensors for Recognizing Eating Activities

Kee-Hoon Kim and Sung-Bae Cho *

Department of Computer Science, Yonsei University, 50 Yonsei-ro, Seodaemun-gu, Seoul 03722, Korea; aruwad.open@gmail.com
* Correspondence: sbcho@yonsei.ac.kr; Tel.: +82-2-2123-2720

Received: 10 October 2017; Accepted: 5 December 2017; Published: 11 December 2017

Abstract: Recently, recognizing a user's daily activity using a smartphone and wearable sensors has become a popular issue. However, in contrast with the ideal definition of an experiment, there could be numerous complex activities in real life with respect to its various background and contexts: time, space, age, culture, and so on. Recognizing these complex activities with limited low-power sensors, considering the power and memory constraints of the wearable environment and the user's obtrusiveness at once is not an easy problem, although it is very crucial for the activity recognizer to be practically useful. In this paper, we recognize activity of eating, which is one of the most typical examples of a complex activity, using only daily low-power mobile and wearable sensors. To organize the related contexts systemically, we have constructed the context model based on activity theory and the "Five W's", and propose a Bayesian network with 88 nodes to predict uncertain contexts probabilistically. The structure of the proposed Bayesian network is designed by a modular and tree-structured approach to reduce the time complexity and increase the scalability. To evaluate the proposed method, we collected the data with 10 different activities from 25 volunteers of various ages, occupations, and jobs, and have obtained 79.71% accuracy, which outperforms other conventional classifiers by 7.54–14.4%. Analyses of the results showed that our probabilistic approach could also give approximate results even when one of contexts or sensor values has a very heterogeneous pattern or is missing.

Keywords: human activity recognition; context-awareness; Bayesian network; mobile application; wearable computing

1. Introduction

Recently, with the rapid development of wearable sensor environments, a human activity recognition (HAR) with consistently collected daily data and various learning classifiers has become a popular issue: a vision-based recognition using a camera [1], recognition of five daily activities with acceleration data from a mobile phone and vital signs [2], and recognition with acceleration data from a chest-wearable device [3], and so on. However, despite mature studies and analyses on simple actions, like walking, standing, or sitting, complex activities that are composed of many low-level contexts and show various sensor patterns with respect to the background contexts have not been deeply studied yet [4].

In this paper, we propose a method which recognizes the eating activities in real life. Providing automatically information related with eating activities, such as the time and duration of eating activities, is crucial for healthcare management systems for people, in general, automatic monitoring for patients, such as diabetics, whose eating activities should be carefully managed, or the elderly who live alone, and so on. Although there are already plentiful studies recognizing simple eating and other daily activities, their approach did not catch the very large variety of activities in real life and are, therefore, difficult to extend to real situations. Eating activities could be a very complicated activity to recognize using sensors, especially with limited low-power sensors, as it could have different sensor patterns with respect to different backgrounds and spatial/temporal contexts. In this paper, we propose a probabilistic method, especially the Bayesian network, which is based on the idea that those complexities might be handled better with a probabilistic approach.

The paper is organized as follows: In Section 2, we provide some analyses to show the complexity of eating activities based on the real-life logging, and specify requirements to deal with those issues. In Section 3, we explore HAR-related works using low-level sensor data, and related theories analyzing components of human activity. In Section 4, we explain how to construct Bayesian networks in further detail, and verify their realistic usefulness in a variety of angles in Section 5. Finally, Section 6 concludes the paper and discusses future works.

2. Background

Before further discussions, we have collected the sensor data of 10 daily activities, including eating activities, from 25 subjects (detailed specifications are provided in Section 5) equipped with the wrist-wearable device and a smartphone with sensors (see Section 4.1), and have analyzed to ascertain the complexity of eating activities and show the requirements for the eating activity recognizer to be useful in the real world.

Table 1 shows the correlation scores of each attribute with respect to the class (darker color indicates higher value). Since we had collected the various eating activities, such as eating chicken with a fork, or a sandwich with a hand, eating activities of a baby, and so on, each attribute itself showed very low correlation scores. Despite the popular adoption and relatively high performance of accelerometers, the scores of 'h_acc's ('h' for a hand, 'acc' for an accelerometer) are considerably low, even lower than those of the environmental attributes ('lux' for illuminance, 'temp' for temperature, 'hum' for humidity), except the 'h_acc_y' which measures the back-and-forth motion of the hand when eating. The scores of 'acc's are considerably high compared to other attributes, but they are also fairly low and largely caused by the constraints that the collection was not done with the user's phone and they usually did not use the phone. Considering many people operate their smartphone while eating, it is rational to expect that those scores would be lower, like 'h_acc's. Table 2 shows the correlation matrix of the attributes (darker color indicates higher value), which also shows very low value, except 'h_acc_x' and 'h_acc_y', and 'acc's. Figure 1 shows a more specific example of a three-axis accelerometer value of the hand of four different eating activities. Even with a glimpse of observation, there are considerably different patterns: 'h_acc_y' of the child is comparably low as the position of the food is higher for them; the variance of all values is low when eating outside, as the user grabbed a sandwich and did not move his hand frequently; 'h_acc_x' is much higher than other cases when eating chicken using a fork, as the user tore on the left and right sides, and so on. In addition to the value of the sensor located on the wrist, the value of the smartphone sensor could be more unpredictable and variable as the smartphone could be anywhere while eating: in the pocket, on the table, in the hand, and so on. These could imply that the recognizer may require (i) manual modeling of activity instead of using the sensor value itself, or automatically extracted features with a learning classifier; (ii) a probabilistic reasoning that infers various kinds of contexts occurring probabilistically. In addition to the precise recognition itself; (iii) the constraint of the power and memory consumption of sensors; and (iv) the obtrusiveness to the user should be considered for the practical usage [5], as a recognizer should collect and recognize continuously without charging and too high a battery consumption could restrict the usage of devices for the original purpose.

Table 1. Correlation scores of each attribute.

Name [1]	Value	h_acc_x [2]	h_acc_y	h_acc_z	h_lux	h_temp	h_hum	acc_x	acc_y	acc_z
Correlation	Pearson correlation coefficient	0.1068	0.2887	0.0819	0.0217	0.0101	0.1379	0.2351	0.2837	0.3997
InfoGain	$\frac{H(C) - H(C\|A)}{H(C\|A)}$	0.0883	0.1866	0.0725	0.0685	0.1202	0.1556	0.4786	0.4604	0.336
GainRatio	$\frac{H(C) - H(C\|A)}{H(A)}$	0.0142	0.0304	0.0137	0.0133	0.0157	0.02	0.076	0.0678	0.0737
SymUncert	$\frac{2(H(C) - H(C\|A))}{H(C) + H(A)}$	0.0245	0.0523	0.023	0.0222	0.0278	0.0354	0.1311	0.1181	0.1208

[1] Correlation coefficient, information gain, information gain ratio, symmetric uncertainty; [2] h = hand, acc = accelerometer, lux = illuminometer, temp = temperature, hum = humidity.

Table 2. Correlation matrix of attributes.

	h_acc_x	h_acc_y	h_acc_z	h_lux	h_temp	h_hum	acc_x	acc_y	acc_z
h_acc_x	1								
h_acc_y	0.32	1							
h_acc_z	0.07	0.1	1						
h_lux	0.04	0.07	0.04	1					
h_temp	0.08	0.16	0.05	0.06	1				
h_hum	0.03	0.07	0.04	0.07	0.09	1			
acc_x	0.09	0.13	0.04	0.17	0.21	0.01	1		
acc_y	0.08	0.19	0.12	0.04	0.23	0.06	0.49	1	
acc_z	0.15	0.21	0.14	0.05	0.22	0.02	0.61	0.77	1

To fulfill those requirements, the proposed method (i) uses only five types of low-power sensors attached to the smartphone and the wrist-wearable device (Figure 2); (ii) is built on the context model of an eating activity which could represent the composition of complex eating activities, based on theoretical background and domain knowledge; and (iii) uses the Bayesian network (BN) for probabilistic reasoning, with a tree-structured and modular design approach to increase the scalability and reduce the cost for inference and management. Our contributions are as follows: (i) obtain and describe the complexity of real activities and the limitations of typical learning algorithms using real complex data; (ii) recognize the activity using only low-power and easily-accessible sensors; (iii) propose the formal descriptive model based on the theoretical background and show its usefulness; and (iv) provide the various experiments and analyses using a large amount of data from 25 different volunteers with 10 activities and various features.

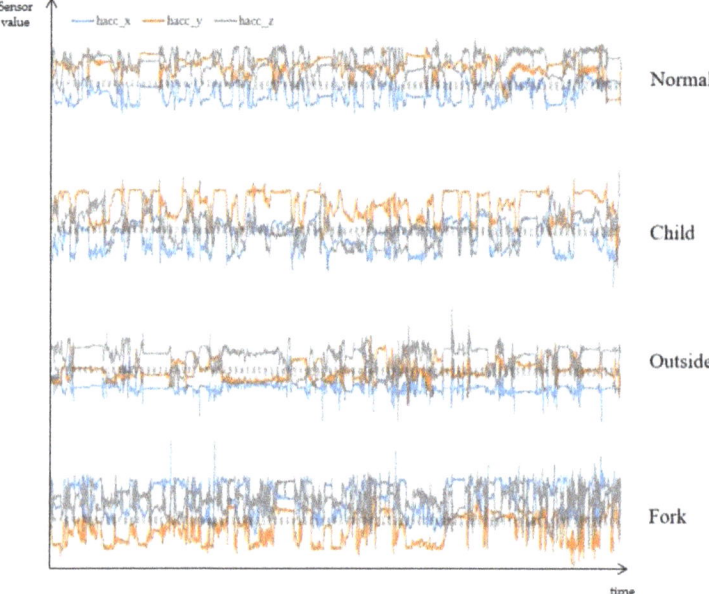

Figure 1. A time-series variation of acceleration sensor data in various activities.

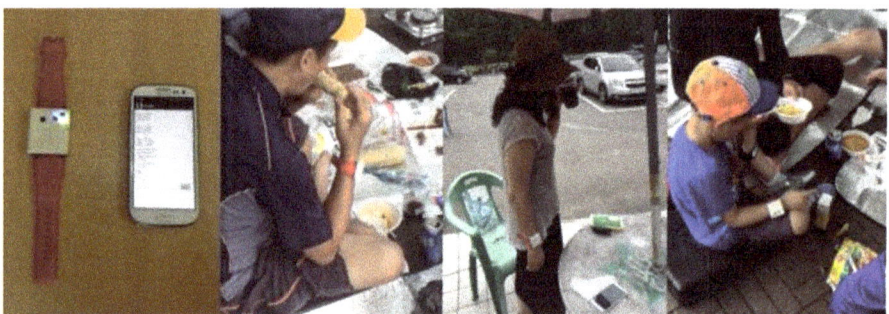

Figure 2. Smartphone and wrist-wearable device for data collection.

3. Related Works

Approaches for human activity recognition can be classified as two categories in terms of the location of sensors: external sensors and internal sensors [5]. Using external sensors, such as surveillance cameras for intrusion detection, a set of thermometers, hygrometers, or motion detectors for a smart home, is a primary approach. However, the internal sensor approach is more suitable for eating activity recognition because (i) the external sensor approach cannot track the user as sensors are generally fixed at a specific location; (ii) a user-centered sensor environment is better than a location-centered sensor environment for personalized context-aware services; and (iii) personal sensor data could be abused for intruding privacy. For these reasons, we have chosen the internal sensor approach using a mobile and wearable device that can be widely used in daily life.

Table 3 shows recent studies of the internal sensor approach for human activity recognition using various sensors and methods. Three-axis accelerometers are most widely used for the activities deeply related with a user's motion. However, accelerometers may not enough for the source of information when a recognizer attempts to recognize a complex activity. Bao et al. tried to recognize 20 daily activities using accelerometers attached to five locations [6]. In his experiment, accuracies of complex activities, such as stretching (41.42%), riding an elevator (43.58%), or riding an escalator (70.58%), were far lower than other simple activities, and showed larger deviations between people, or even in one person. This implies that complex activities with a great variety of different patterns may need more sensors, such as hygrometers or illuminometers, for environmental information. Cheng et al. recognized daily activities including food/water swallowing, using electrodes attached to the neck, chest, leg, and wrist [7]. Although it seems fairly reasonable using electrodes attached to the neck or chest for eating activity recognition, and they recognized various complex activities with better than 70% accuracy, their sensor environment might be uncomfortable in daily life. Obtrusiveness of the user should be concerned for the daily activity recognizer to be practical [8]. If the construction cost of the sensor environment is very high, or a user feels very uncomfortable wearing those devices, the recognizer is difficult to be used, generally. Thus, the composition and location of sensors must be acceptable for daily life. In addition, the energy consumption for sensor data collection should also be reasonable: if a smartphone will be run out of power after recognizing for just a few hours, not many people will want to use it. For this reason, it is difficult to use non low-power sensors, like the Global Positioning System (GPS) or gyroscopes.

Table 3. Sensors, activities, and methods of daily activity recognition works.

Author	Sensors	Activities	Feature Extraction	Classifier
Jatoba et al. [5]	Accelerometer (wrist, elbow, etc.)	Walking, jogging, climbing upstairs, etc.	Step count, mean value of local maxima, angle value, etc.	K-nearest neighbor, naïve Bayes, binary decision tree, etc.
Bao et al. [6]	Accelerometer (wrist, ankle, tight, elbow, hip)	20 daily activities (eating, walking, etc.)	Mean, energy, entropy, etc.	Decision tree, naïve Bayes, nearest neighbor, decision table
Cheng et al. [7]	Electrodes (neck, chest, leg, wrist)	Looking to various sides, bread/water swallowing, etc. (while sitting/walking)	Manual observation, time-domain features	Linear discriminant analysis
Tapia et al. [9]	Accelerometer (right-wrist, tight, ankle), heart rate monitor	Various exercise (walking, running, ascending/descending stairs, cycling, rowing, etc.)	Mean distance, entropy, correlation coefficient, FFT peaks and energy	Decision tree, naïve Bayes
Lee et al. [10]	Accelerometer (wrist, hip)	20 daily activities (dinner, lunch, office work, etc.)	Mean, standard deviation, mean crossing rate	Semi-Markov conditional random field

There are also many issues for feature extraction and classification. A large number of studies used statistical indices directly calculated from the sensor data value, such as the mean, standard deviation, energy, entropy, and so on. For complex activities, like eating or drinking, manual observation for patterns has also been conducted [7]. As shown in Figure 1, and studies in Table 3, sensor values could have a large deviation between people with various ages, genders, cultures, or even in one person. We attempted to find and construct the general context model for activity recognition based on the "Five Ws" (who, what, when, where, and why) and activity theory. The Five Ws are a publicly well-known and self-explanatory method to analyze and explain a situation for humans, so it can give a more understandable result [11]. Marchiori attempted to classify a very large amount of data on the World Wide Web based on Five Ws, and Jang used the Five Ws to define a dynamic status of a resident in a smart home [11,12]. Although the Five Ws give us a systematic and widely-agreed method of describing a situation, it is too abstract to apply directly to low-level sensor data. For example, eating a lunch at a restaurant cannot be directly recognized by acceleration or temperature. It should be embodied in a measurable level like 'correspondence of the space illumination'. Activity theory gives more specific evidence on how an activity should be composed. Nardi compared an activity theory with situated action models and a distributed cognition approach to systemically understand a structure of human activity and situation [13]. According to activity theory, a human activity consists of a subject, which includes human(s) in that activity, an object as a target object of the subject, which induces a subject to a special aim, an action that subject must perform in order to achieve the intended activity, and an unconsciously and repetitively occurring operation while doing an activity [14]. While action theory is primarily to examine the individual's own behavior as an analysis unit, situated action theory focuses on the relevance of actors and environmental factors at the moment of occurrence of the activity [15,16]. According to this theory, defining a human activity systemically should sufficiently consider environmental factors which can fluctuate dynamically [13]. In our proposed model, subject properties represent emergent properties of an eating person, which can be subclassified as an action and an operation. To deal with environmental factors, we use spatial and temporal properties independently.

For the classifiers for human activity recognition, learning approaches, such as decision trees, hidden Markov models, naïve Bayes, and nearest neighbor, are dominant. A large number of studies show a high accuracy for many daily activities (Table 1). However, as an activity becomes complex, or the number of subjects increases, many deterministic classifiers may not give good accuracy: Tapia et al. recognized various exercising activities and obtained over 90% accuracy for one subject, but 50–60% for many subjects. Vinh et al. used a probabilistic approach, a semi-Markov conditional random field, and showed good accuracy for complex activities, including dinner, lunch, and so on [10]. In this paper, we propose the Bayesian network that learns its conditional probability table for the probabilistic approach.

4. Proposed Method

Figure 3 shows the overall system architecture of the proposed method. It has a modular BN that infers the target activity node from a child node, which infers the low-level context, and simple decision trees that infer evidence nodes of the modular BN (see Sections 4.2 and 4.3). When the training process starts and the raw sensor data from nine channels and its class information are entered, the system learns and constructs its decision tree and conditional probability table, as described in the Section 4.3. For the recognition, the trained decision trees obtain raw sensor data continuously and make an inference of the probability of their evidence node, and the modular BN infers gradually from the evidence nodes to the query node, the eating activity. If the probability of the query node is larger than the predefined threshold, the recognition result becomes 'eating'.

4.1. Sensors

As mentioned in Section 1, we only used low-power sensors attached to the smartphone and a wrist-wearable device to consider constraints of power consumption and obtrusiveness of the user. The distribution rate of the wrist-wearable device is much higher than other forms of wearable devices and is in a natural position to collect daily life data consistently. Moreover, as we use our hands to eat something, the wrist is an appropriate position to collect food intake-related movement and the position of hands, and parametric temperature or humidity. We combined the four kinds of sensors for the wrist-wearable device (Figure 2), which are composed of MPU-9250 motion sensor of InvenSense (Seoul, republic of Korea), BME280 environment sensor of Bosch (Seoul, republic of Korea), and APDS-9900 illumination sensor of Avago Technologies (Seoul, republic of Korea). Table 4 shows the type of sensors with their power consumption and collecting frequency. The device can collect data continuously for about 6 h without charging.

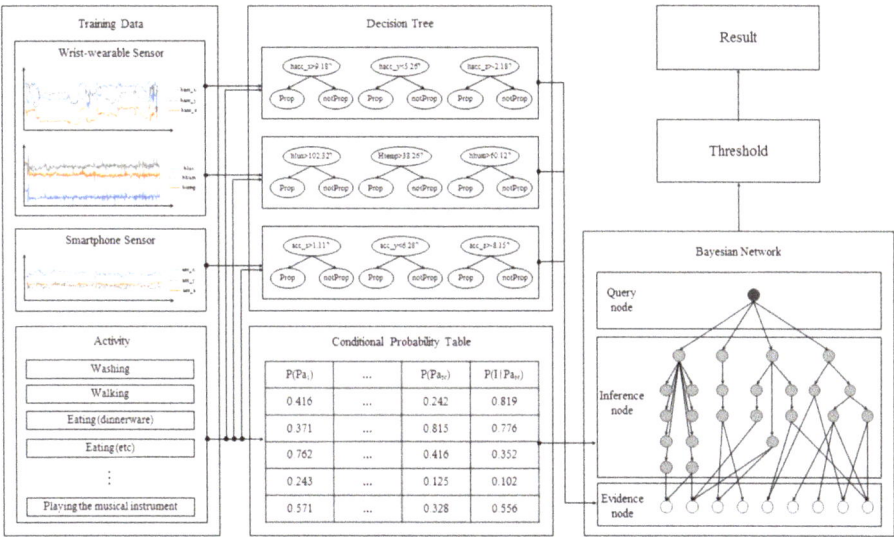

Figure 3. An overview of the proposed method.

Table 4. Sensors attached to wrist-wearable devices for recognition.

Sensor	Abbreviation	Units	Power Consumption	Collecting Frequency
Accelerometer	h_acc	m/s^2	450 µA	20 Hz
Illuminometer	h_lux	lux	250 µA	1 Hz
Thermometer	h_temp	°C	1.0 µA	1 Hz
Hygrometer	h_hum	g/m^3	0.8 µA	1 Hz

4.2. Context Model of Activity

An eating activity is a complex activity which consists of many low-level contexts, such as the spatial and temporal background, movement of the wrist, and temperature. Table 5 shows the web ontology language (OWL) representation of the proposed context model based on the activity theory and the "Five W's", for systemic analysis on an eating activity. Four subclasses represent the components of the Five W's, except 'Why", as this context is considered difficult to measure with the limited sensor environment. A subject property consists of goal-directed processes (actions) and the unconsciously appearing status of the body (body temperature, posture, and so on; operations). Nine properties describe the low-level context of the eating activity. Each intermediate node is linked to leaf nodes, namely, sensors, which are considered as related. Although the movement of the user is the main feature to recognize activities, used for most intermediate nodes, environmental features could also contribute, especially when the movement patterns are diverse. The proposed context model has three other subclasses (object, spatial, and temporal properties) to consider those environmental factors. A temporal property uses the system time for judging one property, whether the current time is appropriate for eating. A spatial property has four properties, such as whether the user is indoors or outdoors, changes of space, and whether the intensity of illumination of the space is appropriate for eating.

Table 5. OWL representation of the context model for eating activity recognition.

Class: Eating activity	subClassOf: Subject property	subClassOf: Activity	subClassOf: Wrist	ObjectProperty: Position of hand
				ObjectProperty: Dinnerware
				ObjectProperty: Movement of hand
			subClassOf: Body	ObjectProperty: Posture
				ObjectProperty: Move/stop
				ObjectProperty: Movement of body
		subClassOf: Operation		ObjectProperty: Body temperature
				ObjectProperty: Posture
				ObjectProperty: Humidity of hand
	subClassOf: Object property	ObjectProperty: Existance of food		
	subClassOf: Spatial property	ObjectProperty: Eating place		
		ObjectProperty: Indoor/outdoor		
		ObjectProperty: Move/stop		
		ObjectProperty: Illuminance of space		
	subClassOf: Temporal property	ObjectProperty: Eating time		

4.3. The Proposed Bayesian Network

A formal definition of the BN and its nodes are as follows.

Definition 1. *A BN is a directed acyclic graph (DAG) with a set of nodes N, a set of edges $E = (N_i, N_j)$, and a conditional probability table (CPT) which represents a causal relationship between connected nodes. Each node represents a specific event on the sample space Ω, and each edge and the value of the CPT represent a conditional relationship between a child node and parent nodes, $P(C = c|P = p)$. Given the BN and evidence e, the posterior probability $P(N|e)$ can be calculated by chain rule, where $Pa(N)$ is the set of parent nodes of N [17]:*

$$P(N|e) = \prod P(N|Pa(N)) \times e = \prod P(N|Pa(N)) \prod_{e_i \in e} e_i, \quad (1)$$

Definition 2. *A set of nodes N consists of the set of query nodes Q, which represents the event user wants to know from the BN a set of evidence nodes V, which observes the sensor data and classifies the properness, and a set of inference nodes I, which infers the probability of related contexts based on a CPT.*

Figure 4 shows the proposed BN. The proposed BN consists of V, I, and Q, where $|V| = 64$, $|I| = 23$, and $|Q| = 1$. Full names of sensors are described in Table 4. Nodes in V are set by nine types of low-level sensor data, the query node in Q represents the recognition result, eating or not, and each intermediate node in I represents the sublevel context of the target activity. By using intermediate nodes, the proposed model is more resistant to overfitting than typical learning models which mainly depend on automatically calculated statistics, such as the mean, deviation, or Fourier coefficients. For example, even if the model is trained only with the eating data using a fork, it could approximately recognize the eating activity using chopsticks if the user eats while sitting and shows the similar pattern of the movement of the hand, and so on. Moreover, in addition to the complex composition of the eating activity itself, there could be many unexpected or omitted sensor values: user may eat while lying down or eat at midnight, or take off the wrist-wearable device or smartphone, where the accelerometer value is omitted. A BN could deal with these issues as it provides the probabilistic approach for recognizing each context, so it can give an approximate answer even if some data are uncertain or missing, compared to other deterministic classifiers which give a wrong answer or cannot give any answer at all.

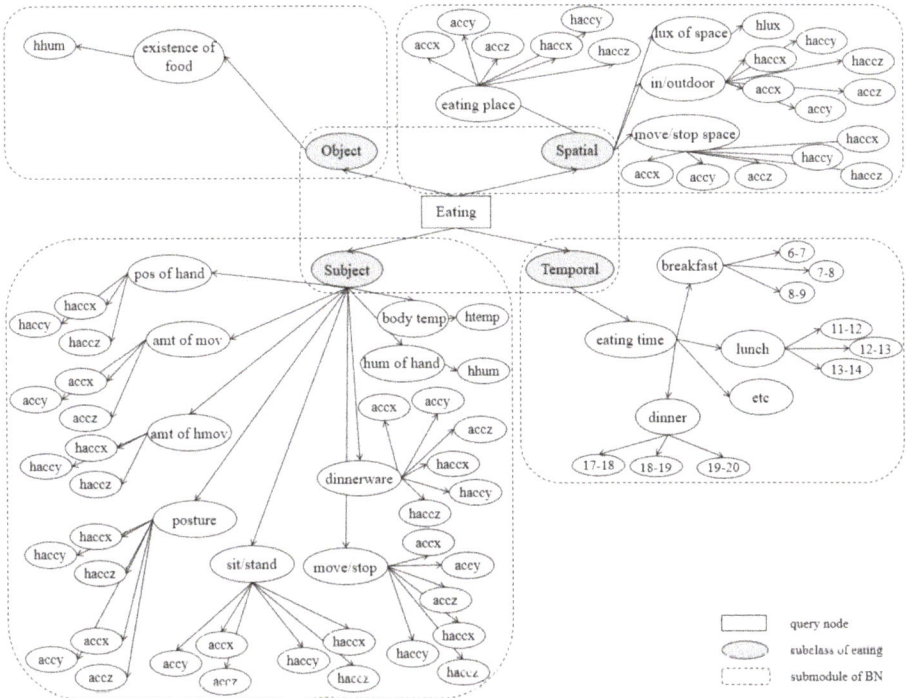

Figure 4. The proposed Bayesian network.

For a structure of the proposed BN, we construct the modular BN with a tree-structured design.

Definition 3. *Modular Bayesian network [18]. A Modular BN (MBN) consists of a set of submodular BNs M and the conditional probability between submodules R. Given BN submodules $\theta_i = (V_i, E_i)$ and $\theta_j = (V_j, E_j)$, the link $R_{i,j} = \{< \theta_i, \theta_j > | i \neq j, V_i \cap V_j = \varnothing\}$ is created. Two submodules are connected and communicate only by shared nodes.*

The proposed MBN has one main module containing a query node and four submodules where each leaf node in a main module (object/spatial/subject/temporal) becomes the root node of each submodule. All submodules are designed by a tree-structured approach, where each module has only one root node, which is also a shared node, and all child nodes have exactly one parent node. By following these design approaches, the proposed model is more explainable as the probability of each shared node could easily be calculated and explain the probability of each context to an individual. Moreover, these design approaches substantially reduce the complexity of the BN to $O(k^3 n^k + wn^2 + (wr^w r^w)n)$; by limiting k to 2 and minimizing the w, where n is the number of nodes, k is the maximum number of parents, r is the maximum number of values for each node, and w is the maximum clique.

Algorithm 1. Learning algorithm for the CPT.

---

for∀D,// D is the input data
increment numOfData by 1;
C := class of D;
for i = 1 to n(I) do
if C includes I_i then
        increment num(I_i) by 1;
        if $\exists\, q \in Q$ s.t. $q \in C$ then increment num($I_i \cap Q$);
for i = 1 to n(I) do
$P(I_i) := \frac{num(I_i)}{numOfData}$;
$$\mathrm{CPT}(I_i) := P(I_i|Q) = \frac{P(I_i,Q)}{P(Q)} = \frac{num(I_i \cap Q)}{num(Q)};$$

To calculate the value of the CPT, the proposed BN learns the data using simple learning algorithm. In the training process, the training data enters into E and I. For evidence nodes in E, there is a simple binary decision tree for each evidence node and it learns a criterion for classification. For inference nodes in I, BN counts the number of occurrences that $C \subset I_i$ for $\forall I_i \in I$ and update the element of the CPT, as shown in Algorithm 1. For example, if $C_k = \{sitting\} \cap \{dinnerware\} \cap \{eating\}$, $C_k \subset I_1 = \{sitting\}$ and $C_k \subset Q_1 = \{eating\}$, so $num(I_1)$ and $num(I_1 \cap Q_1)$ increment, and so on. For this algorithm, the proposed BN needs $O((M + N) \times ND)$ time complexity for learning, where ND is the amount of data, and when either the number of nodes or data is fixed, the time complexity becomes linear.

5. Experimental Results

5.1. Data Specification

For the experiment, we collected 948 min of data from 25 different volunteers for 10 activities. Subjects were asked to wear a wrist-wearable device and have a smartphone, performed activities that they wanted to perform, and tagged the activity they were doing on the smartphone when the new activity started. They were also asked not to perform more than one activity simultaneously to collect accurate sensor data for each class. If they performed another activity that were not supposed to be collected, such as moving to another place or getting a phone call, collection was temporarily stopped. To collect as much real-life data as possible, we did not request them to come to a certain place; instead, we went to where they lived while performing their daily activities and collected the data. When a self-tagging was difficult, like for a baby or the elderly who are not familiar with a smartphone, we observed and tagged their activities simultaneously. Each subject performed, at most, four different activities and each activity was prolonged for, at most, 20 min to prevent a small number of subjects from dominating most of the data. A specific distribution of each item is shown in Table 6, and indices of activities and jobs are shown in Table 7. We attempted to balance the gender of the subjects, and chose the list of activities by referencing Activities of Daily Livings (ADLs) which is known as a proper method describing the functional status of a human, performing an important role in a healthcare service [19]. 'Etc' in the job includes a four-year old baby. An eating activity consists of 47.27% (448 min out of 948 min), so the data is well-balanced in terms of the eating activity.

Table 8 shows a brief comparison of the collected data with other popular open data for HAR: Opportunity dataset [20] and Skoda dataset [21]. Note that as our approach is supposed to recognize various real eating activities with people with various contexts, we focused on collecting the data from a sufficiently large number of subjects, so the length of collected data for each subject is relatively small, which is supposed to capture short intervals of daily life, mainly including eating activities. Additionally, note that we tried to use very limited sensors and devices, which are supposed to only include low-power sensors that are easy to use in daily life.

Table 6. Data specification.

Activity	Count	Job	Count	Gender	Count
1	1 (4%)	1	3 (12%)	M	12 (48%)
2	2 (8%)	2	2 (8%)	F	13 (52%)
3	1 (4%)	3	1 (4%)	Age	Count
4	11 (44%)	4	6 (24%)	0~10	2 (8%)
5	6 (24%)	5	1 (4%)	20~30	9 (36%)
6	3 (12%)	6	8 (32%)	30~40	2 (8%)
7	2 (8%)	7	3 (12%)	40~50	3 (12%)
8	5 (20%)	8	1 (4%)	50~60	8 (32%)
9	1 (4%)			60~	1 (4%)
10	1 (4%)				

Table 7. Index of activities and jobs.

Index	Activity	Job
1	Washing	Undergraduate
2	Walking	Graduate
3	Housework	Student
4	Eating (dinnerware)	Houseworker
5	Eating (etc.)	No job
6	Conversation	Office worker
7	Driving	Businessman
8	Sedentary work	etc.
9	Subway	
10	Playing the piano	

Table 8. Comparison of our dataset with another open dataset for HAR.

	Number of Subjects	Number of Instances	Length	Activities	Sensors
Our dataset	25	379,013	16 h	10 daily activities	Three-axis accelerometers (2), hygrometer, illuminometer, thermometer
Opportunity	4	96,667	6 h	17 simple activities	Inertial measurement unit (7), three-axis accelerometers (12)
Skoda	1	179,853	3 h	10 gestures	Three-axis accelerometers (20)

5.2. Accuravy Test

Tables 9 and 10 show the result of the 10-fold cross-validation of the proposed BN. The proposed BN produced 76.86% accuracy with the threshold value of 0.6. The specificity of the proposed BN (83%) was higher than the sensitivity (76.05%), which means that the proposed BN classifies better in the non-eating activity than the eating activity. Figure 5 shows the ROC (receiver operating characteristic) curve as the threshold for the eating probability decreases. The cost for decreasing the threshold was the smallest at the point 'threshold = 0.6', and where the threshold is lower than 0.2, the BN classified all activities as an eating activity. As shown in Figure 5, the AUC (area under curve) is fairly large, which supports the usefulness of the BN. Figure 6 shows the accuracy, sensitivity, and specificity of the various typical learning classifiers. We used the Weka 3.8.0 tool (of the university of the Waikato, Hamilton, New Zealand) to analyze the results. Five classifiers have a large deviation between tests, as they tend to be overfitted to the train data; when the test data is composed mostly of similar data with the train data, their performance is very high, but in the other case, they are very low. The proposed BN, LR, and RF showed smaller deviations. The accuracy of the proposed BN was 7.54–14.4% higher than other classifiers. In the case of naïve Bayes and Adaboost, sensitivities are very high (96.15% and 95.91%, respectively), but specificities are also very low (37.68% and 53.77%, respectively), which means that the two classifiers classified most cases as an eating activity. For the multilayer perceptron (MLP), it showed good results among five other classifiers, but the time to build the model and classify was much higher than other methods. For the one-sample t-test, suppose the population has a normal distribution, and let the null hypothesis $H_o = \prime accuracy < 0.8\prime$. With $\overline{X} = 0.7854, s = 0.386, t = -0.0378 > -2.262$, and H_o is rejected. When $H_o\prime =\prime accuracy > 0.9\prime$, $t = -0.2969 < -2.262$, so $H_o\prime$ is rejected and the proposed model is expected to have an accuracy of 0.8–0.9 for the population.

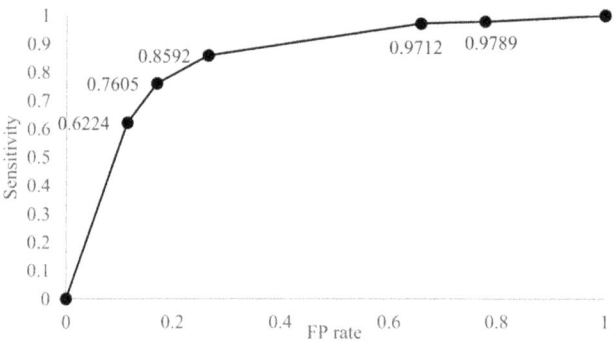

Figure 5. ROC curve for the proposed BN.

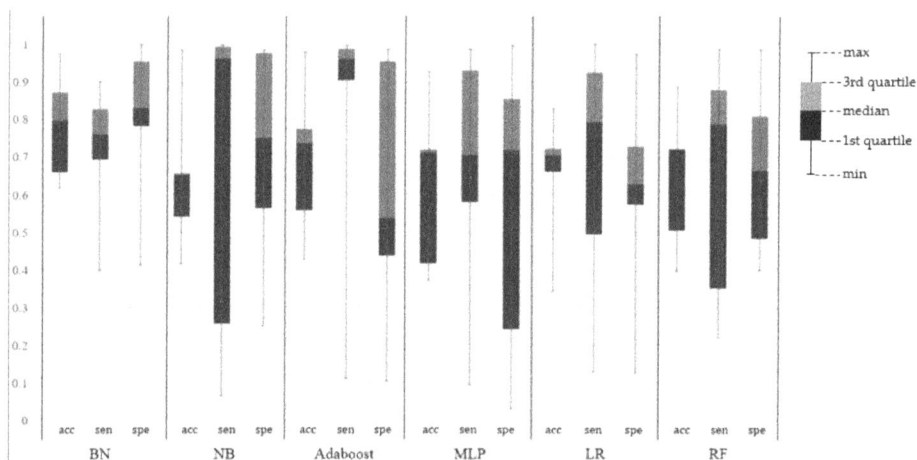

Figure 6. Ten-fold cross-validation for other typical classifiers (accuracy, sensitivity, specificity).

Table 9. Confusion matrix of the proposed BN.

	Positive	Negative
True	TP = 136,354	FN = 42,937
False	FP = 33,949	TN = 165,773

Table 10. Statistical indices of the results.

Index	Value
Accuracy	$\frac{TP+TN}{TP+TN+FP+FN} = 79.71\%$
Precision	$\frac{TP}{TP+FP} = 80.07\%$
Sensitivity	$\frac{TP}{TP+FN} = 76.05\%$
Specificity	$\frac{TN}{FP+TN} = 83\%$

5.3. Error Case Analysis

Figure 7 shows the proportion of each activity to the whole error case, and Figure 8 shows the error rate of each activity. The index of each activity is shown in Table 7. Eating with dinnerware shows the highest proportion (40%), followed by sedentary work (30%) and conversation (10%). However, due to the proportion of eating with dinnerware being far greater than that of sedentary work, the error rate is much larger with respect to sedentary work (0.424). As sedentary work and conversation generally show similar patterns in the amount of movement of the hand, and usually happens indoors, the same as with the eating activity, the two activities show a higher error rate than any other activities. However, in the case of walking, as it is typically a dynamic activity easily distinguished from the eating activity, it showed a very low error rate (0.004%; 174 lines out of 39,822 lines). For driving and subway activities, differences of movement and spatial properties make those activities' error rates low.

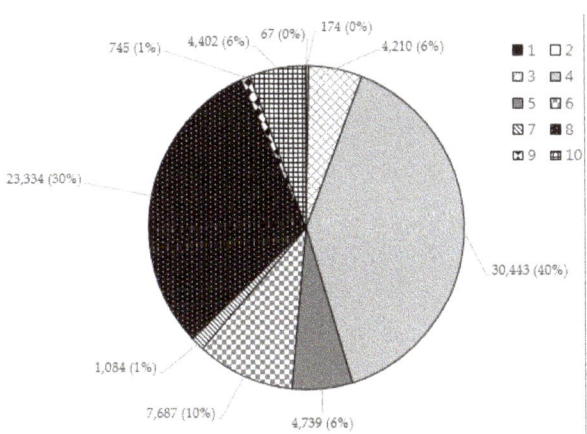

Figure 7. Proportion of the error case.

Figure 9 shows the specific case, which is the eating activity of a left-handed person, who wore the wrist-wearable device on the right wrist and mainly used the left hand to eat, but also used the right hand for moving food, using a smartphone, gesturing in conversation, and so on. Compared to the right-handed person (Figure 1), the accelerometer shows a different pattern, such as a much lower and steady value for the *x*-axis and a higher and irregular pattern of the *y* and *z*-axis, as they used their right hand for various purposes in addition to eating. As a result, the probability of using dinnerware shows very low and high deviance. However, as the person ate in a normal environment like other subjects, the spatial property compensating the final recognition and overall eating probability shows acceptable results. This means that the proposed BN could approximately recognize the complex eating activity when one of the contexts or sensor values has a very different pattern or is even omitted. Note that the proposed method might approximately recognize these cases without incorporating information of which hand the person uses and applying different algorithms. This is important since, in the real world, the person might use different hands for various situations; one might prefer to use the left hand to drink coffee, while using the right hand to eat chicken.

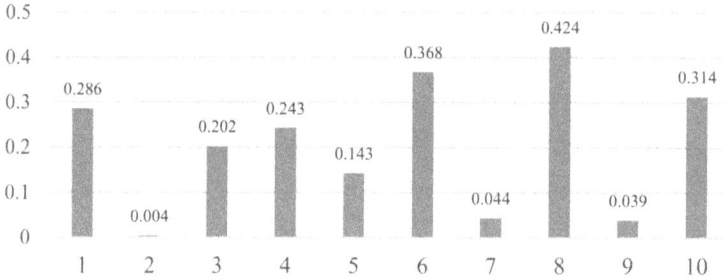

Figure 8. Error rate of each activity.

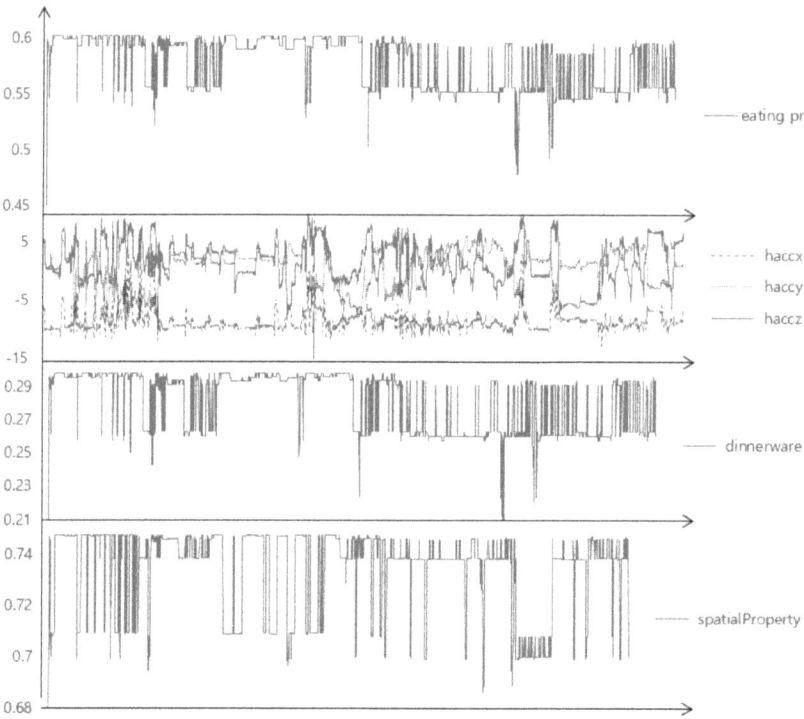

Figure 9. Eating activity of a left-handed person.

6. Conclusions

In this paper, we proposed the eating activity recognition method based on a Bayesian network, using low-power sensors attached to a smartphone and a wrist-wearable device. Contributions of this paper are as follows: (i) obtain and describe the complexity of real activity and limitations of typical learning algorithms using real complex data; (ii) recognize it using only low-power and easily-accessible sensors with low time complexity; (iii) propose the probabilistic model based on the theoretical background; and (iv) provide the various experiments and analysis using large data from 25 different volunteers for 10 activities and various features, showing the usefulness of the proposed method. The proposed method showed an accuracy of 79.71%, which is higher than other learning classifiers, with of 7.54–14.40% better accuracy. We analyzed the error case and the results show that the proposed method could approximately give the answer even when some of contexts or sensor values are very different. Future works include the collection of much larger and representative data, the construction and evaluation of the proposed method for various complex and daily activities, and the evaluation of the proposed method with open data.

Acknowledgments: This work was supported by an Electronics and Telecommunications Research Institute (ETRI) grant funded by the Korean government (17ZS1800, Development of self-improving and human-augmenting cognitive computing technology).

Author Contributions: Sung-Bae Cho devised the method and guided the whole process to ccreate this paper; Kee-Hoon Kim implemented the method and performed the experiments; and Kee-Hoon Kim and Sung-Bae Cho wrote the paper.

Conflicts of Interest: The authors declare no conflict of interest.

References

1. Testoni, V.; Penatti, O.A.B.; Andaló, F.A.; Lizarraga, M.; Rittner, L.; Valle, E.; Avila, S. Guest editorial: Special issue on vision-based human activity recognition. *J. Commun. Inf. Syst.* **2015**, *30*, 58–59. [CrossRef]
2. Tian, L.; Sigal, L.; Mori, G. Social roles in hierarchical models for human activity recognition. In Proceedings of the Computer Vision and Pattern Recognition, Providence, RI, USA, 16–21 June 2012.
3. Casale, P.; Pujol, O.; Radeva, P. Human activity recognition from accelerometer data using a wearable device. In Proceedings of the Pattern Recognition and Image Analysis, Las Palmas de Gran Canaria, Spain, 8–10 June 2011.
4. Liu, L.; Peng, Y.; Wang, S.; Liu, M.; Huang, Z. Complex activity recognition using time series pattern dictionary learned from ubiquitous sensors. *Inf. Sci.* **2016**, *340*, 41–57. [CrossRef]
5. Jatoba, L.C.; Grossmann, U.; Kunze, C.; Ottenbacher, J.; Stork, W. Context-aware mobile health monitoring: Evaluation of different pattern recognition methods for classification of physical activity. In Proceedings of the IEEE Annual Conference of Engineering in Medicine and Biology Society, Vancouver, BC, Canada, 20–25 August 2008.
6. Bao, L.; Intille, S.A. Activity recognition from user-annotated acceleration data. In Proceedings of the Pervasive Computing, Vienna, Austria, 18–23 April 2004.
7. Cheng, J.; Amft, O.; Lukowicz, P. Active capacitive sensing: Exploring a new wearable sensing modality for activity recognition. In Proceedings of the Pervasice Computing, Helsinki, Finland, 17–20 May 2010.
8. Lara, O.D.; Labrador, M.A. A survey on human activity recognition using wearable sensors. *IEEE Commun. Surv. Tutor.* **2013**, *15*, 1192–1209. [CrossRef]
9. Tapia, E.M.; Intille, S.S.; Haskell, W.; Larson, K.; Wright, J.; King, A.; Friedman, R. Real-time recognition of physical activities and their intensities using wireless accelerometers and a heart rate monitor. In Proceedings of the IEEE International Symposium on Wearable Computers, Boston, MA, USA, 11–13 October 2007.
10. Lee, S.; Le, H.X.; Ngo, H.Q.; Kim, H.I.; Han, M.; Lee, Y.-K. Semi-Markov conditional random fields for accelerometer-based activity recognition. *Appl. Intell.* **2011**, *35*, 226–241.
11. Marchiori, M. W5: The Five Ws of the World Wide Web. In Proceedings of the International Conference on Trust Management, Oxford, UK, 29 March–1 April 2004.
12. Jang, S.; Woo, W. Ubi-ucam: A unified context-aware application model. In Proceedings of the Modeling and Using Context, Stanford, CA, USA, 23–25 June 2003.

13. Nardi, B.A. *Context and Consciousness: Activity Theory and Human-Computer Interaction*; Massachusetts Institute of Technology: Cambridge, MA, USA, 1995; pp. 69–102.
14. Leont'ev, A.N. The problem of activity in psychology. *Sov. Psychol.* **1974**, *13*, 4–33. [CrossRef]
15. Suchman, L.A. *Plans and Situated Actions: The Problem of Humanmachine Communication*; Cambridge University Press: Cambridge, UK, 1987.
16. Ghahramani, Z. Learning dynamic Bayesian networks. In *Adaptive Processing of Sequences and Data Structures*; Giles, C.L., Gori, M., Eds.; Springer: Berlin/Heidelberg, Germany, 1992; pp. 168–197.
17. Korb, K.B.; Nicholson, A.E. *Bayesian Artificial Intelligence*, 2nd ed.; CRC Press: Boca Raton, FL, USA, 2010; pp. 29–54.
18. Lim, S.; Lee, S.-H.; Cho, S.-B. A modular approach to landmark detection based on a bayesian network and categorized context logs. *Inf. Sci.* **2016**, *330*, 145–156. [CrossRef]
19. Hong, Y.-J.; Kim, I.-J.; Ahn, S.C.; Kim, H.-G. Mobile health monitoring system based on activity recognition using accelerometer. *Simul. Model. Parct. Theory* **2010**, *18*, 446–455. [CrossRef]
20. Roggen, D.; Calatroni, A.; Rossi, M.; Holleczek, T.; Förster, K.; Tröster, G.; Lukowicz, P.; Bannach, D.; Pirkl, G.; Ferscha, A.; et al. Collecting complex activity data sets in highly rich networked sensor environments. In Proceedings of the 7th IEEE International Conference on Networked Sensing Systems (INSS), Kassel, Germany, 15–18 June 2010; pp. 233–240.
21. Zappi, P.; Lombriser, C.; Farella, E.; Roggen, D.; Benini, L.; Tröster, G. Activity recognition from on-body sensors: Accuracy-power trade-off by dynamic sensor selection. In Proceedings of the 5th European Conference on Wireless Sensor Networks (EWSN), Bologna, Italy, 30 January–1 February 2008; pp. 17–33.

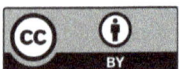

© 2017 by the authors. Licensee MDPI, Basel, Switzerland. This article is an open access article distributed under the terms and conditions of the Creative Commons Attribution (CC BY) license (http://creativecommons.org/licenses/by/4.0/).

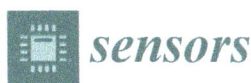

Article

Smart Device-Based Notifications to Promote Healthy Behavior Related to Childhood Obesity and Overweight

Gustavo López [1,*], Iván González [2], Elitania Jimenez-Garcia [3], Jesús Fontecha [2], Jose A. Brenes [1], Luis A. Guerrero [1] and José Bravo [2]

1. Research Center for Communication and Information Technologies (CITIC), University of Costa Rica, San José 11501, Costa Rica; joseantonio.brenes@ucr.ac.cr (J.A.B.); luis.guerrero@ecci.ucr.ac.cr (L.A.G.)
2. MAmI Research Lab, University of Castilla-La Mancha, 13071 Ciudad Real, Spain; ivan.gdiaz@uclm.es (I.G.); jesus.fontecha@uclm.es (J.F.); jose.bravo@uclm.es (J.B.)
3. Faculty of Engineering, Architecture and Design, Autonomous University of Baja California, Ensenada 21100, Mexico; ejimenez@uabc.edu.mx
* Correspondence: gustavo.lopez_h@ucr.ac.cr; Tel.: +506-2511-8030

Received: 29 October 2017; Accepted: 12 January 2018; Published: 18 January 2018

Abstract: Obesity is one of the most serious public health challenges of the 21st century and it is a threat to the life of people according to World Health Organization. In this scenario, family environment is important to establish healthy habits which help to reduce levels of obesity and control overweight in children. However, little efforts have been focused on helping parents to promote and have healthy lifestyles. In this paper, we present two smart device-based notification prototypes to promote healthy behavior with the aim of avoiding childhood overweight and obesity. The first prototype helps parents to follow a healthy snack routine, based on a nutritionist suggestion. Using a fridge magnet, parents receive graphical reminders of which snacks they and their children should consume. The second prototype provides a graphical reminder that prevents parents from forgetting the required equipment to practice sports. Prototypes were evaluated by nine nutritionists from three countries (Costa Rica, Mexico and Spain). Evaluations were based on anticipation of use and the ergonomics of human–system interaction according to the ISO 9241-210. Results show that the system is considered useful. Even though they might not be willing to use the system, they would recommend it to their patients. Based on the ISO 9241-210 the best ranked features were the system's comprehensibility, the perceived effectiveness and clarity. The worst ranked features were the system's suitability for learning and its discriminability.

Keywords: ubiquitous computing; health; human-centered computing

1. Introduction

Obesity is one of the most serious public health problems of the 21st century and it is a threat to people's lives [1]. Obesity is influenced by several factors. At a personal level, simple things such as eating alone or in the presence of other people can affect a person's food intakes. Moreover, nutritional habits are also important factors influencing children obesity and overweight. For instance, restrictive eating practices are associated with weight gain [2]. Furthermore, people that insist on excessively control their eating behaviors show less ability to self-regulate food and energy intake across meals.

Not only human factors affect people's behavior, there are also non-appropriate environments that impact on human beings at a social level. For instance, when people operate in contexts that offer larger than necessary food portions, that have a high availability of energy-dense foods, or strong influence for sedentary behaviors, living a healthy life becomes harder.

Several efforts have been conducted to prevent and delay the growth of this issue. Mobile devices, heart rate monitors, chest pins and other devices are used for lifestyle monitoring and self-control. Moreover, many interventions have been developed over the years to determine the proper way to promote healthy behaviors. Lau et al. described that when technological applications or devices are used for these purposes, the results are either as effective as other ways of intervention. The only exception is face to face interventions [3].

Many efforts have been put into using mobile technology to promote healthy behavior. External memory aids play an important role in supporting habit development; they are useful when they refer to the target behavior and the situation in which it needs to be executed. Even though the effectiveness and relevance of reminders decrease with time, reminders keep people engaged and help them to repeat the behavior, and in some cases, could support the start of the new habit, as the new behavior might develop faster than the decay of effectiveness of the reminder [4].

The effects of mobile-based notifications have been established in previous works. The amount of notifications received in a mobile phone is now unmanageable for users [5,6]. Therefore, we believe that combining mobile applications with pervasive computing through smart devices could have more impact in the people and enhance their user experience.

By smart devices we mean: instruments, equipment or machines that have their own computational capacity. These electronic devices are connected to a network and interact autonomously with other devices and users [7]. Moreover, smart devices also refer to devices that have properties of ubiquitous computing.

In this paper, we describe a smart device-based system that helps to promote healthy behaviors with the aim of preventing overweight and obesity in children. Moreover, we present findings and suggestions for future developments obtained during the implementation and evaluation processes. The system has been applied in two scenarios; the first one intended to support parents in having a healthy snack routine, based on a nutritionist suggestion; the second scenario to deal with the problem of forgetting the required equipment on sports days, through notification reminders in the form of visual cues at proper timing. Both scenarios are focused on families with children between the ages 6 and 12, since it is important to take care of obesity in the early ages of the child as a strategy to promote healthy life, when physiology is more malleable [8]. Furthermore, the effects of the implemented actions are likely to be long-lasting. The goal of the system is to help people to establish routines that lead to healthier habits. Additionally, we want to use the proper technology and functionality to minimize user interaction and intrusion.

The system presented in this paper is developed in the context of a larger research with the goal of testing a conceptual framework to develop smart device-based notifications [9,10]. Moreover, the prototypes presented in this paper are developed using the knowledge gathered through the development of more than ten similar prototypes applied in four case studies.

The system uses different technologies including low cost microcontrollers, sensors and simple actuators to deliver information to the users, a NoSQL database to model people and devices into the system, and a lightweight messaging protocol to allow the devices to work with low processing capabilities consuming small amounts of energy.

The system was developed in the context of an international collaboration between Spain, Mexico and Costa Rica researchers. Moreover, the evaluation includes the perspectives of specialists in nutrition and physical activity from these three countries.

2. Related Work

Health and obesity problems related to physical activity and diet have been studied in the past. Moreover, some interventions have been conducted to assess the impact of reminders in these domains. This section presents related works to the one described in this paper. Even though there are many works focusing on comparing results of weight change, eating habits and physical activity in different contexts [11–13], we will only consider related works that use some kind of device or notification as a reminder for people.

In 2011, Monteiro et al., described a randomized controlled trial lifestyle intervention. Authors focused on nutrition and physical activity. Their study focused on mothers with young children (0–5 years old). The designed intervention used face to face workshops, emails and Short Message Service (SMS) reminders as notification mechanisms [14].

Also in 2011, Winett et al., described a program to assess nutrition, physical activity and body weight outcomes applying a social cognitive theory to health. This was a web-based intervention. Authors selected sedentary participants between 18 and 63 years old. With this intervention authors concluded that a simple web-based program can help people to comply with healthy behaviors [15].

Other studies focus more on behavior changing. For instance, in 2015, Hattar, Hagger and Pal, described a randomized control trial study protocol that developed psycho-education using implementation intentions and mental imagery (through videos). In this work authors developed and presented the protocol to evaluate the HEALTHI (Healthy Eating and Active LifesTyle Health Intervention) program. This is a theory-based intervention with the goal of changing dietary intake and physical activity behaviors in overweight people. Authors also propose the use of SMS in this work [16].

In 2016, Quintiliani and Whiteley, conducted a randomized trial to examine the feasibility of a nutrition and physical activity behavioral intervention. In this work, the communication mechanisms used were motivational phone calls from trained peer counselors. Even though authors reported no statistical differences between the control and intervention groups, the overall satisfaction with the program was high [17].

Finally, a category that has been study is the use of mobile apps to improve diet, physical activity and sedentary behavior. From studies combining SMS, emails, apps and websites [18], pregnant women using mobile phone as reminder and a Fitbit (Fitbit International Limited., San Francisco, CA, USA) as a control mechanism [19], textual and auditory cues delivered through a mobile app to increase fruit and vegetable intake and health literacy in general [20], all the way to mobile games using an activity trackers Tractivity (Kineteks Corp., Mainland, Vancouver, BC, Canada) as input to promote physical activity in children [21].

From the literature review conducted, we could not identify studies that used smart device-based notifications to promote healthy behaviors regarding snacking and physical activity to avoid or reduce overweight and obesity levels.

3. System Description

The user interface of our system consists of simple smart devices with embedded screens and visual LED cues that provide important information to the users in the right place at the right time. The idea behind these smart devices is that they are normal objects such as fridge magnets or cabinet drawer hooks that also have the capability of delivering information. The system has some key functions including: storing and processing data from the users, generating notifications and dispatching them to the properly smart device(s).

The two prototypes described in this paper were designed and built following a conceptual framework for smart device-based notifications [9]. This framework proposes a modular conception of the system and defines guidelines for the decisions during the design process. The following sections describe the main components of the system.

Many of the design decisions of the two devices described in this paper are the result of lessons learned through the construction of several smart devices (included in the conceptual framework). One of the most important characteristics is the use of visual cues. Even though sound cues (auditory notifications) were strongly suggested by developers during the design process, the use of the framework lead to the decision of avoiding such notifications. The main reason to avoid sound notifications is that this type of notifications can easily become overwhelming. Moreover, visual recognition memory is superior to auditory recognition memory [22]. Furthermore, encoding messages in sounds is a difficult task; therefore, auditory notifications would have to present the full text of the notification to be effective.

3.1. Main Components

Our system is comprised of six main technological components. The first component, the physical activity tracker, is a device that family members use to gather their physical activity data and store it in the database. Activity bracelets attached to the wrist of children during the week provide information about steps, activity time, distance, calories burned, and quality of sleep among other features. Analysis of these data is later used to determine, for example, proper times of notification in conjunction with general information, food habits and anthropometric measurements that are manually collected. Recognition of parameters from activity bracelets can be performed in an automated and transparent. However, since we are using Xiaomi 1S (Xiaomi Inc., Haidian District, Beijing, China) smart wristband this process is semi-automated (i.e., data are synchronized with a smartphone via Bluetooth connection and requires a manual script).

Physical activity data was collected using the activity band during a week. The data obtained was daily activity such as steps, activity time (hh:mm), distance (km), burned calories (cal) by day as well as the breakdown of all the activities carried out during the day. One week later the band was removed, the data was synchronized to the Band App and finally we used a script to transfer the data to our database.

All the gathered data are stored in a central database (2nd component). In this project, we have used a non-structured document database built using MongoDB v3.6. The purpose of this is to take advantage of the flexibility and scalability provided by this technology. Another reason to build this system using MongoDB has been the necessity of adaptability during the development and evaluation of the solution. Depending on the user's characteristics, the available data differs. Therefore, a traditional structured approach is not appropriate.

The third technological component is the notification generator. The conceptual framework applied in the development of this system was conceived to be applied in several contexts. The name notification generator specifies a piece of software that uses the gathered information and environment conditions to generate notifications. However, these notifications do not have to be automatically generated. In the case of our system the notifications that are delivered through the prototypes are generated based on the recommendations of specialists in nutrition and physical activity (i.e., the information and parameters for delivery of each notification are predefined). However, the system could be used to generate automatic notifications based predefined conditions and the information gathered and stored in the central database.

The notification generator, in our system, is a piece of software developed to use the predefined information stored in the central database to create a notification. Moreover, this part of the system includes the parameters for delivery, also predefined, to establish the delivery interval of each notification in accordance with the timing specified by the specialists. Generated notifications are stored in the central database, because the notification dispatcher extracts notifications from this centralized repository to be delivered.

For the specific purposes of the implementations of the framework described in this paper, the notifications are listed and specified by specialists in nutrition and physical activity. This list of notifications is stored in the database and specific parameters are established to determine when the reminder should be delivered. Moreover, all the available information (stored in the database) is used to determine if the notification can be delivered through the predefined device (i.e., fridge magnet, cabinet drawer or other available devices). An example of the use of this information is the use of sleep patterns to determine an appropriate time to display notifications. The use of a non-structured document database allows different types of data to be stored and used in whichever way the notification requires. A more detailed explanation of the notifications delivered is described in Section 4 (Application Domains).

The fourth component is the notification dispatcher. This is a software component in charge of serving notifications to their final recipient devices. The notification dispatcher functions as a link between the system and each dedicated device. This approach is required to address the problem of standardization in the smart device domain. Each smart device offers different functionalities; therefore, different ways to deliver notifications must be implemented.

The notification dispatcher allows communication between the database and the smart notification devices through the Message Queuing Telemetry Transport (MQTT) protocol. MQTT is a publish-subscribe-based lightweight messaging protocol that runs on top of the TCP/IP protocol. Publish-subscribe is a communication pattern where senders of messages, called publishers (e.g., notification dispatcher), do not route messages to be sent directly to subscribers (e.g., notification devices), but instead characterize messages into topics and publish/post them on a broker. The subscribers then receive the messages from the broker depending on the settings of their connection and the topics they are subscribed on. The broker (5th component) consists of a dedicated server placed between publishers and subscribers to manage message dispatching and to ensure delivery through different quality of service (QoS) strategies that reinforce the delivery mechanisms of the TCP/IP protocol.

The use of a MQTT broker between the notification dispatcher and the notification devices, instead of a direct link, was a deliberate decision. QoS level 1 and QoS level 2 policies ensure that messages (notifications in this case) reach the target device/s. If a target (notification) device is unreachable at a time, for instance, due to an accidental disconnection or because it has no power, the MQTT broker will store undelivered notifications and will serve them, when the device is available again. In addition, advanced QoS strategies play an important role in energy saving enabling the use of power save configurations in the notification devices. Thus, the duty cycle percentage, which is power demanding, may be substantially reduced in the notification devices by entering deep sleep mode periodically. If there are notifications attempts while target devices are sleeping, they will be forwarded by the MQTT broker and received in the upcoming duty cycles.

Finally, the last components are the smart devices used for notification delivery. In the present work, two dedicated devices have been created from scratch. Currently, there are several smart devices available for purchase. However, these devices do not provide the proper functionalities to deliver information and gather responses from users as it is intended with our system. A review of available IoT devices was conducted before deciding to implement the two smart devices described in this paper. Even though we found more than 85 smart devices (with different functionalities) none was sufficiently customizable or provided all the functionalities that the developed prototypes offer. Appendix A shows the list of smart devices studied before deciding to develop the dedicated prototypes.

The two prototypes of notification devices that have been built in the present work are equipped with a low-cost System on a Chip ESP8266-12E (Espressif Systems Inc., Shanghai, China), which integrates a 32-bit RISC Tensilica Xtensa LX106 micro-controller and an 802.11 B/G/N Wi-Fi transceiver to support wireless communication and Internet access through the TCP/IP protocol stack built in the firmware. MQTT client code supporting publications and subscriptions to topics with QoS level 1 has been implemented and compiled to run on top of the TCP/IP protocol. In addition, the ESP8266-12E enables Inter-Integrated Circuit and SPI (Serial Peripheral Interface) serial communications to connect different sets of sensors and actuators.

Both prototypes have been specifically designed to deliver notifications that promote healthy behaviors in children. The most complex consists of a fridge magnet that includes a 0.96-inch monochrome OLED graphic display, which has been connected through the SPI bus to the micro-controller. It has 128×64 pixels that can be used to display static or dynamic monochromatic images and text messages. Furthermore, this prototype is equipped with a single InvenSense MPU-6050 6-DOF IMU (InvenSense Inc., San Jose, CA, USA) wired through the I2C interface. It has been included to support feedback actions in notifications, such as "opened/closed fridge door alarm", among others. This prototype is focused on delivering notifications that promote healthy eating behaviors through the fridge door, as it is a right place to do it. This decision is since kitchen surfaces, particularly fridge doors, are frequently used as reminder systems at home-specific locations [23]. Shopping lists, to-do lists, tailored messages, and paper reminders are often left on the fridge. In this context, emphasis is placed on the importance of fridge magnets as they are seen to contribute to a fluidity and configurability that make fridge surfaces unique to provide contextual cues to the users [24]. Therefore, fridge doors are appropriate places to deliver proactively notifications that support habit formation and behavior changes [25]. Specifically, the magnet prototype is well-suited to provide notifications in the form of visual cues which persuade users to prepare snacks in advance promoting healthy eating. The hardware scheme of this first prototype can be seen in Appendix B.

On the other hand, the second prototype for notification delivery focuses on promoting physical activity in children, another factor to reduce overweight and obesity levels. It has no display and it relies on a simplest resource for providing notification awareness. In this case, the prototype consists of a five RGB LED array with integrated drivers from Adafruit (Adafruit Industries Inc., New York City, NY, USA). A relevant keyword ("Sports Day") is carved out on the prototype 3D printed plastic case, so that it allows the light to pass through the letter gaps highlighting the keyword. Furthermore, this prototype is equipped with a push button not to turn the notification LED lights off, but to give feedback to the system so that the notification has been attended by the end users.

It has been designed in the form of a cabinet drawer hook, as it is a right place for sportswear reminders. This assertion is supported by two basic arguments. The first is that the cabinet is de facto a usual place to store sportswear so that visual cues on sports days, at proper timing, ensure that the notification has been seen. The second reason is purely technical; since the prototype incorporates a built-in Wi-Fi transceiver intended for its use at home settings. The prototype is designed to remain static in the context of the household. An overview of the system including main actors, software components and technological infrastructure is depicted in Figure 1.

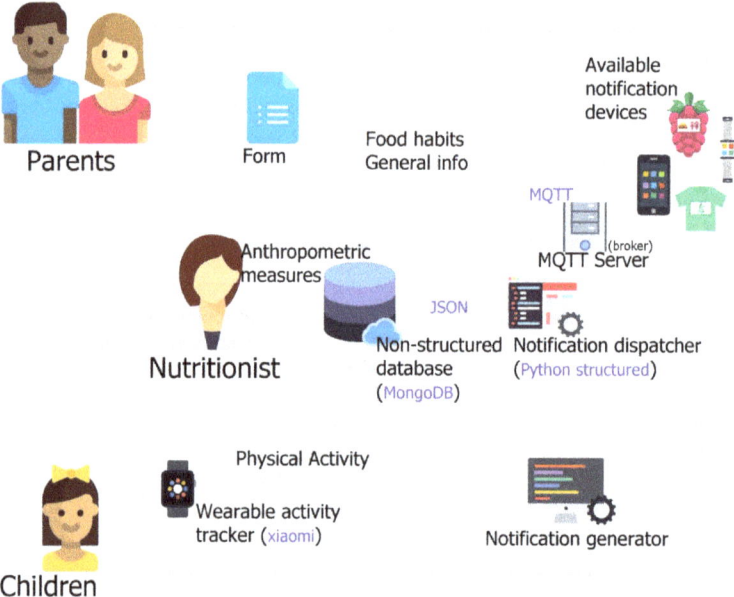

Figure 1. System overview including: main actors, software components, and technological infrastructure.

To the best of our knowledge, there are no further studies that attempts to persuade users to not forget their sportswear promoting physical activity through notification reminders in this context. In 2015 Lau, Wong, Luk and Kwok [26], described the problem of forgetting important items depending on the daily school schedule. It was addressed through a reminder system based on near field communication. Particularly, this system was integrated into a school bag and it provided reminders about items such as lunch boxes and sportswear, among others. Nevertheless, the prototype in [26] is considered for mobility beyond the household.

The hardware scheme of our second prototype focuses on promoting physical activity in children through sportswear notification reminders can be seen in Appendix C.

Both prototypes use 3.7 volts lithium polymer batteries and they are complemented by a regulator circuit to provide stable 3.3 volts to the different modules, together with a charge controller that regulates the charge process and avoids the complete discharge of the battery during use. Moreover, both prototypes have 3D printed cases. Table 1 overviews detailed specifications of these two prototypes.

Table 1. Dedicated devices hardware characterization.

Characteristic	Healthy Eating Behaviors	Physical Activity Reminder
Communications	802.11 B/G/N Wi-Fi connection with Internet access/Lightweight client implementation of the MQTT protocol with QoS level 1 publish/subscribe services	802.11 B/G/N Wi-Fi connection with Internet access/Lightweight client implementation of the MQTT protocol with QoS level 1 publish/subscribe services
Processor Power	32-bit RISC micro-controller, 80 MHz CPU clock speed, light/deep sleep power modes	32-bit RISC micro-controller, 80 MHz CPU clock speed, light/deep sleep power modes
Memory	160 KB RAM, 4 MB external SPI flash	160 KB RAM, 4 MB external SPI flash
Operating Voltage	3.0–3.6 V (3.3 V LDO voltage regulator)	3.0–3.6 V (3.3 V LDO voltage regulator)
Power Consumption	Reduced time in deep sleep mode (interrupted by MPU-6050 IMU readings to sense fridge door) Deep sleep power < 10 µA During transmission in duty cycle ~120–140 mA	Longer time in deep sleep mode (waking by a 1 to 10-min timer is enough) Deep sleep power < 10 µA During transmission periods in duty cycle ~120–140 mA
Functionality	Show graphical notifications in a monochrome OLED screen/Sense fridge door	RGB LED array ON and OFF actions/Push button to indicate notification awareness
Cost	$35	$30

3.2. Modeling the Notification Message Structure

As stated in the Main Components section, the notification generator can build customized notifications and plan their delivery by using the information stored in the non-structured database. Notifications are dispatched to the proper smart devices thanks to the notification dispatcher and the MQTT broker. In addition, the recipient devices also have the technical ability to send acknowledgement notifications to the dispatcher (if required).

To build a flexible and scalable system, the notification message structure has been modeled to be independent of the notification mechanism, the application's context and the target device.

Notifications are encapsulated within MQTT messages and therefore, both, the notification devices and the notification dispatcher should implement the MQTT stack and operate as MQTT clients. While the notification devices use an embedded lightweight version of the MQTT client which can be loaded into the memory of the microcontroller; the notification dispatcher, for its part, implements a full-featured standalone client.

Since the non-structured database and the logic that governs the notification generator and the notification dispatcher work with JSON data, the notification has also been modeled as a JSON object which can be enclosed in the MQTT message, instead of using plain text. The JSON syntax provides a flexible mechanism to build a general notification scheme that can be adapted to many application's contexts and notification devices.

The use of this notification model is very valuable. When the notification is defined and queued to be delivered, the generator does not know which device would be used to deliver the notifications. Therefore, a flexible format allows storing the notification content independently to other metadata. Moreover, the same notification can have content in different formats (e.g., audio, text, and figure) and that information would be used depending on the device that is selected to deliver the notification.

4. Application Domains

The primary requirement pursued in the developed system has been to make it easy to use and accessible. Therefore, the two prototypes have been designed to interact with the user through very simple visual cues as mechanisms to address notification delivery regarding promotion of healthy life in terms of reducing obesity and overweight in children population. By helping with eating habits, the first prototype promotes a healthy snacking behavior; by implementing a visual reminder for sportswear, the second prototype prevents self-sabotage or simply forgetting the required equipment to practice physical activity when it is sport day.

4.1. Healthy Snacking Behavior

Meal frequency and timing patterns are two of the most important factors that affect obesity rates [27]. Snacking is an important part of the eating habits around the world. A snack could consist of chips, nuts, cheese, yogurt, cookies or biscuits, vegetables, fresh fruit, chocolate or other foods. Snacks are supposed to be an in-between meals food. The 2014 Nielsen global snacking report [28] stated that nutrition is the most important reason to eat snacks, followed by getting an energy boost. Therefore, healthy snacks are important.

There are two types of snackers. The first are planners, those who prepare or purchase their snacks in advance. These types of snackers are usually very selective. Second, the spontaneous snackers. These snackers often eat snacks as soon as they buy or prepare them without previously planning. The latest usually lack a regular eating pattern, not considering the health and nutritional aspect of the snack.

Getting healthy snacks in a spontaneous purchase without a steady provider is a difficult task. Normally, when you buy snacks on the street they are not healthy. In this context, the purpose of our system is to provide a reminder for snack planners and for spontaneous snackers who want to plan their meals and adopt regular snack eating patterns, taking care of nutritional and healthy aspects and making this behavior extendable to the entire family unit.

Our prototype is a snack reminder developed to deliver personalized notifications to support parents in remembering snack preparation and reminding them to deliver the snacks to their children before they leave the house. As a fridge magnet, this device is supposed to be an ornament. However, the embedded hardware makes it capable of delivering graphical notifications to anyone with access to the fridge. Figure 2 shows the prototype and the aspect of one of the notifications delivered.

The system works based on the recommendations of a nutritionist. Either through a generic snack diet or a personalized diet depending on the circumstances. Given a diet proposal, the system sends a list of required ingredients for the week snacks. Then, graphical cues to remind parents which snacks they are supposed to give their children are daily delivered.

The notification delivery mechanisms could also be used to send visual cues as reminders the day before if parents require to prepare the snack in advance.

The way in which these notifications are defined is justified by the fact that for overweight children, programs that involve the parents and the home setting are better to promote healthy eating habits. Moreover, presumably the childhood period has a strong influence on the weight through life [29]. To provide some of the rationale for these notifications, we used The Five W's, shown in Table 2.

To summarize, the healthy snacking behavior prototype provides notification based on recommendations of specialists in nutrition that create a list of snacks per family member (specially focused on children). These notifications are delivered through a smart device (fridge magnet) during the morning. The intention of the notification is to reinforce parents desire to prepare healthy snacks and to avoid forgetting to pack the snacks for their children. The snack recommendations are stored through simple web form interface.

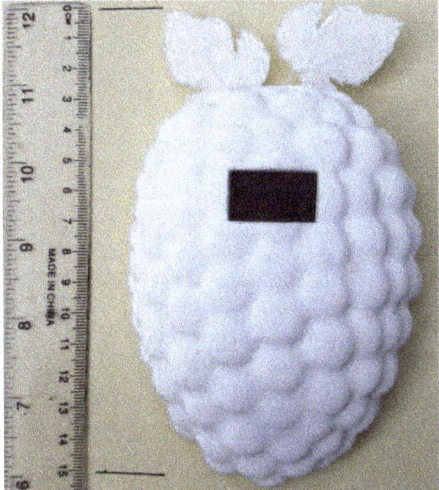 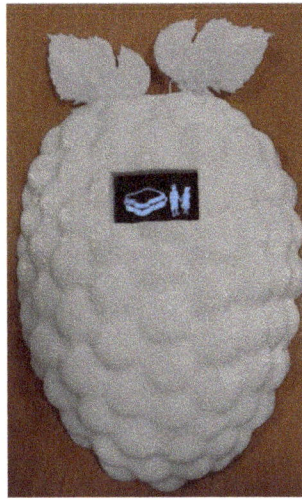

Figure 2. Prototype developed to promote healthy snack behavior and one example of notification delivered. (**Left**) Prototype powered-off and case, ruler for reference; (**Right**) Prototype powered-on, displaying a sandwich notification for two children.

Table 2. Five Ws description of snacking behavior notifications.

Five Ws	Description
Who will receive notifications	The snack notifications are directed to parents who want to either prepare healthy snacks or avoid forgetting to give the snacks to their children.
What will be notified	In the case of preparation notifications, parents will be reminded of the type of snack their children are supposed to take to school. The other notifications help parents to avoid forgetting to provide the snacks, therefore they show which snack corresponds to each family member.
When will the notifications be delivered	These notifications are delivered early in the morning or one day in advance to help people remind that they should prepare snacks. The notifications are also present when someone is supposed to leave the house depending on their daily routine.
Where will the notifications be displayed	The smart device for these notifications should be placed in the fridge. As it is a fridge magnet. This allows people to associate the notifications with food and seemingly forces them to act immediately as they are already in the right place to prepare or pack their snacks.
Why will the notifications be delivered	These notifications help people who usually do not prepare their snacks to do it. Also, they avoid that parents forget to pack their snacks. This leads to a healthier eating behavior.

To deliver the notifications all the information stored in the database is considered and a set of rules and scripts define the time slots in which each notification should be delivered. The system also includes a feedback mechanism that is activated when someone opens and closes the fridge door.

4.2. Physical Activity (Sportswear)

There are always those days in which people intend to do something, but they search for any excuse to avoid it. For physical activity, one of those is to forget sportswear. Getting to do sports with your children or going to the gym requires preparation and habits if people want it to become part of their routine. Figure 3 shows the prototype.

Willpower is also a limited resource [30]. If people continuously forget something necessary for their physical activity, a change is required to avoid it. People could also use little reminders (for example post-its), however, this will require them to place the post-its somewhere. Furthermore, post-its provide static information; this means that they do not dynamically adapt the information contained to the actual context (in this case to the current day of the week). That is why this system uses visual cues to remind a person that today is a day for physical activity or not.

Using a small dedicated device that can be hooked, for example, in a cabinet drawer our system delivers a notification that help users remind carrying sportswear. This may also be combined with the snack notification device to remind users to carry water bottles or other required snacks for hydration and energy recovery. Table 3 shows the rationale for this notification.

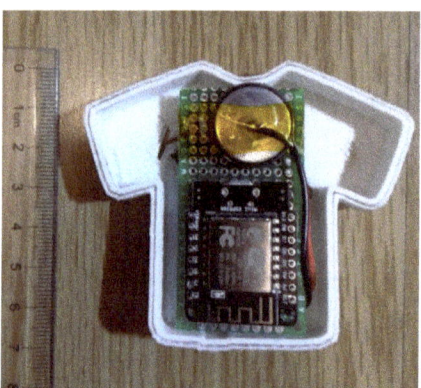 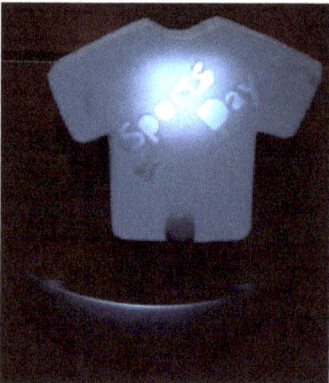

Figure 3. Prototype developed to remind people of sportswear to promote physical activity. (**Left**) Dedicated device and case, ruler for reference; (**Right**) Device powered-on.

Table 3. Five Ws description of sportswear notification.

Five Ws	Description
Who will receive the notification	In this case the notification could either be directed to the children or the parents.
What will be notified	This notification will only show an illuminated case with the word "Sports Day". The idea is that this notification will provide enough information to remember that it is a sports day.
When will the notification be delivered	This notification will be delivered on days that are planned to be sports days. This is decided by the parents and configured in the system (notification generator).
Where will the notification be displayed	The device will be placed in a closet drawer of either the parents or the children.
Why will the notification be delivered	Forgetting sportswear is one of the most common excuses to avoid physical activity [30]. Therefore, having this constant reminder on sports day would make people less likely to forget unconsciously.

5. Evaluation

The evaluation was conducted through a series of interviews with specialists in nutrition and physical activity from three different countries: Spain (one male and two females), Mexico (two males and one female) and Costa Rica (one male and two females).

For each interview, a physical prototype and a storyboard were presented to the participant and a series of questions were asked. In each session, the same interview protocol was used. The protocol consisted of three main parts: participants' information, prototype usefulness and prototype usability/ergonomics. The questions in the protocol are detailed in Appendix D.

The goal with this evaluation was to assess the system's perceived usefulness and usability. Moreover, the thoughts of the specialists were gathered and added to the prototypes.

The system was presented using the physical device and storyboards [31]. Using storyboards, we presented the main use cases for the prototypes and their benefits. Participants were presented with two storyboards, one for healthy eating behaviors and the other for sportswear reminders.

The developed interview protocol and questionnaire was designed using two main references: The first set of questions (focused on the prototype) were based on different scales [32] with the intention of gather the perspective of the participants on the usefulness of the system. The second part was based on the standard ISO 9241-210:2010 Ergonomics of human-system interaction [33].

To provide a better understanding we will describe our interpretation of the ISO 9241-210:2010 terminology. By effectiveness we mean the accuracy and completeness with which users achieve specified goals. By efficiency we mean resources expended in relation to the accuracy and completeness with which users achieve goals. By satisfaction we mean freedom from discomfort and positive attitudes towards the use of the product.

Conciseness, consistency and self-descriptiveness deal with the amount of information required to deliver the message and the way in which this data is displayed every time. The characteristics of presented information (i.e., detectability, legibility, discriminability, clarity and comprehensibility) are related to freedom from distraction and interpretability.

Finally, suitable for individualization means that, users can modify interaction and presentation of information to suit their individual needs and suitable for learning means that the system conforms to user's expectations and it prevents or tolerates errors.

6. Results and Discussion

In this section, we present the results of the interviews. The evaluation protocol was explained in the Evaluation Section. All results are positive. However, some of the evaluators provided feedback and improvement opportunities that we will also discuss. We asked the evaluators to use three words to describe the system. Figure 4 shows the results of this exercise. The most common word used to describe the system was useful (5 out of 9) followed by simple (4 out of 9).

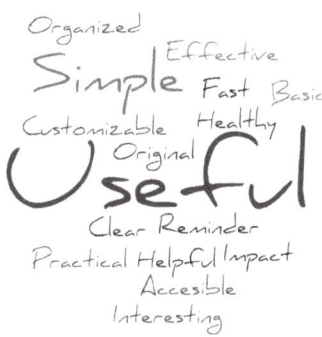

Figure 4. Word cloud of main characterizers used by evaluators.

Some words caught the interviewer's attention. For instance, when a reviewer used the word "accessible", we followed up to determine that she was referring to the possibility of many people to reach the information on the device. This includes everyone in the household and since the system uses graphical representations it is also accessible for children that do not know how to read or write.

One of the interviewees also used the word "basic" we followed up to determine that she saw potential to add other functionalities to the device. Therefore, the version presented was too basic. Another word was "organized" delving in this we determined that the characterization was for the users and not the system. Therefore, organized people are potential users of the system.

Two questions were asked to the evaluators to assess their willingness to either use the system or to recommend it to their friends, family or patients. Figure 5 shows the answers to this question. It is interesting to observe that nine out of nine evaluators (specialists in nutrition and physical activity) are somewhat interested in using the system. However, eight out of nine evaluators consider that they would recommend the system. To further explain this, we must note that usually specialists in nutrition and physical activity have a healthy lifestyle, therefore they might not see fit to use the system. However, during the interviews most of the evaluators stated that remembering healthy snacks was one of the main problems of their patients.

Some of the evaluators stated that they would not use the system as it is. But they would reconsider if it included some of their feedback (especially screen size and the amount of information that can be delivered through the device). The evaluation had two main focuses, the first one was to assess the evaluator's opinion on the system, the second one was focused on the look and feel of the device (human factors and ergonomics perspective). We asked a question regarding the evaluators' satisfaction with the look and feel of the devices. All the answers were positive (5 somewhat satisfied, 3 very satisfied and 1 extremely satisfied). Figure 6 shows the responses to this question.

Most of the improvement opportunities mentioned by the evaluators include: enlarging the device screen and making it in color, changing the shape of the case, adding sound to the notifications, and adding text to the notification and not only images. This were the main concerns regarding the device.

One of the evaluators recommended to add text, this text would be used to provide information about the ingredients of the snack. In Costa Rica, the two of the evaluators asked to change the shape of the snack reminder case to an apple as it is traditional in Costa Rica to have an apple shaped magnet fridge.

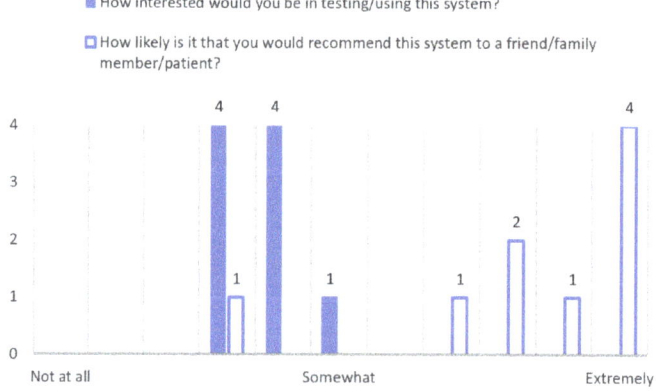

Figure 5. Likelihood to use the system or recommend the system.

Another important observation was that some of the evaluators compared the system with mobile applications with similar functionalities. Other evaluator requested for the system to sync with mobile applications.

Delving on the device functionalities, most of the comments were focused on the snacking reminder device. The first recommendation was to add reminders not only to people to carry their snacks but also to prepare them in advance. This would be helpful to assure that the snacks are ready to go when they are required. One evaluator recommended to use only one device with more information (i.e., combining both devices).

The last part of the evaluation focused on the ergonomics of human-system interaction. In this section, 13 characteristics of the system were assessed by the evaluators. Figure 7 shows the results of this evaluation segmented by country. Table 4 shows the five-number summary and a reliability analysis of the data depicted in Figure 7.

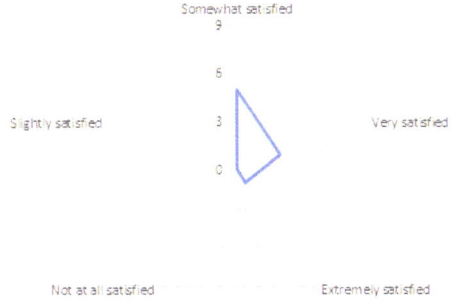

Figure 6. Evaluator's satisfaction with the look and feel of the system. Scale (0, 3, 6, 0) represents the number of participants in each category.

An interesting finding of this evaluation is that both Mexico and Costa Rica on average consider the system good (4.3 out of 5 points). However, in Spain, the opinions were less positive (3.9 out of 5 points). We do believe that being Latin-American countries, Costa Rica and Mexico share opinions on how the system could be used.

In general, the best ranked categories were system's comprehensibility, the perceived effectiveness and clarity (4.5 out of 5 points). The worst ranked categories are the system's suitability for learning and it discriminability (3.7 out of 5 points).

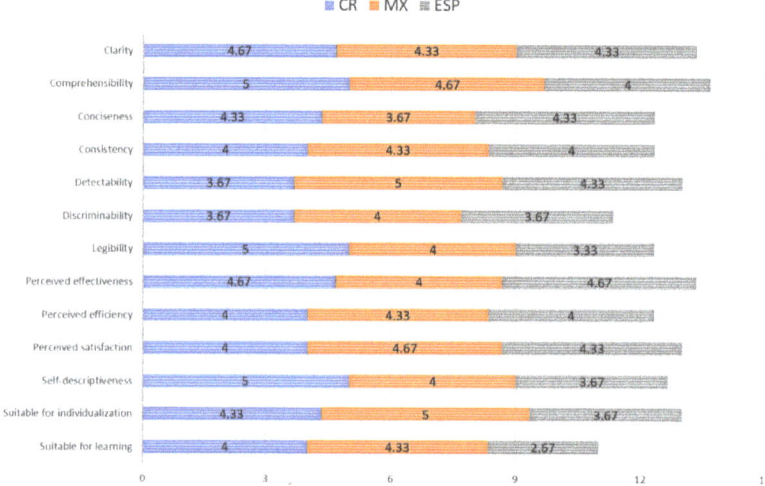

Figure 7. Evaluation of system characteristics based on the standard ISO 9241-210:2010.

Table 4. Minimum, maximum, quartiles and reliability analysis for Likert scales depicted in Figure 7. All items Cronbach Alpha: 0.8307, Std. Alpha: 0.8431. Reliability analysis calculated using [34].

Characteristic	Min	1st Quartile	2nd Quartile	3rd Quartile	Max	Cronbach Alpha
Clarity	4	4	4	5	5	0.8350
Comprehensibility	3	4	5	5	5	0.8106
Conciseness	3	4	4	4	5	0.8157
Consistency	3	4	4	4	5	0.8139
Detectability	3	4	4	5	5	0.8425
Discriminability	3	3	4	4	5	0.8186
Legibility	2	3	5	5	5	0.8056
Perceived effectiveness	3	4	5	5	5	0.8391
Perceived efficiency	3	4	4	4	5	0.7919
Perceived satisfaction	4	4	4	5	5	0.7981
Self-descriptiveness	3	3	5	5	5	0.8051
Suitable for individualization	3	4	4	5	5	0.8412
Suitable for learning	1	4	4	4	5	0.8135

A system is suitable for learning when it supports and guides the user in learning to use the system. In our case since the notification and device are supposed to share little information the suitability for learning suffers. To be able to learn to use the system a simple guide should be provided. The discriminability problem is mostly related to the device screen size and resolution. The implemented prototype used a 0.96-inch monochrome OLED graphic display; to improve this, a bigger screen should be used. Moreover, images that avoid ambiguity could be used. Enlarging the screen would also allow for text to be shown, improving discriminability of the notifications.

The final improvement opportunities for the system are focused on the notifications. One evaluator suggested adding personalization based on the user's data and preferences (already considered in the system). However, she added the possibility to add diseases and allergies into the notifications. Another evaluator suggested the necessity of creating profiles (also considered in the system), but he requested to be able to change between profiles using the device.

In general, one recommendation is to add more nutrition facts of the snacks. For instance, alimentary groups, portion sizes and water consumption.

One confronted opinion between evaluators was if the personalization should be performed by the user or if the definition of snacks should be personalized by the nutritionist. One of the evaluators suggested that she would like to be able to specifically set the food characteristics for a given day in their patient's device. Another evaluator suggested doing a consumption analysis of the user. However, this would require sensing capabilities that the system does not provide as it is designed for notifications.

The last opinion on the system is that two evaluators would prefer this to be a mobile application rather than a physical device. The main reason provided is that most people already have a mobile device. During the design phase of this system, this discussion was carried.

One of the main arguments to avoid push notifications on smart devices is that the indiscriminate use of these notifications is causing people to stop paying attention to them. Social media notifications, dedicated apps (e.g., Netflix, Yelp, and Amazon), email, and other mobile phone notifications are just some examples of this overwhelming amount of notifications.

Finally, all evaluators highlighted the positive effect of using these devices in day to day to prevent overweight and obesity if activities and tasks associated with notifications are carried out properly.

7. Conclusions and Future Work

In this work, we presented the design, implementation and expert evaluation of two smart devices used to promote healthy behaviors (i.e., healthy snacking and physical activity). We presented the technical details of the device implementation and software architecture based on a framework to develop smart device-based notifications.

The prototypes were evaluated by nine specialists in nutrition and physical activity from three countries (i.e., Spain, Mexico and Costa Rica). Results show that the system is well received by the experts, and that they will be willing to recommend the system to their friends, family or patients.

The system was evaluated applying a standard categorization for ergonomics in human-system interaction. The best ranked categories for this evaluation were comprehensibility, effectiveness and clarity. This leads us to think that the system will be usable, and it will provide a nice user experience. The worst ranked categories were suitability for learning (i.e., the system does not teach the user how to use it) and discriminability. The discriminability problem is mainly due to the use of a small graphic display in the prototype.

Furthermore, we observed that the degree of satisfaction in Mexico and Costa Rica are the same. However, evaluators from Spain are more reluctant about the system. According to the expert evaluators (eight out of nine), the system proposed in this paper would be useful to promote healthier behaviors in the system users. The only negative response believes that providing the notification is not sufficient, but also more control should be provided by the system.

In future work, we will improve the system based on the expert suggestions and evaluate it with families in their households, integrating the analysis of physical activity parameters to support the enrichment of adapted notifications provided by the system.

Furthermore, we will investigate how human activities are affected by this kind of smart device based notifications. Also, if users make responsible and proper use to achieve what smart devices pretend by adding new functionalities regarding persuasion and motivation focused on other domains of application, not only childhood obesity and overweight.

Although this research was prepared and executed carefully, it still has some limitations. First, the evaluation sample size (nine specialists in nutrition and physical activity) is reduced. This is due to the difficulty to personally work with specialists. Researchers considered applying an online survey to reach a larger sample; however, the final decision was to conduct personal interviews to focus the evaluation in the prototypes usefulness and its usability/ergonomics. Another limitation is that the evaluators are from different countries. Therefore, they might have different perspectives and points of view. However, the selection of three Spanish-speaking countries with cultural similitudes was a key factor to conduct the research as it is described in this paper.

Acknowledgments: This work was partially supported by CITIC at Universidad de Costa Rica, Grant No. 834-B8-165, by MICITT and CONICIT of the government of Costa Rica, and by the Plan Propio de Investigación from Castilla-La Mancha University.

Author Contributions: Gustavo López and Luis A. Guerrero defined the framework applied in this project. Gustavo López designed the evaluation instrument. Iván González designed the technical components of the smart devices. The evaluations were performed by Gustavo López and José A. Brenes (Costa Rica), Elitania Jimenez-Garcia (Mexico), Iván González, Jesús Fontecha and José Bravo (Spain). The work was also based in a previous work developed by Elitania Jimenez-Garcia, Jesús Fontecha and José Bravo.

Conflicts of Interest: The authors declare no conflict of interest.

Appendix A

This appendix lists the smart devices considered before deciding to develop from scratch two dedicated devices.

Table A1. List of smart devices revised durin the development of this research.

Smart Devices		
Kolibree	Breeze: Wireless breathalyzer	CubeSensors
iBGStar Blood Glucose Meter	TP-Link: Multicolor smart wi-fi	AwairGlow
CINDER: Sensing cooker	Mimo: Smart baby monitoring	Wemo Mini: Wifi smart plug
Vessyl Cup	UP3: Health tracker	Honeywell Lyric T5
Tagg Plus: Pet tracker collar	Ring: Video doorbell pro	SmartMat: Intelligent yoga mat
Cue	Misfit Wearables: Shine 2	Nest Cam: Outdoor
HAPIfork	June: Intelligent oven	Foobot: Indoor air quality monitor
TAO	Apple TV: Apps and voice control	August: Smart Keypad
Keen Home: Smart vent	Philips Hue Bridge: Homekit ready	Philips Hue: Dimmer switch
Fitbit Surge: Fitness tracker	Osmo: Gaming system for iPad	Samsung Family Hub Refrigerator
Flip 2: Wearable for kids	Deeper: Smart portable fish finder	Bluesmart: Connected Carry-On
Withings: Wireless blood pressure monitor	Garmin Vivosmart: Fitness band and smartwatch	Luna: Turn your bed into a smartbed
Talkies: A new way to chat with kids	iBaby Monitor: Digital video monitor with night vision	ShutterEaze: Automate your plantation shutters
FitBark: Activity tracking for your pet	Olive: Intelligent bracelet that helps you manage	Google Home: Speaker with Google Assistant
Google Daydream: Virtual reality headset	Samsung Galaxy View: Connected screen	Logitech Pop: Smart button controller
Logi Circle: Portable Wi-Fi video camera	Onyx: Wearable communication device	Ray Super Remote: Touchscreen universal
AWS IoT Button: Programmable dash button	MOTA SmartRing: Connectivity at your	CUJO: Smart firewall for the smart home
MUZO Cobblestone: Wireless music receiver	Aether Cone: The thinking music player	Xiaomi Yeelight: Indoor connected night light
Awair: Smart air quality monitor	August: Smart lock	iRobot Mirra: Pool cleaning robot
Refuel: Smart propane tank gauge	Kinsa: Smart thermometer	Roku 3: Streaming media player
Belkin WeMo: Insight Switch	Click & Grow: Smart herb garden	Amazon Echo Dot: 2nd Generation
Amazon Tap: Portable voice controlled speaker	Prodigio: Connected Nespresso machine	Solu: Smallest general-purpose computer
Google Chromecast: Second generation	Amazon Dash Button: Smart home shopping	Philips Hue Go: Portable connected lighting
Singlecue: Gesture control for connected home	TAH: Bluetooth device for Internet of things	Valta: Simple home energy management
Netatmo Welcome: Smart camera with face	Lutron Caseta: HomeKit-enabled smart lighting kit	Sengled Pulse: LED light + wireless speakers
Roost: Smart battery for smoke alarms	Point: A softer take on home security	Scout Alarm: Simple connected home security
LIFX: White 800 connected light bulb	Ambi Climate: Smart add-on for your air conditioner	Allure EverSense: Proximity based thermostat
Rico: Turn your smartphone into a smarthome device	Highfive: Video conferencing you can actually love	Smappee: Smart home energy manager
Chamberlain: Garage connectivity Kit	OpenSprinkler: Automate your sprinklers	

Appendix B

This appendix presents the hardware scheme of the notification device for promoting healthy eating behaviors.

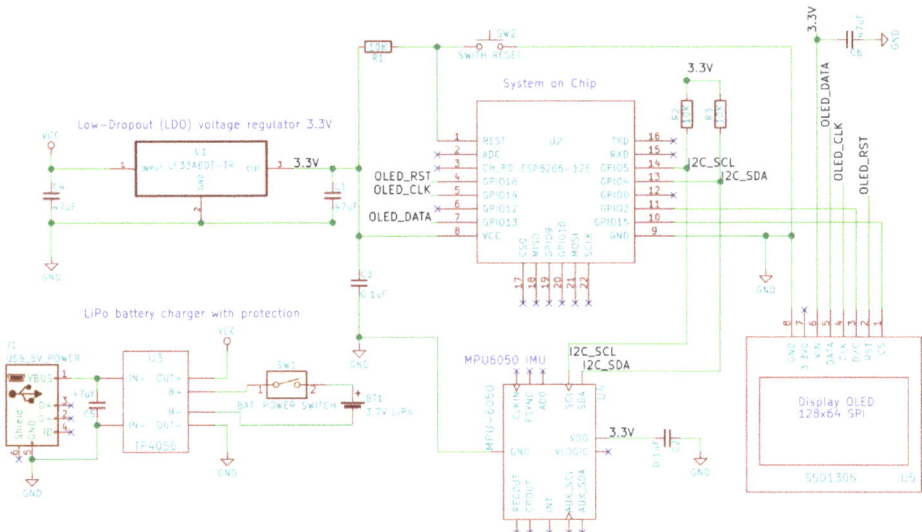

Figure A1. Hardware scheme of the smart device for healthy eating behaviors.

As indicated in Section 3 the prototype developed to promote healthy eating behaviors has been equipped with a monochrome 0.96" 128 × 64 OLED graphic display using the driver chip SSD1306 from Adafruit (Adafruit Industries Inc., New York City, NY, USA). The OLED display (U5 component in the schematic diagram) has been connected through a SPI 4-wire interface to the ESP8266-12E System on a Chip (U2 component). The ESP8266 also keeps an I2C two-wire serial communication with the tri-axial accelerometer + tri-axial gyroscope InvenSense MPU-6050 IMU (U4 component). These three components are supplied with a 3.3 V regulated DC voltage provided by the LF33ABDT-TR 3.3 V Low-Dropout regulator (STMicroelectronics Inc., Geneva, Switzerland) (U1 component). A low-cost TP4056 micro USB single-cell lithium battery charger with cut-off protection (NanJing Top Power ASIC Corp., Nanjing, Jiangsu, China) has been used to properly adjust the charging current supplied to the 3.7 V LiPo battery and to prevent its total discharge. The TP4056 is represented by the U3 component in the schematic diagram.

Appendix C

This appendix presents the hardware scheme of the notification device for promoting physical activity in children. It is a simpler hardware scheme than the previous one from Appendix B. It keeps the LF33ABDT-TR 3.3 V LDO regulator, the ESP8266-12E and the TP4056 lithium battery charger which correspond to the components U1, U2 and U3, respectively. There are no OLED display and no IMU in this hardware scheme. Instead, a 5 RGB LED array (component U4) with integrated drivers from Adafruit is connected to the ESP8266-12E through the GPIO2 pin to provide visual cues. Lastly, this notification device also incorporates a feedback switch button (SW3 component) connected to the GPIO5 through a pull-up resistor. It is used to provide feedback to the system so that the notification has been attended by the end users.

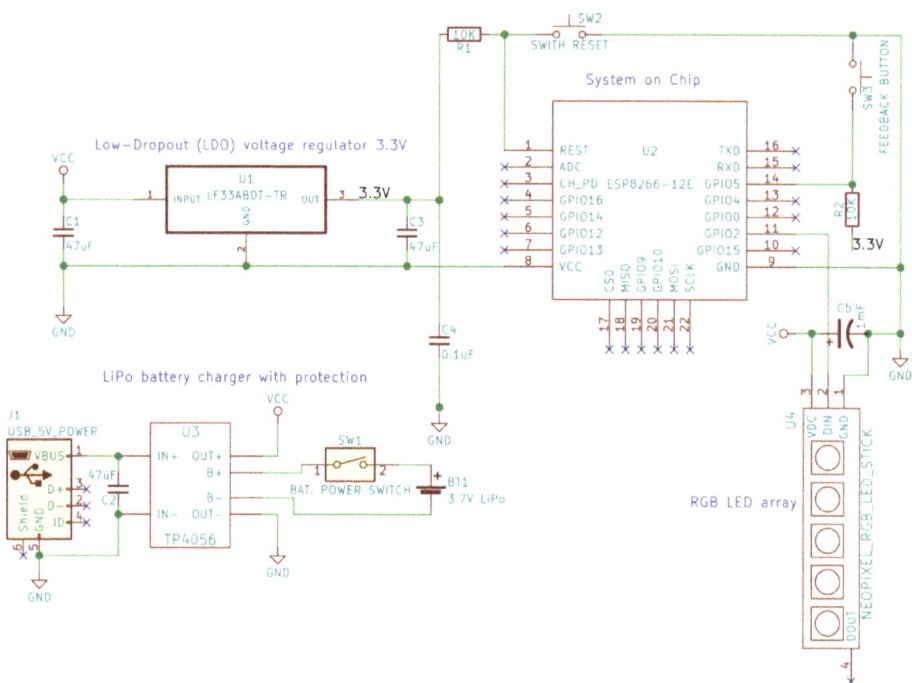

Figure A2. Hardware scheme of the smart device for promoting physical activity.

Appendix D

This appendix describes the questions asked to each evaluator and the scale used for each question.

1. Participant information

    a. Name
    b. Professional background

2. Prototype

    a. What do you think is the main goal of the system? (open question)
    b. How hard would it be to use the system? (0–10 scale)
    c. How interested would you be in testing/using this system? (5pt Likert scale)
    d. How satisfied are you with the look and feel of this system? (5pt Likert scale)
    e. Would you buy this system? Why? (Yes/No and open question)
    f. Do you have any thoughts on how to improve this system? (open question)
    g. In three words, describe this system (open question)
    h. Will this system be a good tool to promote healthy behaviors? (Yes/No and open question)
    i. How likely is it that you would recommend this system to a friend/family member/patient? (0–10 scale)

3. Ergonomics of Human-System Interaction

    a. For each category select a response (5pt discrete scale)

        • Perceived effectiveness

- Perceived efficiency
- Perceived satisfaction
- Clarity
- Discriminability
- Conciseness
- Consistency
- Detectability
- Legibility
- Comprehensibility
- Self-descriptiveness
- Suitability for individualization
- Suitability for learning

b. Is there anything else you would like to share? (open question)

References

1. Robertson, A. *Food and Health in Europe: A New Basis for Action*; Academic Search Complete; WHO Regional Office for Europe: Kobenhavn, Denmark, 2004; ISBN 9789289013635.
2. Faith, M.S.; Scanlon, K.S.; Birch, L.L.; Francis, L.A.; Sherry, B. Parent-Child Feeding Strategies and Their Relationships to Child Eating and Weight Status. *Obes. Res.* **2004**, *12*, 1711–1722. [CrossRef] [PubMed]
3. Lau, P.W.; Lau, E.Y.; Wong, D.P.; Ransdell, L. A Systematic Review of Information and Communication Technology–Based Interventions for Promoting Physical Activity Behavior Change in Children and Adolescents. *J. Med. Internet Res.* **2011**, *13*, e48. [CrossRef] [PubMed]
4. Stawarz, K.; Cox, A.L.; Blandford, A. Beyond Self-Tracking and Reminders. In Proceedings of the 33rd Annual ACM Conference on Human Factors in Computing Systems—CHI '15, Seoul, Korea, 18–23 April 2015; ACM Press: New York, NY, USA, 2015; pp. 2653–2662.
5. Böhmer, M.; Lander, C.; Gehring, S.; Brumby, D.P.; Krüger, A. Interrupted by a Phone Call: Exploring Designs for Lowering the Impact of Call Notifications for Smartphone Users. In Proceedings of the 32nd Annual ACM Conference on Human Factors in Computing Systems—CHI '14, Toronto, ON, Canada, 26 April–1 May 2014; ACM: New York, NY, USA, 2014; pp. 3045–3054.
6. Grandhi, S.A.; Jones, Q. Knock, knock! Who's there? Putting the user in control of managing interruptions. *Int. J. Hum.-Comput. Stud.* **2015**, *79*, 35–50. [CrossRef]
7. Dolui, K.; Mukherjee, S.; Datta, S.K. Smart device sensing architectures and applications. In Proceedings of the International Computer Science and Engineering Conference, Bangkok, Thailand, 4–6 September 2013; IEEE Computer Society: Washington, DC, USA, 2013; pp. 91–96.
8. World Health Organization. *Report of the Commission on Ending Childhood Obesity*; World Health Organization: Geneva, Switzerland, 2016.
9. López, G.; Guerrero, L.A. Ubiquitous Notification Mechanism to Provide User Awareness. In *Advances in Ergonomics in Design*; Advances in Intelligent Systems and Computing; Rebelo, F., Soares, M., Eds.; Springer International Publishing: Cham, Switzerland, 2016; Volume 485, pp. 689–700, ISBN 978-3-319-41982-4.
10. López, G.; Guerrero, L.A. Supporting User Awareness Using Smart Device-Based Notifications. In *Ubiquitous Computing and Ambient Intelligence*; García, C.R., Caballero-Gil, P., Burmester, M., Quesada-Arencibia, A., Eds.; Springer International Publishing: Cham, Switzerland, 2016; pp. 333–340, ISBN 978-3-319-48746-5.
11. Watts, A.W.; Mâsse, L.C.; Naylor, P.-J. Changes to the school food and physical activity environment after guideline implementation in British Columbia, Canada. *Int. J. Behav. Nutr. Phys. Act.* **2014**, *11*, 50. [CrossRef] [PubMed]
12. Lindvall, K.; Jenkins, P.; Scribani, M.; Emmelin, M.; Larsson, C.; Norberg, M.; Weinehall, L. Comparisons of weight change, eating habits and physical activity between women in Northern Sweden and Rural New York State- results from a longitudinal study. *Nutr. J.* **2015**, *14*, 88. [CrossRef] [PubMed]

13. Romeike, K.; Abidi, L.; Lechner, L.; de Vries, H.; Oenema, A. Similarities and differences in underlying beliefs of socio-cognitive factors related to diet and physical activity in lower-educated Dutch, Turkish, and Moroccan adults in the Netherlands: A focus group study. *BMC Public Health* **2016**, *16*, 813. [CrossRef] [PubMed]
14. Monteiro, S.M.; Jancey, J.; Howat, P.; Burns, S.; Jones, C.; Dhaliwal, S.S.; McManus, A.; Hills, A.P.; Anderson, A.S. The protocol of a randomized controlled trial for playgroup mothers: Reminder on Food, Relaxation, Exercise, and Support for Health (REFRESH) Program. *BMC Public Health* **2011**, *11*, 648. [CrossRef] [PubMed]
15. Winett, R.A.; Anderson, E.S.; Wojcik, J.R.; Winett, S.G.; Moore, S.; Blake, C. Guide to health: A randomized controlled trial of the effects of a completely web-based intervention on physical activity, fruit and vegetable consumption, and body weight. *Transl. Behav. Med.* **2011**, *1*, 165–174. [CrossRef] [PubMed]
16. Hattar, A.; Hagger, M.S.; Pal, S. Weight-loss intervention using implementation intentions and mental imagery: A randomised control trial study protocol. *BMC Public Health* **2015**, *15*, 196. [CrossRef] [PubMed]
17. Quintiliani, L.M.; Whiteley, J.A. Results of a Nutrition and Physical Activity Peer Counseling Intervention among Nontraditional College Students. *J. Cancer Educ.* **2016**, *31*, 366–374. [CrossRef] [PubMed]
18. Partridge, S.R.; McGeechan, K.; Hebden, L.; Balestracci, K.; Wong, A.T.; Denney-Wilson, E.; Harris, M.F.; Phongsavan, P.; Bauman, A.; Allman-Farinelli, M. Effectiveness of a mHealth Lifestyle Program With Telephone Support (TXT2BFiT) to Prevent Unhealthy Weight Gain in Young Adults: Randomized Controlled Trial. *JMIR mHealth uHealth* **2015**, *3*, e66. [CrossRef] [PubMed]
19. Choi, J.; Lee, J.H.; Vittinghoff, E.; Fukuoka, Y. mHealth Physical Activity Intervention: A Randomized Pilot Study in Physically Inactive Pregnant Women. *Matern. Child Health J.* **2016**, *20*, 1091–1101. [CrossRef] [PubMed]
20. Elbert, S.P.; Dijkstra, A.; Oenema, A. A Mobile Phone App Intervention Targeting Fruit and Vegetable Consumption: The Efficacy of Textual and Auditory Tailored Health Information Tested in a Randomized Controlled Trial. *J. Med. Internet Res.* **2016**, *18*, e147. [CrossRef] [PubMed]
21. Garde, A.; Umedaly, A.; Abulnaga, S.M.; Robertson, L.; Junker, A.; Chanoine, J.P.; Ansermino, J.M.; Dumont, G.A. Assessment of a Mobile Game ("MobileKids Monster Manor") to Promote Physical Activity Among Children. *Games Health J.* **2015**, *4*, 149–158. [CrossRef] [PubMed]
22. Cohen, M.A.; Horowitz, T.S.; Wolfe, J.M. Auditory recognition memory is inferior to visual recognition memory. *Proc. Natl. Acad. Sci. USA* **2009**, *106*, 6008–6010. [CrossRef] [PubMed]
23. McGee-Lennon, M.; Wolters, M.; Brewster, S. Designing Reminders for the Home—The Role of Home Tours. In *Include*; Royal College of Art: London, UK, 2011.
24. Swan, L.; Taylor, A.S. Notes on fridge surfaces. In Proceedings of the CHI '05 Extended Abstracts on Human Factors in Computing Systems—CHI '05, Portland, OR, USA, 2–7 April 2005; ACM Press: New York, NY, USA, 2005; p. 1813.
25. Pinder, C.; Vermeulen, J.; Wicaksono, A.; Beale, R.; Hendley, R.J. If this, then habit: Exploring context-aware implementation intentions on smartphones. In Proceedings of the 18th International Conference on Human-Computer Interaction with Mobile Devices and Services Adjunct—MobileHCI '16, Florence, Italy, 6–9 September 2016; ACM Press: New York, NY, USA, 2016; pp. 690–697.
26. Lau, S.; Wong, Y.W.; Luk, F.W.; Kwok, S.S. The effectiveness of a smart school bag system for reminding students of forgotten items and reducing the weight of their bags. *Springerplus* **2015**, *4*, O2. [CrossRef]
27. Mattson, M.P.; Allison, D.B.; Fontana, L.; Harvie, M.; Longo, V.D.; Malaisse, W.J.; Mosley, M.; Notterpek, L.; Ravussin, E.; Scheer, F.A.J.L.; et al. Meal frequency and timing in health and disease. *Proc. Natl. Acad. Sci. USA* **2014**, *111*, 16647–16653. [CrossRef] [PubMed]
28. The Nielsen Company. *Snack Attack: What Consumer Are Reaching for around the World*; The Nielsen Company: New York, NY, USA, 2014.
29. Casazza, K.; Fontaine, K.R.; Astrup, A.; Birch, L.L.; Brown, A.W.; Bohan Brown, M.M.; Durant, N.; Dutton, G.; Foster, E.M.; Heymsfield, S.B.; et al. Myths, Presumptions, and Facts about Obesity. *N. Engl. J. Med.* **2013**, *368*, 446–454. [CrossRef] [PubMed]
30. Carter, C. *The Sweet Spot: How to Find Your Groove at Home and Work*; Random House Publishing Group: New York, NY, USA, 2015; ISBN 9780553392043.

31. Truong, K.N.; Hayes, G.R.; Abowd, G.D. Storyboarding: An Empirical Determination of Best Practices and Effective Guidelines. In Proceedings of the Conference on Designing Interactive Systems, University Park, PA, USA, 26–28 June 2006; ACM Press: New York, NY, USA, 2006; pp. 12–21.
32. Fox, J.E.; Fricker, S.S. Beyond words: Strategies for designing good questionnaires. In Proceedings of the Usability Professionals' Association Annual Conference, Baltimore, MD, USA, 19 June 2008.
33. International Organization for Standardization. *Ergonomics of Human-System Interaction—Part 210: Human-Centred Design for Interactive Systems*; International Organization for Standardization: Geneva, Switzerland, 2010.
34. Wessa, P. Cronbach Alpha (v1.0.5) in Free Statistics Software 2017. Available online: https://www.wessa.net/rwasp_cronbach.wasp (accessed on 1 December 2017).

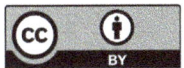

© 2018 by the authors. Licensee MDPI, Basel, Switzerland. This article is an open access article distributed under the terms and conditions of the Creative Commons Attribution (CC BY) license (http://creativecommons.org/licenses/by/4.0/).

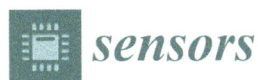

Article

Creating Affording Situations: Coaching through Animate Objects

Chris Baber [1,*], Ahmad Khattab [1], Martin Russell [1], Joachim Hermsdörfer [2] and Alan Wing [3]

1. School of Engineering, University of Birmingham, Birmingham B15 2TT, UK; in06khattab@gmail.com (A.K.); m.j.russell@bham.ac.uk (M.R.)
2. Department of Sport and Health Sciences, Technische Universität Munchen, 80992 Munchen, Germany; joachim.hermsdoerfer@tum.de
3. School of Psychology, University of Birmingham, Birmingham B15 2TT, UK; a.m.wing@bham.ac.uk
* Correspondence: c.baber@bham.ac.uk; Tel.: +44-121-414-3965

Received: 14 July 2017; Accepted: 3 October 2017; Published: 11 October 2017

Abstract: We explore the ways in which animate objects can be used to cue actions as part of coaching in Activities of Daily Living (ADL). In this case, changing the appearance or behavior of a physical object is intended to cue actions which are appropriate for a given context. The context is defined by the intention of the users, the state of the objects and the tasks for which these objects can be used. We present initial design prototypes and simple user trials which explore the impact of different cues on activity. It is shown that raising the handle of a jug, for example, not only cues the act of picking up the jug but also encourages use of the hand adjacent to the handle; that combinations of lights (on the objects) and auditory cues influence activity through reducing uncertainty; and that cueing can challenge pre-learned action sequences. We interpret these results in terms of the idea that the animate objects can be used to create affording situations, and discuss implications of this work to support relearning of ADL following brain damage or injury, such as might arise following a stroke.

Keywords: tangible user interface; affordance; multimodal cueing; animate objects; activities of daily living

1. Introduction

In this paper we consider 'coaching' in terms of encouraging people to act. Broadly, coaching involves a set of processes which are aimed at helping an individual (or group of individuals) improve, develop or learn skills. Often coaching will involve a dialogue between the individual and their coach. Replacing a (human) coach with a digital counterpart, therefore, raises some interesting questions concerning the ways in which to determine the improvement, development or learning by the individual, and the ways in which 'dialogue' could occur. Ensuring that the coaching is tailored to the abilities of the individual is essential for digital coaching [1]. From this, a basic specification for a digital coach would include the ability to recognize the actions performed by the individual, to evaluate these actions (against some quality criterion), and to provide advice and guidance that could lead to improvement (or alteration) in the performance of the actions (Table 1).

Table 1. Support for coaching.

Features of Coaching	Requirements for Support
Help improve, develop, learn skills	Define goal performance
Monitor and evaluate activity	Recognise actions and predict errors
Define targets for improvement	Define measures of effectiveness
Dialogue to discuss targets and plan programme of training	Determine route from current performance to goal
Tailoring programme to individual	Modify route to cater for individual capability
Evaluate progress	Recognise action against performance goal

For example, assume that you will make a hot drink by boiling a kettle and then pouring boiling water into a mug into which you have already added coffee granules. This can be decomposed into a sequence of steps; each step has a set of successive steps which are more likely to lead to the goal. When a person appears confused, e.g., when they fail to act, or when they make an error, i.e., when they perform an action which is not one of the recommended ones, then they might require a prompt. The challenge is to prompt actions in a sequence in order to either correct the sequence, or prevent further errors, and in order not to distract or frustrate the person.

Within the EU-funded project *CogWatch* (http://www.cogwatch.eu/, Figure 1) we developed technology that supported Activities of Daily Living (ADL) through recognition of activity and cueing to reduce errors [2,3].

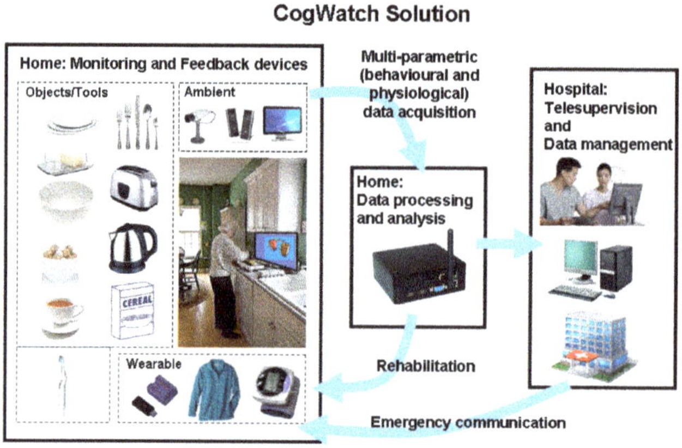

Figure 1. Schematic of the *CogWatch* concept.

Figure 2 shows the *CogWatch* system being used. When a person performs a sequence of actions, such as making a cup of tea, each action they perform is recognized and compared with a set of plausible actions. If an action is not part of this plausible set it could be defined as an error, e.g., because an action is repeated or because it was not appropriate at that point in the sequence. If this occurs then the user receives a prompt on the visual display.

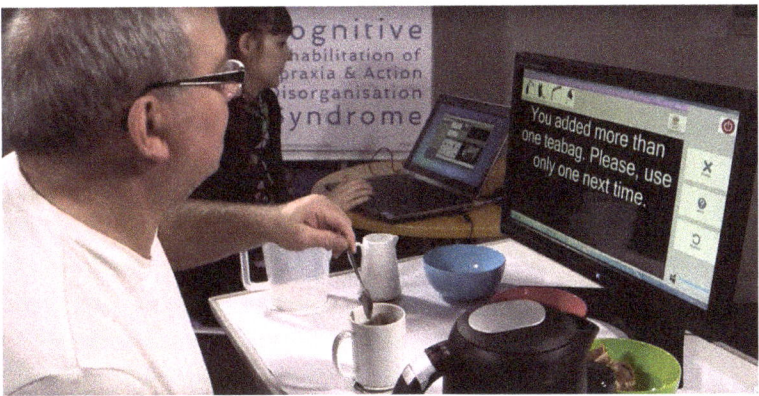

Figure 2. Interacting with the *CogWatch* system.

Sensors (accelerometers and force sensitive resistors, FSRs) on the objects detect the actions that a person makes with them. Data from the sensors, together with hand tracking using Microsoft Kinect, are used to create Hidden Markov Models for activity recognition [4]. In order to determine when to provide a cue to the user, the activity recognition output is compared with the prediction of the actions which would be appropriate for a goal. The prediction is based on Partially-Observable Markov Decision Process (POMDP) models of task sequence [5,6].

In trials conducted with stroke patients, as part of the *CogWatch* project, it was found that, without support, patients struggle to complete ADL, such as tea-making. Under such conditions, most of the patients tested failing to complete the task successfully. Even when patients were able to consult printed instructions on the step-by-step sequence of actions, they still failed to complete the tasks. We believe that this shows that printed support is ineffective with this particular task and population. Some stroke victims have concomitant cognitive problems in addition to difficulties in executing, and some of these relate to language ability. While efforts were made to select patients with similar impairments, some participants in these trials could have found the printed instructions challenging.

In contrast, almost all of the trials with *CogWatch* support resulted in patients successfully completing the tea-making tasks [2]. However, even in these *CogWatch* trials, patients tended to make errors (which they were able to correct) and took significant time to complete the activity. While the *CogWatch* project demonstrated that patients were able to respond effectively to the cues presented to them, the system relied on the use of a visual display to provide these cues as shown in Figure 2. While Figure 2 shows text instructions (which could create similar problems to those noted for the printed instructions) we also showed guidance using video, and this still led to problems. Another explanation of the time and errors in these trials is that patients might have found it difficult to divide their attention between the physical actions involved in performing the tasks using the objects, and the more abstract task of reading instructions and relating these to their actions. Consequently, in this paper, we explore whether the cues could be provided by the objects themselves.

Designing Intelligent Objects

Objects can be designed to provide visual, tactile or auditory cues to the user [7]. This develops prior work on Tangible User Interfaces (TUIs) or Ambient Displays [8] which involve the development of 'smart objects' [9]. A smart object typically has awareness (defined as the ability to sense where it is, how it is being used etc.), representation (defined as the ability to make sense of its awareness), and interaction (defined as the ability to respond to the user or other objects). In *CogWatch*, as discussed previously, awareness was achieved through the integration of sensors on objects and representation was through the developed on HMM and POMDP. In order to support interaction, we extend the design of these objects to present information to users.

The development of TUIs over the past two decades has been dependent on the availability of miniature sensors and processors. Much of this work has focused on the development of objects as input devices or objects as forms of ambient display. Contemporary work, particularly at MIT [10], has been exploring ways in which objects can be physically transformed. In terms of the healthcare domain, an ambient display has been developed to alert teenagers with Attention Deficit/Hyperactivity Disorder (ADHD) to support everyday activity planning [11]. Similarly, ambient displays can be used to provide reminders to patients concerning the time to take medication [12,13], and a Rehabilitation Internet of Things (RioT) [14] uses wearable sensors to advise on the physical activities of individuals wearing these devices. For *CogWatch*, objects used in ADL were kept as normal as possible in appearance and function, to avoid causing further confusion to the patients. This meant that the sensors had to be small and discrete. For several of the objects used in the archetypical ADL of making a cup of tea, we developed an instrumented coaster. This design allowed us to package the sensors and circuitry (Figure 3). The resulting device can be fitted to the underside of the object, where it has very little visual impact and does not obstruct the use of the object. This is inspired by the well-known MediaCup concept [15].

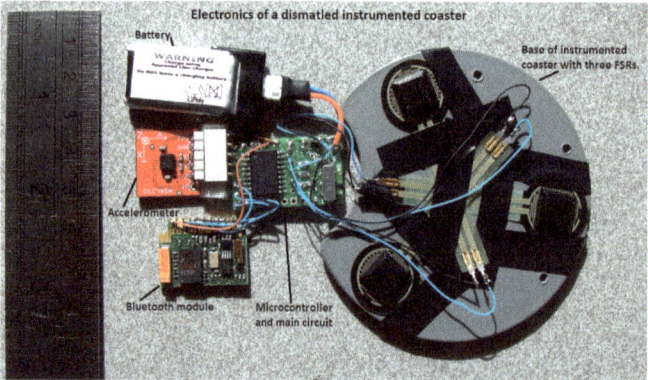

Figure 3. *CogWatch* coaster.

The coaster is fitted with Force Sensitive Resistors (FSRs) which are used to not only determine when the object is on the table or lifted, but can also be used to estimate how much liquid is being poured into a container. In addition to FSRs, triaxial accelerometers are used to record movement. The sensors are controlled by a Microchip dsPIC30F3012 microcontroller, which has an integrated 12 bit analogue digital converter (ADC). The microcontroller is programmed to digitize, compress and prepare the sensor data and manage the transmission of the data via Bluetooth. The data are buffered on the microcontroller so that they can be re-transmitted (avoiding data loss) if the wireless connection is interrupted for a short period. An ARF7044 Bluetooth module is used to transmit the sensor data to a host computer via a Bluetooth wireless connection (Figure 4).

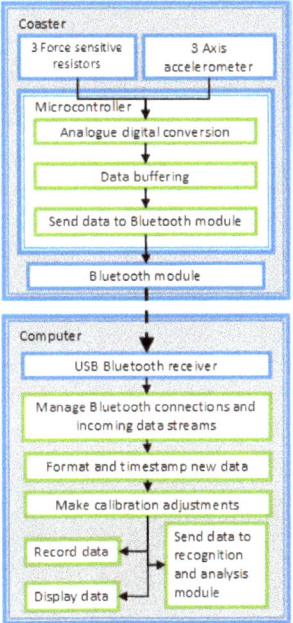

Figure 4. Coaster system design.

As Poupyrev et al. [16] note, there is a tendency for TUIs to respond to users primarily through visual or auditory displays and there has been less work on displays which can change their physical appearance. The development of small, easy-to-use actuators makes it possible for shape-changing objects to be created.

In addition to cueing when to perform an action, it is possible to influence the ongoing performance of an action in order to correct or compensate the manner in which the action is performed. For example, Figure 5 shows a commercial product which is designed to compensate for tremors, such as might arise from Parkinson's disease.

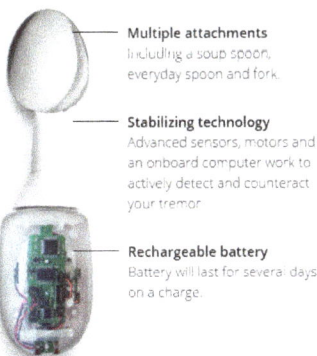

Figure 5. Stabilizing Spoon (https://www.liftware.com/).

Having the object change its physical behavior, e.g., through vibration, could cue the user to which object to pick up (by making the object wobble on the table) as well as compensating for the movements performed by the user. For example, we experimented, with an arrow on the lid of a jug which would point to the direction in which the person should move the jug (the arrow was connected to a servomotor driven by a magnetometer which responded to magnets placed on the table or in other objects). In order to indicate the state of an object, one can use visual cues to show its temperature or whether it is turned on or off, or open or closed. For example, one could use a Light-Emitting Diode (LED) in the handle of a drawer to alert a person to this drawer [17]. The light could indicate that this particular drawer contains the saucepan that the person needs for making a sauce.

Figure 6 shows a set of animate objects used in our initial experiments. The jug has an accelerometer and an LED strip. A Force Sensitive Resistor (FSR), on the base of the jug, is used to detect when the jug has been picked up. A tilt sensor, triggered at an angle of 30°, is used to determine when it is poured, and an MP3 player (SOMO II) and speaker are used to play sounds from an SD card. Finally, we reused the laser position assembly from a DVD drive as the mechanism for raising and lowering of the handle of the jug. The spoon has an accelerometer, vibration motor, data logger and an LED strip. The cups have LED strips. All objects connect to the Wi-Fi network (and for these trials, were controlled via an app running on an Android phone).

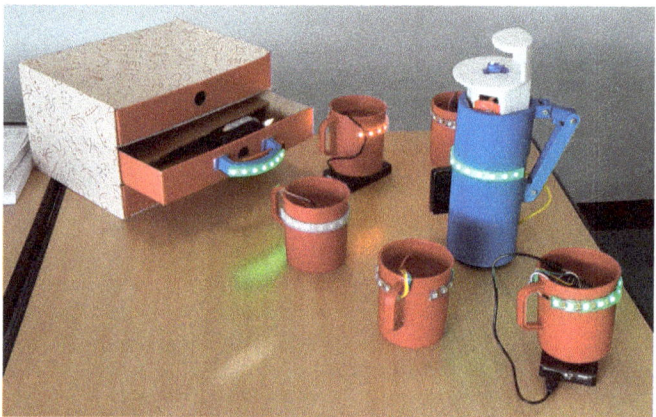

Figure 6. A collection of animate objects.

Note that, in Figure 6, some of the objects have green lights and one mug has red lights. We recognize that green and red may be problematic for color-blind people and this could be reconfigured in later designs. However, in our initial trials we do not tell participants what the lights mean but rather wait to see what interpretation the participants provide. The intention is that the behavior of the objects can both attract the attention of the user and also cues which action to perform. For example, in one trial we place the jug in front of the participant and raise the handle. If the participant does not respond to the handle rising, then the LED strip on the jug turns green. After this, an auditory cue (of the sound of pouring water) is played to draw their attention to the jug and prompt a lift and pour action, and if this fails to elicit a response a verbal prompt (with a voice recording of the phrase 'pick me up') is played.

For communications, Wi-Fi was chosen due to its scalability, lack of infrastructure and the ability to control the experiment from a mobile phone. This also allows devices to communicate with each other and change state based on another device's sensor. All the objects are fitted with an Arduino with built in Wi-Fi (Adafruit Feather M0 Wi-Fi). This Arduino has built in battery management and an SD card shield for data logging. The Wi-Fi server was programmed using Blynk.

Figure 7 shows a user interface, running on an Android mobile telephone that was used to control the objects and record data from the trials. The server's IP address must remain constant in order to ensure all devices connect to it, but the server must be able to connect to other networks (e.g., the university). This requires a DHCP reservation to be made. The server allows multiple phones to connect so multiple phones can control the experiment, but also provides some security in the connections. A local router could be implemented on a Raspberry Pi Zero which can host both the server and the local network. This raspberry pi is small enough to fit inside the jug which will result in no extra equipment needed other than the jug, spoon, cups. The network enables expansion to other objects.

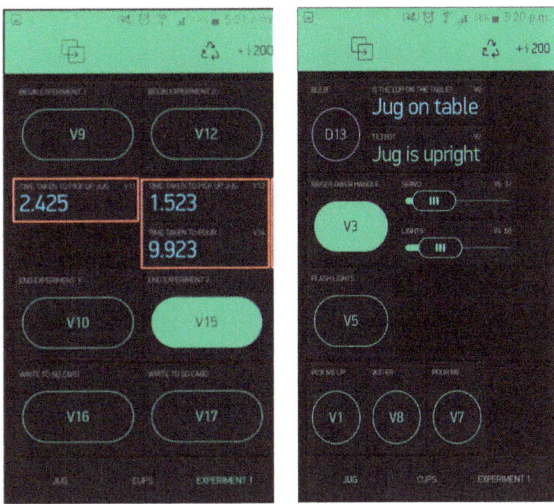

Figure 7. Screenshots of app showing timings for experiments 1 and 2.

2. Evaluation and Initial User Trials

In this section, we report three small-scale user trials in which participants were asked to perform simple tasks using the animate objects. The aim of this was to explore the ways in which the behavior of the objects could be used to cue actions, and how easily people could interpret and respond to these cues. In these user trials, all participants are neurotypical and were recruited from students in the Engineering School. Thus, we are not considering the question of how patients might react to the objects in these studies.

2.1. Participants and Trial Design

All participants gave their informed consent for inclusion before they participated in the study. The study was conducted in accordance with the Declaration of Helsinki, and the protocol was approved by the School of Engineering, University of Birmingham Ethics process. 23 participants (mean age: 25; 19 male, six female). Participants had no prior experience of the equipment or experimental tasks, and received minimal prior instruction as the aim was to see how they would respond on their first encounter with the objects. They were told that the aim of the trials was to allow them to interact with 'animate objects' and that they were to perform an action that they believed would be appropriate on an object as soon as they were confident in the opportunity to act. All participants performed three trials, with each trial involving 6–8 repetitions. In total, this produced 650 records, and $7\frac{1}{2}$ hours of video.

The timings, for the first two trials, were taken from the data recorded from the sensors on objects (FSR and tilt switch). This gave a resolution of 1 ms. Timings for trial 3 were taken from video data. To ensure timings were consistent for all participants, video analysis was performed by two people independently, and were tested to be within 20% tolerance, otherwise the video analysis was repeated. To ensure consistency of video capture, the camera was situated in the same position throughout the whole experiment and was not in the field of view of the participant in order to provide minimal disruption. In this experiment, the independent variables were lights, sounds and the dependent variables were time (pick up jug, spoon, pour, open drawer) and number of mistakes.

2.2. Trial One: Multimodal Cueing of Object State and Required Tasks

The use of simple visual cues, such as LEDs, have been shown to be robustly encoded in an action frame of reference [18], which means that the presence of an illuminated LED can be sufficient to guide a person's attention (and reach) to that location. Interestingly, in a study of reaching to buttons cued by LEDs, patients with right stroke show improvement with practice (suggesting a beneficial effect of such cueing) while patients with left stroke do not show such improvement [19]. This suggests that, as a form of cueing, visual information, such as LEDs, could be useful for right stroke patients, but not so useful for left stroke patients. In terms of ADL, Bienkiewicz et al., showed that the noise made during the performance of a task (such as the sound of a saw, the sound of pouring water, or of stirring with a spoon) can support apraxic patients in recalling a motor program which is otherwise not accessible [20]. We presume that the effect of the cue is even stronger if the object itself emits the biological sound. For example, asking patients with Parkinson's Disease to walk in time to the (prerecorded) sound of footsteps on gravel can lead to better support with gait problems than walking in time to a metronome [21]. This suggests that there is some element of the 'natural' sounds which, in addition to the marking of time, can improve performance. In terms of Tangible User Interface, early pioneers of this area referred to these as 'graspable' user interfaces [22], which implies that the physical form of an object would encourage physical interaction with it.

2.2.1. Procedure

Participants began the experiment with both hands on the table. The experimenter then activated the handle of the jug (using the Blynk app as described previously). The jug's handle then rose from the side of the jug. When the handle was fully raised, the LED strip on the top of the jug turned on dimly and a timer began. If the jug had not been picked up after three seconds, the LED strip turned on at full brightness. If the jug had not been picked up after six seconds, the LED strip flashed and the audio prompt of "Pick me up" was played. Once the jug had been picked up (determined by the FSR going to zero), the timer stored this time and reset. Once the participant had picked up the jug, a cup lit up and the audio prompt "pour me" was played. The timer ended when the jug was poured (tilt switch that triggered at an angle of 30°). This procedure was repeated using either the dominant or the non-dominant hand, using LED to indicate correct or distraction cups, and using two different sounds: a "pour me" voice command and the sound of the water pouring. This was done to test the effectiveness of different types of audio prompts. In terms of the 'correct or distraction' using LEDs, when the participant was about to perform an action with an object, another object cued the participant to use it instead. For example, when a participant was about to pour into a cup, the LED on the cup turned red and another cup turned green. This tested whether the cues can stop a current action and change an intention. At the end of the eight tasks in this trial, participants were interviewed to ask about their preference for and interpretation of the different cues that were employed, and were asked to explain what decisions they were making during the tasks.

2.2.2. Results

Initially, participants would reach out to grab the jug handle, but appeared uncertain and hesitate, the "pick me up" voice then confirmed their intention. The time taken to pick up the jug was significantly quicker in the no lights case than in the lights case at trial 8 [$t(19) = 1.195$, $p < 0.05$] (Figure 8). The number of attempts before the "pick me up" voice was not required was not different between the lights and the no lights conditions: mean number of attempts for the lights group was 4.18 (± 3.52) and in the no lights group 3.5 (± 1.9). Thus, it took around 4 attempts for participants to be confident that they could pick up the jug when the handle had risen, rather than wait for the audio prompt.

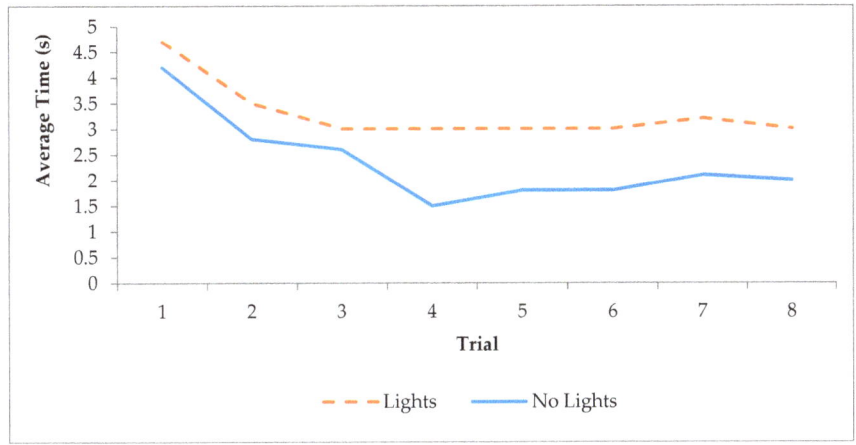

Figure 8. Time to complete tasks in trial one. Times for trials with and without lights are compared to a baseline condition (in which participants picked up the jug as soon as they were instructed by the experimenter).

All participants poured into the cup that was lit up and responded correctly to the vocal prompt. After the cup was lit, some participants would wait for the sound before beginning to pour.

None of the participants poured into an unlit cup and all the participants responded to the distraction correctly, i.e., participants stopped pouring when the light on the cup turned red and poured into another cup that turned green. There was no difference in the time taken to pour between the lights and no lights.

2.2.3. Conclusions

During the post-trial debrief interviews, participants were asked what cued them to pick up the jug. In the lights case, 64% said the handle rising, 18% said the lights on the jug and 18% said the "pick me up" sound. This is in contrast with the no lights case where 90% said the handle rising and 10% said the sound cued to pick up the jug. Participants preferred the "pour me" (69%) sound than the water pouring sound (31%) as a cue to begin pouring. This was because the "pour me" is a clear instruction, whereas the water pouring was unclear. Participants preferred the water pouring sound to be after the "pour me" sound whilst they were pouring. Participants said that the water pouring sound made the experiment more realistic and indicated when they should stop pouring. When the sound stopped, all participants stopped pouring.

When the cup lit up, some participants would wait for the sound before pouring, thus the light is not strong enough as a cue to perform an action, but highlights which object the action should be performed with. Similarly, the lights did not have any effect on the number of attempts needed before the "pick me up" voice was no longer required. Without the lights, participants still picked up the jug as the animation and sound were strong cues. When participants were asked, what cued them to pick up the jug, there was less variation in the responses in the no lights case as there were fewer cues.

Change in the intensity of lights does not prompt an action. The presence of the light cued an action (as seen on the spoon and cups), but changing the brightness did not. Participants stated that when the green light appeared, it meant that an action had to be performed with the object, and they were looking for the simplest possible action. Participants also recognised that the red light meant stop pouring or do not use.

Baseline performance was also recorded. In these trials, participants were asked to complete the pick up and pour actions without waiting for cues. We found that, with the cues, Participants never reached their fastest performance when pouring. In the fastest performance, participants had a clear plan of action with clear instructions. But when cued, participants were waiting for the correct cup to light up before pouring, so there was a clear instruction and introduced a level of uncertainty. This confirms the theory that the action currently being performed is in anticipation of the next action; if the next action is unknown, then participants must wait. Another explanation is that participants were being provided with redundant information.

2.3. Trial Two: Hand and Handle Alignment in Picking up the Jug

We grasp tools according to the intended use [23]. Thus, while we may grasp a hammer in different ways when we want to transport it, we will grasp it at the handle with the thumb towards the heavy part when we want to use it immediately to drive a nail into a wall. Although in apraxic patients a functional grasp does not guarantee the correct use of the tool [24], such a grasp serves as a strong attractor that increases the likelihood of executing the correct gesture [25]. Even for neurotypical participants, people are faster at performing a manual response to an object when they use the hand that is aligned with the handle of a manipulable object compared to its functional end [26]. This suggests that having some means of indicating which part of an object to grasp could be useful. The action could be cued by simple modifications to the handle, e.g., by using LEDs to draw the user's attention to the handle, or by having the handle move to indicate that it could be grasped.

Previous research has shown that people make faster responses, in reaction time tasks, when the orientation of an objects' handle matches the hand which is to be used for the response [27–32]. Trial 2 investigated the question of whether object animation can cue an action, and whether the appearance of the handle on the jug corresponded with the hand used. Relating these tasks to the literature on task sequencing and neurological damage, when patients are asked to demonstrate perform on everyday activities (such as using a coffee machine) they can have difficulty in following multi-step procedures [33]. For patients with right brain damage, the problems related to maintaining position in a sequence of steps (i.e., they could lose track of what they had done and what they might need to do next). For patients with left brain damage, the problems were related to aphasia and retrieval of functional knowledge. This showed that performance of task sequences has different levels of impairment to those observed in the use of single objects (which often relate to difficulties in inferring use from appearance).

2.3.1. Procedure

The experimental protocol was the same as for trial one, except that we only used the jug in this trial. The trials used the same participants as trial 1. Six lifts were performed testing both the dominant and the non-dominant hands. As with trial one, participants were interviewed during debrief following the tasks.

2.3.2. Results

Comparison of first and sixth trial shows a significant reduction in response time: $t(8)$ 2.962, $p = 0.18$ (with mean times reducing from 7.6 ($\pm$3.3)s on trial one to 3.6 ($\pm$2.9) s on trial six). All but 1 of the participants consistently picked up the jug with the hand to which the handle was pointing. This suggests that, for the majority of participants, handle orientation was a reliable cue as to which hand to use. Most participants found it more comfortable to use the aligned hand, and felt that the jug "asked" them to use the aligned hand, even when they might have preferred to use their dominant hand. This suggests that there is a powerful cue of the alignment of the handle. People had to be prompted at the end of the experiment to mention which hand they were picking up the jug. Some participants were using their aligned hand without being aware, as this was something they had thought about. Some said they used their dominant hand, but then they realised the alignment of the handle. One participant mentioned that they used their non-dominant hand one or twice, whereas they had used their non-dominant hand half of the time.

2.3.3. Conclusions

The rising of the handle is a good affordance for determining which hand to use. Participants mentioned after the experiments that they did not notice using the other hand when picking up the jug and they felt it was natural. There was also very little difference between the timings of their non-dominant hand versus their dominant hand which explains the same reasoning.

2.4. Cueing Action Sequences

In previous work, we explored the relationship between LEDs and the state of objects in a simple problem-solving exercise [33]. The objective is to ensure that four boxes had satisfied their goals (Figure 9). The goal of each box was defined by a set of rules known to the box, and defined by the position of the box and its proximity to other boxes. Each box has three LEDs representing its state: one to indicate if the goal has been satisfied, one to indicate 'communication status' (in terms of connection with the table), and one to indicate 'proximity'. We were interested in whether people would try to learn the 'rules' that the boxes were using or whether they would find it easier to learn the pattern, or arrangement of the boxes, and whether the rules or patterns could generalize to new configurations. The argument for this comparison was that the patterns could be considered in terms of 'affordance' [34–37]. Not only were the patterns easier to understand (which suggests that the visual cues provides useful semantic information) but also participants found it easier to generalize patterns than the rules (contrary to our expectations).

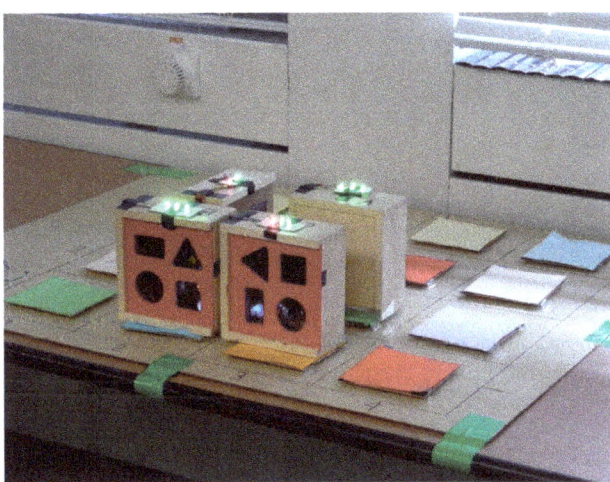

Figure 9. Visual feedback on networked objects [38].

2.4.1. Procedure

The trials used the same participants as trial 1. Cues for stirring and pouring were tested with a combination of lights and sounds (from vibration motor). A sequence of actions similar to making a cup of tea was performed purely from the objects' cues. For a 'team making' task, the experimenter raised the handle of the jug and, once the participant had lifted the jug, the experimenter turned the LED on one of the cups to green. When the participant had poured the jug to the cup, the experimenter turned the LED in the drawer handle green and turned on the vibration motor in the handle of the spoon (inside the drawer). The participant opened the drawer and lifted the spoon, and the experimenter turned the LED on the cup (that had been previously used to pour into) green. The participant put the spoon into the cup (perhaps making a stirring motion) and the task was completed. This constituted the 'logical' sequence of tea making, and was repeated four times. Additionally, an 'illogical' sequence was also repeated four times: this employed the same object activations but had them appear in an order that did not feel correct, e.g., taking the spoon from the drawer and stirring before pouring from the jug.

Each sequence (logical or illogical) was followed by a memory test which entailed placing cards in the same sequence that was performed. The number of mistakes was recorded and participants were not told that they will perform a memory test at the beginning the sequence. Seven cards were used: jug with handle raised, jug tilted (pouring), cup lit green, drawer opened, drawer handle lit green, spoon lit, spoon stirring cup.

Video footage from experiment three (with participant's permission) was analysed using ELAN to obtain timings. The following timings are obtained:

- Time taken to open drawer: Timer begins when light on the handle is on and timer ends when drawer is moved.
- Time taken to pick up spoon: Timer begins when drawer fully opened and timer ends when spoon picked up.
- Time taken to stir: Timer begins when spoon is picked up till head of the spoon is inside the cup.

Midway through the experiment, only one cup lit up. There were no other audible or visual cues. In the experiment with lights on the jug, the majority of participants performed no action when the cup lit up. On the other hand, in the no lights experiment, the majority of participants picked up the jug and poured into the cup even when the jug's handle was not raised, so participants picked up the jug with two hands and poured. As with the previous trials, participants were interviewed at debrief.

2.4.2. Results

When the light on the drawer handle lit up, not all participants opened the drawer, but all participants opened the drawer after the spoon vibrated inside. There was no difference in response between a flashing drawer handle and a steady lit handle. 95% of participants stirred and all participants who did stir, stirred the cup that was lit up.

During the memory recall, participants made exactly double the number of mistakes in the illogical sequence when compared to the logical sequence (Figure 10).

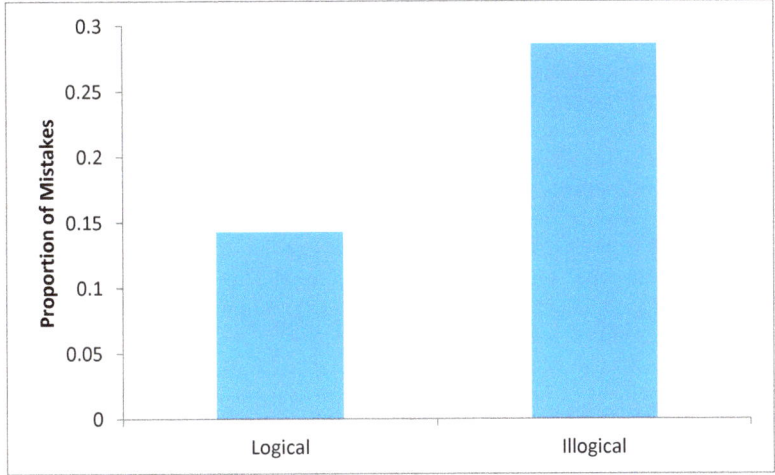

Figure 10. Comparing mistakes made in performing logical and illogical task sequences.

There was a significant difference between the number of mistakes made in the logical and illogical sequence [t(40) = 1.118, $p < 0.05$]. Mean number of mistakes made in the logical sequence was 0.14 (± 0.36) and the illogical sequence was 0.29 (± 0.46).

2.4.3. Conclusions

In terms of performance time, there was no significant difference between the logical and illogical sequences for all actions in the sequence (time taken to open the drawer, pick up spoon and stir). In the illogical sequence, participants found it strange to stir a cup before water was poured, but did so regardless. Flashing lights or a single steady light produced the same effect. If the participant did not respond to a light, a flashing light did not cue an action. An extra level of cueing might be needed, such as sound or animation to prompt an action. For example, a light on the drawer handle did not always cue the participant to open it, whether or not it was flashing or a steady light. However, all participants opened the drawer when the spoon was vibrating and flashing. The animation and sound of the vibration were strong enough for all participants to open the drawer. Bonanni et al. [17] claim is that if lights are placed on objects, people will always respond to the lights. However, our empirical data suggests that people will respond to the light in the context of the action being performed. People may see the light, but do not interpret it as a cue, a light does not guarantee that someone will perform an action. Sound and animation are required too to guarantee an action.

3. Discussion

In this paper we are considered ways in which familiar objects can be adapted to support affording situations. The overall concept is that the action that a person performs will be influenced by the context in which they perform that action. Context will, in turn, be influenced by the person's goals, the previous tasks that they have performed, the objects available to them and the state of these objects. By recognizing the actions that the person has performed we seek to infer their goal (or intention) and from this information we modify the appearance of the objects to cue credible actions in a sequence. Future work will take the notion of cueing further so that, in addition to examining tasks in sequence we will also consider wider contextual definitions of these tasks as the basis for cueing. For example, knowing the time and that the person is walking into the kitchen, we can cue them to open a cupboard (by illuminating the cupboard handle) so that they can take out a mug (which will, once the cupboard door opens, also light up). Once the cup has been retrieved, then we can cue a sequence of steps in the preparation of a drink.

The overall goal of this work is to create, as far as practicable, subtle cues through which actions can be suggested (when this is necessary for a given user). In the case of the recovering stroke patient, the use of these cues might reduce in line with their recovery such that after a few months of using this system, there might be few or no cues presented because the patient has recovered full ability for these tasks. In the case of patients with Alzheimer's or other forms of dementia, the cueing might need to be continued. We note, from [33], that damage to right or left brain impairs the ability to follow action sequences, and such Action Disorganisation Syndrome could be potentially aided by the concepts presented in this paper. We stress that such a claim still requires appropriate clinical testing. However, some previous work does support the idea of using multimodal cues to encourage patients to select an appropriate action in a sequence [20].

We have extended the capability of the objects designed for our prior work by incorporating actuators and displays which can provide the cues outlined in the previous sections. The overall aim is to create affording situations in which the behavior of the person can be cued by the behavior of the object which, in turn, responds to the (inferred) intentions of the user. In this case, coaching will involve building a (computer) model of the intentions of the user (based on the location of the objects, the time of day, previous activity of the person etc.) and a set of criteria for how these intentions ought to be met. The criteria could be learned by the computer or, more likely, could be defined by occupational therapists who would be working with the patient. In this case, the idea would be that a given ADL could be decomposed into specific actions, and each action could be defined in terms of quality of performance. Clearly this work is still in its infancy, and in this paper we are discussing some of the conceptual developments and initial prototypes. None of this work has been exposed to patients and thus we do not know how they might respond and react to lights, sounds or moving parts on everyday objects.

Creating Affording Situations

In Psychology and Human-Computer Interaction, the concept of 'affordance' relates to the ways in which a person's action is performed in response to their perception of the environment [34–37]. Gibson [36] introduced the term affordance into psychology, suggesting that we perceive the world in term of opportunities for action. What an object affords is determined by the physical properties of the objects (e.g., shape, orientation, size), and by the action capabilities of the agent and by the intention that the use of this object will support. Affordance effects for graspable objects can be manipulated by changing the size of the object, orientation, location and congruence. The spatial location of the handle influences stimulus identification in neglect patients, extinction patients and healthy participants. The end state comfort effect can be seen with participants having an uncomfortable grip at the beginning, then ending an action with a comfortable grip [39]. Participants who choose a grasp which was consistent with the end state comfort had a quicker reaction and movement time. Thus, an affordance is the relationship between an individual's ability to act and the opportunities provided to that person in the given situation in pursuit of a given intention. That is, a cup of particular dimensions can be grasped by a person of particular abilities in the context of performing a task with a particular intended goal: a person with hemiparesis might struggle to use a pinch grasp on a small teacup handle; a person with tremor might find it difficult to raise a full cup to their mouth (without spillage). A person laying the table will pick up the cup differently than a person who intends to drink from it.

From this perspective, one can consider coaching in terms of the form of encouragement of, and support for, actions which are appropriate to a given context (defined by objects, person's abilities and intentions). We aim to create 'affording situations' in which the appropriate action is subtly cued by the objects that the person needs to use. In this way, cueing is embedded naturally into the familiar world of the person's home, and coaching is a matter of responding to these cues.

The manner in which a person interacts with an object can be used to infer the physical and cognitive difficulties they might be experiencing in performing the task. As the person interacts with the object, data (from sensors on the object) will be used to define the nature of the atomic tasks being performed and, from these data, the intended outcome can be inferred. Having inferred a possible outcome, objects can modify their state to invite or cue subsequent actions, or provide feedback on the task as it is performed.

The concept of affording situations is intended to highlight the importance of context in understanding affordance; it is not simply a matter of saying that a 'jug affords lifting or pouring'. While these are actions that are, of course, possible with the jug, in order to know that this particular jug can be lifted or poured by this particular person, one also needs to know the capabilities of the person. Furthermore, in order to know whether either lifting or pouring is an appropriate action to make, one also needs to know the intention of the person (or the intention that could be plausible in that situation). Our aim is to develop technology that can recognize and interpret these contextual factors and use these to discern the plausibility of actions in a given sequence. We can then adapt the technology to provide cues that are intended to encourage the user to perform these actions. In this manner, coaching becomes a matter of creating the situations in which users of objects can learn to associate an object with an action, and an action with an intention, and an intention with a desirable outcome.

4. Conclusions

The objects discussed in this paper are all first-order prototypes and have been designed to support experimental evaluation with neurotypical participants, rather than patients. Patients with neurological deficit, as the result of degeneration, damage or injury, can often struggle with Activities of Daily Living (ADL). These problems can range from confusion over the sequence in which tasks should be performed, to forgetting which action can be performed using a given object, to failing to recognize a given object. These errors could involve putting breakfast cereal into a coffee mug (when making coffee) or attempting to pour from a milk container before opening it [40]. Around 1/3 of stroke survivors have difficulty with ADL and the errors that they make in planning and execution of errors can be predicted [41]. If it is possible to predict errors (rather than these being random occurrences) then it is possible to predict *when* an error could be likely to arise and to provide some cueing to either prevent the erroneous action or to encourage a preferred, i.e., non-erroneous, action.

Returning to the basic specification for this paper, for a system to provide coaching for patients with neurological deficit to allow them to perform ADL, we would need to recognize which actions people are performing (which typically means having some means of sensing that an action is being performed), to determine the quality of the performance (which requires not only activity recognition but also some evaluation of how this performance meets some criterion), to evaluate performance in terms of an anticipated outcome or intention, and to provide some means of guiding, cueing or otherwise providing advice and feedback in response to the action and in anticipation of subsequent action.

Author Contributions: Baber wrote the paper and designed the experiments; Khattab (with Baber) designed and built the objects, and conducted the experiments; Khattab and Baber conducted the analysis of the results; Russell, Hermsdorfer and Wing managed on the CogWatch project that contributed to the design concepts and commented on drafts of the paper.

Conflicts of Interest: The authors declare no conflict of interest.

References

1. Op den Akker, H.; Jones, V.M.; Hermens, H.J. Tailoring Real-Time Physical Activity Coaching Systems: A Literature Survey and Model. *User Model. User-Adapt. Int.* **2014**, *24*, 351–392. [CrossRef]
2. Hermsdörfer, J.; Bienkiewicz, M.; Cogollor, J.M.; Russel, M.; Jean-Baptiste, E.; Parekh, M.; Wing, A.M.; Ferre, M.; Hughes, C. CogWatch—Automated Assistance and Rehabilitation of Stroke-Induced Action

Disorders in the Home Environment. In *International Conference on Engineering Psychology and Cognitive Ergonomics*; Springer: Berlin/Heidelberg, Germany, 2013; pp. 343–350.
3. Giachritsis, C.; Randall, G. CogWatch: Cognitive Rehabilitation for Apraxia and Action Disorganization Syndrome Patients. In Proceedings of the Seventh International Workshop on Haptic and Audio Interaction Design, Lund, Sweden, 23–24 August 2012.
4. Jean-Baptiste, E.M.; Nabiei, R.; Parekh, M.; Fringi, E.; Drozdowska, B.; Baber, C.; Jancovic, P.; Rotshein, P.; Russell, M. Intelligent assistive system using real-time action recognition for stroke survivors. In Proceedings of the 2014 IEEE International Conference on Healthcare Informatics (ICHI), Verona, Italy, 5 March 2015; pp. 39–44.
5. Jean-Baptiste, E.M.; Rotshtein, P.; Russell, M. POMDP based action planning and human error detection. In *IFIP International Conference on Artificial Intelligence Applications and Innovations*; Springer International Publishing: Berlin, Germany, 2015; pp. 250–265.
6. Jean-Baptiste, E.M.; Rotshtein, P.; Russell, M. CogWatch: Automatic prompting system for stroke survivors during activities of daily living. *J. Innov. Digit. Ecosyst.* **2016**, *3*, 48–56. [CrossRef]
7. Kortuem, G.; Kawsar, F.; Fitton, D.; Sundramoorthy, V. Smart objects as building blocks for the Internet of Things. In *IEEE Internet Computing*; IEEE Computer Society: Washington, DC, USA, 2010; pp. 44–51.
8. Ishii, H. The tangible user interface and its evolution. *Commun. ACM* **2008**, *51*, 32–36. [CrossRef]
9. Ishii, H.; Leithinger, D.; Follmer, S.; Zoran, A.; Schoessler, P.; Counts, J. TRANSFORM: Embodiment of Radical Atoms at Milano Design Week. In Proceedings of the 33rd Annual ACM Conference Extended Abstracts on Human Factors in Computing Systems, Seoul, Korea, 18–23 April 2015; pp. 687–694.
10. Kortuem, G.; Kawsar, F.; Sundramoorthy, V.; Fitton, D. Smart objects as building blocks for the internet of things. *IEEE Internet Comput.* **2010**, *14*, 44–51. [CrossRef]
11. Zuckerman, O. Objects for change: A case study of a tangible user interface for behavior change. In Proceedings of the Ninth International Conference on Tangible, Embedded, and Embodied Interaction, Stanford, CA, USA, 15–19 January 2015; pp. 649–654.
12. Sung, M.-H.; Chian, C.-W. The Research of Using Magnetic Pillbox as Smart Pillbox System's Interactive Tangible User Interface. In *International Conference on Human-Computer Interaction*; Springer International Publishing: Berlin, Germany, 2016; pp. 451–456.
13. Reeder, B.; Chung, J.; Le, T.; Thompson, H.J.; Demiris, G. Assessing older adults' perceptions of sensor data and designing visual displays for ambient assisted living environments: An exploratory study. *Methods Inf. Med.* **2014**, *53*, 152. [CrossRef] [PubMed]
14. Dobkin, B.H. A Rehabilitation-Internet-of-Things in the Home to Augment Motor Skills and Exercise Training. *Neurorehabil. Neural Repair* **2016**, *31*, 217–227. [CrossRef] [PubMed]
15. Gellersen, H.-W.; Beigl, M.; Krull, H. The MediaCup: Awareness technology embedded in an everyday object. In *Handheld and Ubiquitous Computing 1st International Symposium HUC'99*; Springer: Berlin, Germany, 1999; pp. 308–310.
16. Poupyrev, I.; Nashida, T.; Okabe, M. Actuation and tangible user interfaces: The Vaucanson duck, robots, and shape displays. In Proceedings of the 1st International Conference on Tangible and Embedded Interaction, Baton Rouge, LA, USA, 15–17 February 2007.
17. Bonanni, L.; Lee, C.H.; Selker, T. CounterIntelligence: Augmented reality kitchen. In *CHI'05*; ACM: New York, NY, USA, 2005; p. 45.
18. Howard, L.A.; Tipper, S.P. Hand deviations away from visual cues: Indirect evidence for inhibition. *Exp. Brain Res.* **1997**, *113*, 144–152. [CrossRef] [PubMed]
19. Pohl, P.S.; Filion, D.L.; Kim, S.H. Effects of practice and unpredictable distractors on planning and executing aiming after stroke. *Neurorehabil. Neural Repair* **2003**, *17*, 93–100. [CrossRef] [PubMed]
20. Bienkiewicz, M.N.; Gulde, P.; Schlegel, A.; Hermsdörfer, J. The Use of Ecological Sounds in Facilitation of Tool Use in Apraxia. In *Replace, Repair, Restore, Relieve–Bridging Clinical and Engineering Solutions in Neurorehabilitation*; Springer: New York, NY, USA, 2014.
21. Young, W.R.; Shreve, L.; Quinn, E.J.; Craig, C.; Bronte-Stewart, H. Auditory cueing in Parkinson's patients with freezing of gait. What matters most: Action-relevance or cue continuity? *Neuropsychologia* **2016**, *87*, 54–62. [CrossRef] [PubMed]

22. Fitzmaurice, W.G.; Ishii, H.; Buxton, W. Bricks: Laying the foundations for graspable user interfaces. In Proceedings of the SIGCHI Conference on Human Factors in Computing Systems, Denver, CO, USA, 7–11 May 1995; pp. 442–449.
23. Hermsdörfer, J.; Li, Y.; Randerath, J.; Goldenberg, G.; Johannsen, L. Tool use without a tool: Kinematic characteristics of pantomiming as compared to actual use and the effect of brain damage. *Exp. Brain Res.* **2012**, *218*, 201–214. [CrossRef] [PubMed]
24. Randerath, J.; Li, Y.; Goldenberg, G.; Hermsdörfer, J. Grasping tools: Effects of task and apraxia. *Neuropsychologia* **2009**, *47*, 497–505. [CrossRef] [PubMed]
25. Graham, N.L.; Zeman, A.; Young, A.W.; Patterson, K.; Hodges, J.R. Dyspraxia in a patient with cortico-basal degeneration: The role of visual and tactile inputs to action. *J. Neurol. Neurosurg. Psychiatry* **1999**, *67*, 334–344. [CrossRef] [PubMed]
26. Matheson, H.; Newman, A.J.; Satel, J.; McMullen, P. Handles of manipulable objects attract covert visual attention: ERP evidence. *Brain Cogn.* **2014**, *86*, 17–23. [CrossRef] [PubMed]
27. Tucker, M.; Ellis, R. On the relations between seen objects and components of potential actions. *J. Exp. Psychol. Hum. Percept. Perform.* **1998**, *24*, 830. [CrossRef] [PubMed]
28. Tucker, M.; Ellis, R. The potentiation of grasp types during visual object categorization. *Vis. Cogn.* **2001**, *8*, 769–800. [CrossRef]
29. Craighero, L.; Fadiga, L.; Rizzolatti, G.; Umiltà, C. Visuomotor priming. *Vis. Cogn.* **1998**, *5*, 109–126. [CrossRef]
30. Craighero, L.; Fadiga, L.; Rizzolatti, G.; Umiltà, C. Action for perception: A motor- visual attentional effect. *J. Exp. Psychol. Hum. Percept. Perform.* **1999**, *25*, 1673–1692. [CrossRef] [PubMed]
31. Bub, D.N.; Masson, M.E. Grasping beer mugs: On the dynamics of alignment effects induced by handled objects. *J. Exp. Psychol. Hum. Percept. Perform.* **2010**, *36*, 341. [CrossRef] [PubMed]
32. Roest, S.A.; Pecher, D.; Naeije, L.; Zeelenberg, R. Alignment effects in beer mugs: Automatic action activation or response competition? *Attent. Percept. Psychophys.* **2016**, *78*, 1665–1680. [CrossRef] [PubMed]
33. Hartmann, K.; Goldenberg, G.; Daumüller, M.; Hermsdörfer, J. It takes the whole brain to make a cup of coffee: The neuropsychology of naturalistic actions involving technical devices. *Neuropsychologia* **2005**, *43*, 625–637. [CrossRef] [PubMed]
34. Norman, D.A. *The Design of Everyday Things*; Doubleday: New York, NY, USA, 1990.
35. Gaver, W. Technology affordances. In Proceedings of the SIGCHI Conference on Human Factors in Computing Systems, New Orleans, LA, USA, 27 April–2 May 1991; pp. 79–84.
36. Gibson, J.J. *The Ecological Approach to Visual Perception*; Houghton Mifflin Company: Dublin, Republic of Ireland, 1986.
37. Blevis, E.; Bødker, S.; Flach, J.; Forlizzi, J.; Jung, H.; Kaptelinin, V.; Nardi, B.; Rizzo, A. Ecological perspectives in HCI: Promise, problems, and potential. In Proceedings of the 33rd Annual ACM Conference Extended Abstracts on Human Factors in Computing Systems, Seoul, Korea, 18–23 April 2015; pp. 2401–2404.
38. Cervantes-Solis, J.W.; Baber, C.; Khattab, A.; Mitch, R. Rule and theme discovery in human interactions with an 'internet of things'. In Proceedings of the 2015 British HCI Conference, Lincolnshire, UK, 13–17 July 2015; pp. 222–227.
39. Rosenbaum, D.A.; Vaughan, J.; Barnes, H.J.; Jorgensen, M.J. Time course of movement planning: Selection of handgrips for object manipulation. *J. Exp. Psychol. Learn. Mem. Cogn.* **1992**, *18*, 1058. [CrossRef] [PubMed]
40. Schwarz, M.F.E.; Reed, E.S.; Montgomery, M.W.; Palmer, C.; Mayer, N.H. The quantitative description of action disorganization after brain damage—A case study. *Cogn. Neuropsychol.* **1991**, *8*, 381–414. [CrossRef]
41. Hughes, C.M.L.; Baber, C.; Bienkiewicz, M.; Worthington, A.; Hazell, A.; Hermsdörfer, J. The application of SHERPA (Systematic Human Error Reduction and Prediction Approach) in the development of compensatory cognitive rehabilitation strategies for stroke patients with left and right brain damage. *Ergonomics* **2015**, *58*, 75–95. [CrossRef] [PubMed]

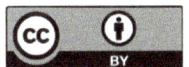

© 2017 by the authors. Licensee MDPI, Basel, Switzerland. This article is an open access article distributed under the terms and conditions of the Creative Commons Attribution (CC BY) license (http://creativecommons.org/licenses/by/4.0/).

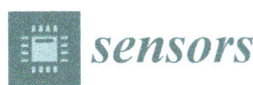

Article

Location-Enhanced Activity Recognition in Indoor Environments Using Off the Shelf Smart Watch Technology and BLE Beacons

Avgoustinos Filippoupolitis *, William Oliff, Babak Takand and George Loukas

Computing and Information Systems Department, University of Greenwich, Old Royal Naval College, Park Row, London SE10 9LS, UK; william.oliff@gre.ac.uk (W.O.); b.takand@gre.ac.uk (B.T.); g.loukas@gre.ac.uk (G.L.)
* Correspondence: a.filippoupolitis@gre.ac.uk

Academic Editors: Oresti Banos, Hermie Hermens, Chris Nugent and Hector Pomares
Received: 2 April 2017; Accepted: 19 May 2017; Published: 27 May 2017

Abstract: Activity recognition in indoor spaces benefits context awareness and improves the efficiency of applications related to personalised health monitoring, building energy management, security and safety. The majority of activity recognition frameworks, however, employ a network of specialised building sensors or a network of body-worn sensors. As this approach suffers with respect to practicality, we propose the use of commercial off-the-shelf devices. In this work, we design and evaluate an activity recognition system composed of a smart watch, which is enhanced with location information coming from Bluetooth Low Energy (BLE) beacons. We evaluate the performance of this approach for a variety of activities performed in an indoor laboratory environment, using four supervised machine learning algorithms. Our experimental results indicate that our location-enhanced activity recognition system is able to reach a classification accuracy ranging from 92% to 100%, while without location information classification accuracy it can drop to as low as 50% in some cases, depending on the window size chosen for data segmentation.

Keywords: activity recognition; wearable devices; inertial sensors; Bluetooth beacons; machine learning

1. Introduction

Knowledge of context, with respect to the activity performed by a user, promotes the efficiency of human-centric technologies. Especially in an indoor setting, human activity recognition is beneficial for applications such as personalised health monitoring, building energy management, security and safety. Most activity recognition approaches use custom devices in order to gather data related to the activity performed. As we discuss in Section 2, these specialised devices are either worn on multiple body parts or are installed in various locations inside the building, forming a wireless sensor network. This can include a network of pressure, temperature, humidity and acoustic sensors installed in the area [1], proprietary sensors attached to objects within specific areas [2,3], optical monition capturing systems [4] and RFID tags [5].

These approaches, however, are obtrusive and suffer in terms of practicality, as multiple specialised devices have to be installed on various objects and in different locations inside the area. This also affects integration and user acceptance, as most of the times, these devices use communication protocols (e.g., ZigBee) that are not compatible with devices such as a mobile phone carried by a typical user. The goal of this research is to accurately recognise activities related to specific areas in an indoor space by only using commercial off-the-shelf devices and investigate the effect that information related to the user's location has on the system's performance.

To achieve this, we have designed and developed a system that is composed of a smart watch, BLE beacons, a mobile phone and a server. The system collects and processes data coming from these devices, without relying on specific or customised implementations, which results in enhanced flexibility. The popularity of wearable devices has significantly increased in recent years [6], while BLE beacons have become extremely popular, and there is a wide range of commercial offerings available from multiple manufacturers [7]. In previous work [8], we investigated the feasibility of activity recognition using commercial smart watches. Here, BLE beacons are used to enhance our activity recognition system in an unobtrusive way with information regarding the location of the occupants. In particular, in this work, we investigate our system's performance when we fuse the inertial data coming from a commercial smart watch with data coming from BLE beacons. We have also evaluated different classification algorithms, feature types and segmentation window sizes. Our evaluation is based on real-world experiments, using our proposed system, that took place in an indoor laboratory environment.

In particular, the first contribution of this work is the development of an activity recognition system that incorporates commercial off-the-shelf BLE beacons in conjunction with wearable devices to enhance the system's performance. As we discuss in Section 2, the majority of existing approaches either rely solely on wearable sensors or they use specialised infrastructure. The second contribution is the development of a data collection and labelling framework, which integrates the wearable devices and the BLE beacons and allows for the creation of labelled datasets to be used with activity recognition algorithms. Finally, the third contribution is the evaluation of our activity recognition system's classification accuracy when using different classification algorithms and feature types and the comparison of its performance to that of systems that only rely on wearable devices.

We should note that the focus of this work is to evaluate the effect of location enhancement in recognising human activities. However, instead of only providing our experimental results for the location-enhanced system, we also present results for the case where only a wrist-worn device (i.e., a smart watch) is used by the participants. This provides the baseline that can help us compare the performance of the location-enhanced system to that of systems that only use wearable devices, as discussed in Section 2.

The remaining of this paper is structured as follows. In Section 2, we discuss related literature in the area of human activity recognition using wearable devices, both commercial and custom. We continue in Section 3 with a description of our system's architecture, while Section 4 elaborates on the design of our activity recognition chain. The details of our experimental setup are presented in Section 5. In Section 6, we present our experimental results and discuss the performance of our system before we summarise our conclusions in Section 7.

2. Related Work

In the research field of Human Activity Recognition (HAR), there has been a growing trend of wrist-worn wearable devices (e.g., smart watches) with Inertial Measurement Units (IMUs) containing a host of different sensors. This was highlighted by a recent survey conducted in [9], which showed an even bigger trend in the use of IMUs with accelerometers, gyroscopes and magnetometers. The increased usage and interest of wrist-worn devices is not surprising, given the global acceptance of these devices in our daily lives. According to Statista [6], the number of worldwide sales for smart watches was five million in 2014, predicted to exceed 75 million in 2017, an increase of 1500% in three years.

There has also been a large amount of research conducted in the field of HAR that uses body-worn sensors, as highlighted by [10]. Body-worn approaches have been shown to have slightly better accuracy [11–14] than approaches that use only wrist-worn devices. However, body-worn approaches currently have the draw-back of being more obtrusive than their wrist-worn counterparts. Prolonged use of body-worn wearable devices may interfere with users' daily lives, thus interfering with how the user performs activities. Moreover, body-worn wearables may become uncomfortable, limiting the devices to only being worn for short periods of time, rendering them less viable for monitoring daily activities. Wrist-worn approaches are less obtrusive and have less impact on the users' daily lives, allowing the devices to be worn for longer periods of time. The literature presented is primarily focused on recent work that involves the use of wrist-worn wearables in the context of HAR.

We have provided some key details of related work in this area, as shown in Table 1. The details given in the table are:

- Indoor space: The type of indoor space the activity recognition experiments were carried out in, such as a home, a laboratory or another environment.
- IMU sensors: The different IMU sensors that were used by a classifier to infer a participant's activity.
- Classification approach: What machine learning classification algorithms were used in the approach to estimate the activity performed by a participant.
- Commercial-Off-The Shelf (COTS): Whether the devices used in the experiments are widely accessible and available to an end user.

Furthermore, we classify captured activities into two general categories, low and high level activities. Low level activities are the ones that require whole body movement in order to be performed, such as walking, running and jumping. High level activities involve interaction with objects as described by [9] and daily activities being performed, as categorised by [10].

2.1. Activity Recognition Using COTS

A number of researchers are now incorporating COTS wrist-worn wearables into their approach for activity recognition rather than creating custom devices, as shown in Table 1. Additionally, COTS smart watches are usual paired with a smartphone, which also contains its own IMU. Therefore, this creates an optional data source that can be used if required, unlike their experimental wearable device counterparts.

The LG G Watch has been used in a couple of approaches [13,15], producing a reasonable level of accuracy. The authors in [15] use an LG G Watch coupled with a Samsung Galaxy S4 smartphone to identify eating activities for different foods. Their approach features a total of eighteen activities (six low and twelve high level) with seventeen participants. A range of classifiers (ANN with Multilayer Perceptron (MLP), NB and RF) are used, and the authors show that RF produces the best overall accuracy of 93.3% in personal classification. However, we should note that the authors do not provide evaluation for the other classifiers. Similarly, in [16], the authors propose a diet monitoring system that uses a smart watch device to detect fourteen eating and seven non-eating activities with a DT classifier. Using the accelerometer and gyroscope data from the smart watch, the authors show that the proposed system achieves an accuracy of 92% for detecting an eating episode. Furthermore, the authors in [13] use the accelerometer data from an LG G Watch for comparing activity estimation between sensor placement on the wrist and elbow (Myo armband) using KNN, DT, RF and bagging classifiers for eight high level gestures. The presented results show that the smart watch, with an accuracy varying between 86.5% and 96.2% depending on the classifier, does provide an 8% better overall accuracy over the armband, but not for every participant.

Another smart watch that has been shown to give good activity classification [17,18] is the Moto 360. The authors in [17] attempt to derive the activity of a shopper by capturing accelerometer and gyroscope data form a Moto 360 and a smartphone for high and low level activities respectively. Their approach achieves a precision accuracy of 92.26% for the high level activities when using an HMM and DT with Conditional Random Field (CRF) classifiers. The main aim in [18] is to increase the energy efficiency of a smart watch with the classification algorithm running locally. The authors not only use a Moto 360 (Motorola Mobility LLC., Libertyville, IL, USA), but also use a Samsung Galaxy Live (Samsung, Daegu, South Korea), Sony S3 (Sony Corporation, Tokyo, Japan) and LG G Watch R (LG Electronics, Seoul, Korea) for various evaluations throughout their work. The proposed system also provides a novel approach for semantic abstraction with NB, SVM, DT and LR classifiers, which delivers a good recall accuracy, averaging at 75% over the classifiers. However, it performs poorly in terms of precision accuracy, with the NB and DT classifiers producing 66% and 55%, respectively. Though, the authors do successfully demonstrate that semantic abstraction does improve overall accuracy.

Additionally, the researchers in [19] use a Microsoft Band smart watch for the purpose of identifying the activities of participants in a basketball game. A wide range of different classification algorithms (SVM, KNN, NB, DT and RF) is used. The authors use a personal classifier first used to distinguish the activity of the participant, and then, a collaborative classifier is used to identify the actual participant. With 10-fold cross-validation, the SVM classifier was shown to produce the best precision and recall accuracies of 91.34% and 94.31%, respectively.

The authors in [20] use the GENEActiv [21], which is a more specialised watch featuring a triaxial accelerometer and is geared towards research applications for free-living, sports research and clinical trials. The watch is available commercially and, therefore, still considered COTS technology. The approach in [20] is focused on classification of seven high level daily activities using HMM and CRF algorithms with leave-one-day-out cross-validation for the 21 days of data collected from two participants. It achieves accuracies ranging between 70% and 77% with the use of sub-classing and highlights that the GENEActiv is a feasible device for activity recognition.

A slightly more unorthodox approach is the one used by the authors in [22], who use two Samsung Galaxy S2 smartphones, with one at the pocket position and the other mounted at the wrist position. As a general rule, a smartphone weighs more than a smart watch. As a result, the device will potentially have a higher centre of gravity, which can affect how a participant performs activities. This aside, the authors in [22] do show that good classification accuracy of seven low level and six high level activities can be achieved using KNN, NB and DT classifiers. Additionally, they also show that using accelerometer and gyroscope data from the smartphone at the pocket position does improve the classification of static activities such as standing and sitting.

2.2. Activity Recognition with Custom Devices

There have been numerous works that use a custom made wrist-worn wearable device for the purpose of activity recognition. A custom wearable device removes any potential limitation that may be imposed by a COTS wearable device, such as adding additional sensors or collecting other information that a COTS wearable device API may not expose. Furthermore, HAR approaches that feature custom wearables devices commonly use additional on-body sensors or wearables to enhance activity classification performance.

One interesting use of a custom wrist-worn wearable device is the approach proposed in [23], where a wrist-worn device is coupled with wearable inertial rings to aid in increasing the accuracy of nine high level activities using DT and SVM classification algorithms. The approach is successful, as using only the wrist-worn device provides an accuracy of 68.85% for DT and 65.03% for SVM, while the whole system provides an accuracy of 89.06% for DT and 91.79% for SVM. Similarly, the authors in [24] use custom wearables at the elbow and wrist positions for the training phase for RF and CRF classifiers for smoking and eating sessions. For three high level smoking activities, the authors demonstrate that using the additional sensor at the elbow position results in an accuracy of 93% for RT and 95.74% for CRF. Furthermore, in [14], the authors evaluate and compare wrist- and body-worn sensors for DT, RT, NB, SVM and KNN classification algorithms with accelerometer data, in the context of fall detection. They show that RF achieves the best overall accuracy among the classifiers while the wrist worn device achieves 72% accuracy, which was marginally better than devices worn on other body locations such as the elbow and chest, which achieved 67% accuracy when classifying ten basic activities. However, sensors positioned at the ankle, knee and belt achieved an accuracy of 77%. This is also shown in the work conducted by [11], who compare hip and wrist sensor placements with an LR classifier using accelerometer data to classify seven basic activities. The authors demonstrate that the hip position provides better accuracy for four activities with an overall accuracy of 91%, while the wrist position provides better accuracy for the remaining three activities with an overall accuracy of 88.4%.

Other approaches using custom wearable devices at the wrist position exclusively include the work conducted by [25], who investigate how the combination of six classification algorithms (NB, SVM, DT, ANN with MLP, KNN and RF) can achieve better accuracy. The authors show that a combination of KNN and RF classifiers for four basic activities only using accelerometer data gives the best accuracy. Furthermore, the authors in [26] compare the ANN with MLP, NB and SVM classifiers using a custom wrist-worn wearable featuring a nine-axial IMU, showing the MLP-based ANN to be the best classifier for their approach. Similarly, the authors in [27] compare the performance of four classifiers (NB, ANN, DT and LR) for identifying eight basic sporting activities, when using a single wrist-worn custom wearable device fitted with a single accelerometer. They show that ANN is the best classifier, achieving an accuracy of 86.7%. The authors in [28] use Emerging Pattern (EP), which is a threshold classifier. EP has low computation requirements, allowing the authors to run the classification algorithm locally on the custom wearable device, which provided an overall accuracy of 86.2% when attempting to classify four basic activities. Lastly, in [29], the authors develop their own classification algorithm that is based on sign-of-slope and threshold evaluation to be used in conjunction with their custom wearable device featuring an accelerometer. They also compare their custom wearable against other COTS devices, specifically the iPhone 6 smartphone, Mi band and SKT smartbands and the Moto360 and Samsung Gear S smart watches. Though the authors' approach is shown to provide better accuracy, it should be noted that data gathering for all of the COTS devices was performed simultaneously, with the participant holding the smartphone and wearing all four COTS devices. This could potentially prevent the participant from performing the activities under a real-life scenario due to the combined weight of the wearables.

2.3. Location-Enhanced HAR

The concept behind location-enhanced activity recognition is to use the location of a person as a feature of an activity. It is reasonable to assume that certain activities can only be performed in certain areas or locations. For example, in a home setting, food preparation would take place in the kitchen, while brushing your teeth would be performed in the bathroom. A recent survey conducted in [30] highlights how the location characteristic, as well as other characteristics (e.g., time, conditions, duration) of an activity can aid in the living of elderly people. Moreover, in [31], the authors show how having these additional characteristics can result in enriching activity modelling and recognition in providing assisted living in smart homes, resulting in activity classification estimates ranging from 88.26 to 100% for basic activities. Furthermore, gaining knowledge of a persons location can be used as an alternative method of improving activity classification as shown by [32], where the authors concluded that adding location awareness aides in activity recognition. Finally, the use of location-enhanced activity recognition grants the benefit of being a more unobtrusive approach as highlighted by [33] than other approaches that use more on-body sensors, as discussed in Section 2.2.

Table 1. HAR publication details.

Publication	Indoor Space			IMU Sensors			Classification Approach										COTS
	Home	Lab	Other	Acc	Mag	Gyro	SVM	KNN	LR	ANN	HMM	NB	DT	RF	CRF	Other	
[22]		X		X		X		X				X	X				X
[23]	X			X		X	X						X				
[25]		X		X			X			X		X	X	X			
[15]		X		X		X		X		X		X		X			X
[11]		X		X					X								
[16]	X			X		X							X				X
[28]		X		X												X	
[17]				X							X		X				X
[24]		X	X	X	X	X						X	X	X	X		
[18]		X		X			X		X			X	X		X		X
[20]	X			X		X	X				X		X				X
[26]		X		X	X	X	X			X		X	X	X			
[27]		X		X					X	X		X	X	X			
[14]		X		X			X	X					X	X			
[13]		X		X				X					X	X			X
[19]			X	X		X	X	X				X	X	X		X	X
[29]	X			X												X	

Legend. IMU sensors: Acc, Accelerometer; Mag, Magnetometer; Gyro, Gyroscope; Classification approach: SVM, Support Vector Machines; KNN, k-Nearest Neighbours; LR, Logistic Regression; ANN, Artificial Neural Network; HMM, Hidden Markov Model; NB, Naive Bayes; DT, Decision Trees; RF - Random Forest; CRF, Conditional Random Field; COTS, Commercial-Off-The-Shelf.

3. System Architecture

Figure 1 illustrates the architecture of our system, detailing the inter-dependencies between its building blocks. Our system can accommodate any wearable device that provides an open API, while there is practically no limitation with respect to BLE beacons as we can adapt our approach to any commercial implementation.

To initiate the system operation, the user runs our mobile application on his/her smartphone, which begins gathering data from the smart watch and the BLE beacons. More specifically, the data are periodically read from the respective devices and transmitted back to the mobile phone using BLE. When the mobile phone has collected the necessary number of samples, which depends on the size of the segmentation window, it transmits them to the server, which uses a trained classifier to recognise the respective activity.

As processing takes place on the server, our system's flexibility increases since we do not require mobile phones with high computational power or storage. The only requirement is to first conduct a data gathering phase, in order to build the dataset, which will be used for the supervised learning classification algorithms, as we further discuss in Section 4.

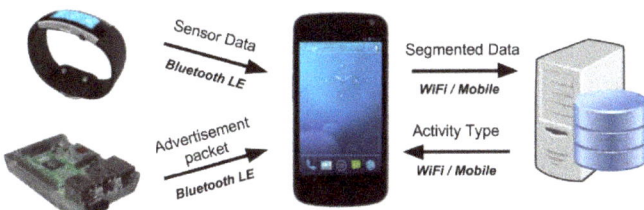

Figure 1. Overall system architecture.

3.1. Smart Watch

There has been an increase in the popularity of wrist-worn sensors, such as smart watches and bands, in recent years. The majority of these devices use inertial sensors, such as accelerometers, in conjunction with health monitoring sensors, such as galvanic skin response and heart rate sensors. In this work, we have chosen to use the Microsoft Band 2. This is a "smart band" type of device and is equipped with a wide range of sensors, including three-axis accelerometer, gyrometer, optical heart-rate sensor, Galvanic Skin Response sensor (GSR), ambient light sensor, ultraviolet light exposure sensor and skin temperature sensor. The device offers a choice among three sampling periods for the accelerometer, namely 16, 32 and 128 ms. During our experimental procedure, we selected a sampling period equal to 32 ms, which results in a sampling frequency of 31 Hz approximately. This is appropriate for our application area, since the frequency required to assess daily physical activities is 20 Hz [34].

3.2. BLE Beacons

The requirement of being able to infer the location of people within a building has been a long-standing problem, mainly due to more traditional localisation services signals such as Global Navigation Satellite System (GNSS) being unable to reach the devices of users, especially in the context of large-scale buildings. BLE beacons have been successfully used in a wide range of location-aware applications, including remote healthcare monitoring [35,36], indoor navigation [37], tourism [38] and transportation [39]. Here, we decided to use a building occupancy detection approach [40–42].

This approach requires a reduced number of Access Points (AP) compared to other Indoor Positioning Systems (IPSs), resulting in a lower deployment cost and a more unobtrusive deployment. Furthermore, the battery life of these devices ranges from 6 to 24 months [7], which minimises maintenance requirements. Finally, the beacons use the BLE protocol, which is also used by most smart watch devices, and are able to communicate with the majority of mobile phones.

To construct the BLE beacons for our system, we used off-the-shelf Bluetooth Low Energy (BLE) technology based on Apple's iBeacon protocol. As shown in Figure 2, our beacons are based on a Raspberry Pi 2 Model B with an attached Bluetooth 4 LE module via a USB interface. The Raspberry Pis uses the BlueZ package to emulate a beacon and allow the customisation of the BLE advertising data being transmitted. Our beacons act as transmitters and broadcast a preset BLE advertising packet at set time intervals.

To separate our beacons from other unassociated Bluetooth traffic and to be able to identify the beacons individually, a small hierarchy was introduced, which made use of the different identifiers available in the beacon packet structure, as illustrated in Figure 3. The Universally Unique Identifier (UUID) is used to define a universal group between all beacons; thus, giving the ability of being able to distinguish the BLE packets being used in our experiments from other Bluetooth traffic. The major number is used to define local groups of beacons who's geographical locations are loosely connected. For example, beacons deployed on certain floors or buildings will have the same major number. Lastly, the minor number is used to identify each individual beacon within its local group.

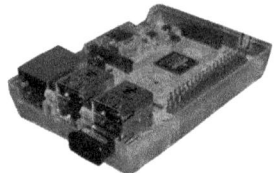

Figure 2. Raspberry Pi-based beacon.

Prefix	UUID	Major	Major	TX
[9 Bytes]	[16 Bytes]	[2 Bytes]	[2 Bytes]	[1 Byte]

Figure 3. BLE beacon advertising packet structure.

3.3. Mobile Application

An Android mobile application was developed to gather the sensor data from the Microsoft Band and the BLE advertising data packets being broadcasted from the BLE beacons. During the system operation, the mobile device is paired with the Microsoft Band and receives the incoming sensor data stream. Furthermore, all BLE traffic the mobile device is in range of is being filtered, so only our beacon advertising data packets are being captured. Then, the respective beacon identifiers and the measured RSSI of each packet are stored. To filter out any unwanted data, the application firstly looks to see if the captured packet is structured in accordance to the iBeacon protocol by checking for the prefix (see Figure 3), and then, it will attempt to find the UUID being used by our beacons.

The application was designed with a modular approach, to allow it to be used with other wearable devices easily without the need to change the core program; thus granting the ability to integrate new wearable devices quickly and efficiently. During the data gathering phase of our experiments, a session is created for every participant. When performing a data capture, the activity about to be performed is selected from a drop down list. Then, during a data capture operated by the start/stop button on the application interface, sensor data from the smart watch and BLE advertising data from the beacons are collected simultaneously and stored locally before being sent to a server once the capture has finished.

3.4. Server

Mobile computing platforms have limited processing power and storage capacity compared to desktops and workstations. In particular, the processing power of wearable devices, such as smart watches and smart bands, is only adequate for their typical tasks, which include visual notifications, data collection and wireless communications. Smart phones offer improved processing power and memory capacity, but they still lag behind server-class computing solutions. To overcome these limitations, we have adopted a cloud-based solution for our system, which involves a server being responsible for the computationally-intensive tasks. More specifically, the role of the server is to process the data sent from mobile devices and then recognise the activity being performed. Initially, the classifiers that run on the server need to be trained using the data gathered during the data gathering phase. In normal operation mode, the server uses the trained classifiers to recognise the activities being performed by the users.

4. Activity Recognition Chain

Figure 4 illustrates the procedure we followed to perform activity recognition. To simplify the illustration, we show the signal from one accelerometer axis for the smart watch and the RSSI from one beacon. During real-world operation, our system uses three accelerometer signals (one for each axis) and eight RSSI signals (one for each of the eight beacons deployed). For the smart watch, we have also experimented with both accelerometer and gyroscope signals, but this did not result in a noticeable improvement in performance.

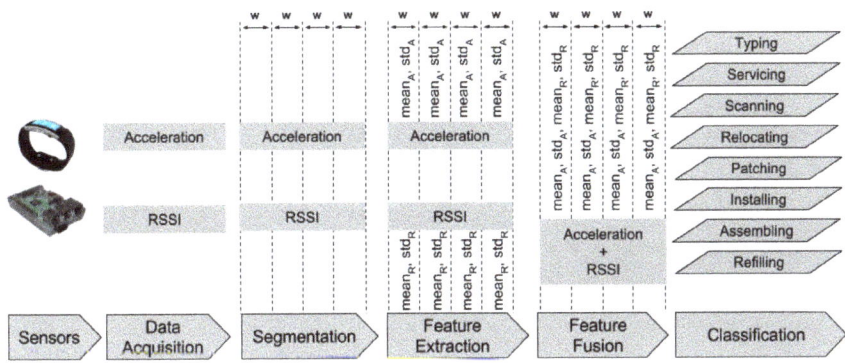

Figure 4. Overview of the activity recognition chain implemented in our system.

The data acquisition phase is performed using our mobile application. When in training mode, where data need to be labelled for using them in the training of the classifiers, the participant has to select the activity he/she is performing from a list of available activities. This guarantees that incoming data will be labelled accordingly.

Our data segmentation approach involves the use of a non-overlapping sliding window. As we further discuss in Section 6.1, we have evaluated our system using window sizes of 1 to 5 s with a 1-s increment, as the window size has been shown to affect the performance of activity recognition [10,43,44]. We have used the same windowing mechanism for the BLE beacon data as it has been shown to benefit multipath mitigation [45].

With respect to feature extraction in the case of the accelerometer data from the smart watch, we have opted for two feature types:

- Type 1: mean and standard deviation.
- Type 2: mean, standard deviation, minimum, maximum and mean crossing rate.

These features are most appropriate for human activity recognition, as shown in the analyses in [43,46,47]. For the beacon data, we used one feature type, mean and standard deviation, based on our previous work on occupancy detection using BLE beacons [41,42]. As we are using a three-axis accelerometer, the total number of smart watch features for Type 1 is six, while for Type 2 it is 15. Similarly, since we have deployed eight beacons, the total number of beacon features is 16.

The next stage of our activity recognition chain is feature fusion [48,49]. In Section 6, we demonstrate that this significantly enhances the performance of our system. We must note, however, that our system can also operate using only the data coming from the smart watch accelerometers.

To better illustrate how feature fusion is implemented, let us define the RSSI signal value corresponding to beacon i at time t as: $r_i^{(t)}$, where $i \in \mathbb{Z} \cap [1, K]$. In our case, there are $K = 8$ beacons.

Thus, at time t, the RSSI signal values corresponding to the eight beacons are: $r_1^{(t)}, r_2^{(t)}, \ldots, r_8^{(t)}$. Similarly, the accelerometer signal values for each axis at time t are: $a_x^{(t)}, a_y^{(t)}, a_z^{(t)}$.

In the data segmentation stage, the signals from each sensor are partitioned into non-overlapping data windows w_s, where s denotes the type of sensor. Consequently, we have:

$$w_{r_1} = (r_1^{(t_1)}, \ldots, r_1^{(t_n)})$$
$$\ldots$$
$$w_{r_8} = (r_8^{(t_1)}, \ldots, r_8^{(t_n)})$$
$$w_{a_x} = (a_x^{(t_1)}, \ldots, a_x^{(t_m)})$$
$$w_{a_y} = (a_y^{(t_1)}, \ldots, a_y^{(t_m)})$$
$$w_{a_z} = (a_z^{(t_1)}, \ldots, a_z^{(t_m)})$$

We must note that, since the transmission frequency of the BLE beacons and the sampling rate of the smart watch are different, the number of samples in the respective windows also differ, as denoted by t_n and t_m. For each window, we extract a set of features, which are then fused into a single feature vector x. For example, if we use the first feature type (mean and standard deviation) for the smart watch data, the fused feature vector for $K = 8$ beacons will be:

$$x = \Big(mean(w_{r_1}), std(w_{r_1}), \ldots, mean(w_{r_8}), std(w_{r_8}),$$
$$mean(w_{a_x}), std(w_{a_x}), mean(w_{a_y}), std(w_{a_y}), mean(w_{a_z}), std(w_{a_z})\Big)$$

The feature vector x is then used as the input to the classifier. For the classification of activities, we have chosen four classifiers that have been successfully used in human activity recognition research, as discussed in Section 2. More specifically, we have chosen k-Nearest Neighbours (KNN), Logistic Regression (LR), Random Forest (RF) and Support Vector Machines (SVM). We partitioned our dataset into 80% training set and 20% test set and used 10-fold cross-validation for hyper-parameter tuning. For SVM, we have chosen the radial basis function kernel, as the number of features is small compared to the number of instances, and mapping our data to a higher dimensional space improves the classification performance [50].

We should note that when the system is used in normal operation mode with a trained classifier residing in the server, as depicted in Figure 1, the mobile phone is responsible for the stages up to and including segmentation. The data are then transmitted to the server where feature extraction, fusion and classification take place.

5. Experimental Setup

In this section, we present the approach we adopted for deploying our BLE beacons and conducting our activities. We first give the details of the indoor space where our experiment took place. We then elaborate on the types and durations of activities performed.

5.1. Beacon Deployment

Eight beacons were deployed inside the University of Greenwich computer laboratory. We have used a virtual grid to map the experimental area and illustrate the geographical positions of the beacons, as depicted in Figure 5.

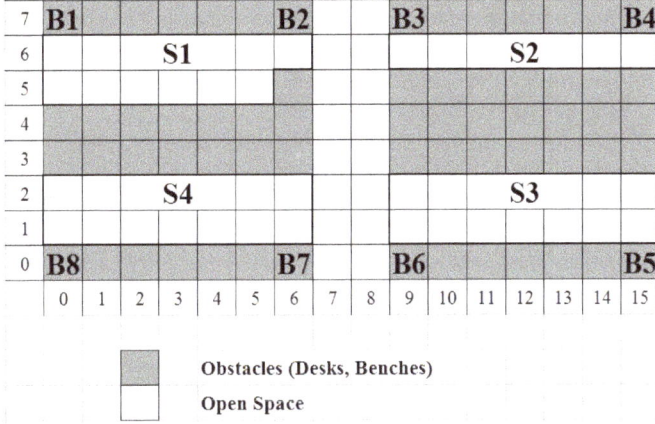

Figure 5. Beacon deployment.

Each grid block represents a 1 m × 1 m area. Grey blocks represent an area that a participant cannot reach (in terms of location) due to an obstacle, whereas the white blocks represent accessible area to the participants. Additionally, the floor plan shows the four sectors within the laboratory. Sectors 2 to 4 are computer bays, and Sector 1 is the technical support staff laboratory area. Throughout the experiments, all of the beacons were configured with an advertising data packet frequency of 7 Hz. This deployment density, as our previous work [41] has shown, provides sufficient performance with respect to location accuracy.

5.2. Laboratory Activities

Using our framework described in Section 3, we collected data for eight different activities that would be typically performed by a technical support staff member. Table 2 illustrates the relationship between area sectors (shown in Figure 5) and activities that can take place inside each sector.

Table 2. Activity codes.

Activity Code	Activity Name	Sector Codes
A1	Typing	S2, S3, S4
A2	Servicing	S2, S3, S4
A3	Scanning	S1
A4	Relocating	S1
A5	Patching	S2, S3, S4
A6	Installing	S1, S2, S3, S4
A7	Assembling	S2, S3, S4
A8	Refilling	S1, S2

This mapping is based on the layout of the experimental area and provides an increased level of realism to our experimental process. For example, refilling printer cartridges takes place in Sectors 1 and 2, since this is the location of the two printers, while the scanning activity only takes place in Sector 1, as this is the location of the barcode scanner. We should also note that each activity was performed in different locations within the same sector, among participants and repetitions. For example, the network switch during the patching activity was positioned in various locations along the benches inside Sectors 2, 3 and 4. Figure 6 illustrates the activities being performed by a participant, while a detailed description of each of the activities is given below:

- Typing: When conducting this activity, the participants used a standard desktop-style computer located in the laboratory, as depicted in Figure 6a. The computer was prepared with randomly-chosen excerpts at the top of the screen with a word processing application at the bottom of the screen. Then, the participants simply needed to type the text into the word processor.
- Servicing: In this activity, the participants were performing servicing tasks on computer equipment by removing and replacing service panels and changing over individual components. This is illustrated in Figure 6b. More specifically, the participants were exchanging components in the network router units by unscrewing the service panels.
- Scanning: For this activity, depicted in Figure 6c, the participants were asked to scan large amounts of small embedded components (LCD screens, keypads, sensors units, etc.) with applied bar codes using a hand-held scanner. This activity would be typically performed when loaning equipment to students or staff or when taking a stock check. Additionally, the participants were only asked to use their dominant hand to hold the scanner when performing this activity.
- Relocating: This activity consisted of moving large volumes of equipment from one storage location to another, as shown in Figure 6d. When performing this activity, the participants were only told to move one piece of equipment at a time. All equipment relocated by the participants could be grasped using only one hand.
- Patching: Within this activity, the participants were presented with multiple network switches accompanied by enough Ethernet cables to be inserted into every port of the switches. Figure 6e illustrates this setup. Each participant was instructed to patch in the Ethernet cables across the multiple switches in any way he/she wished. Additionally, the supplied Ethernet cables were not of equal length.
- Installing: This activity involved the installation of various software packages on a laptop, as shown in Figure 6f. Moreover, the laptop was turned on and was prepared with none of the software packages installed. Then, each participant was supplied with a USB flash drive containing the installers for the software packages and was only instructed on the order in which the packages should be installed.
- Assembling: When conducting this activity, depicted in Figure 6g, the participants were presented with a small dismantled vehicular robot with brief assembling instructions and a basic toolkit. Only required parts and tools were supplied; no additional equipment was given. The only instruction given to each participant was to assemble the robot using the tools and instructions provided.
- Refilling: In this activity, the participants were performing maintenance on two printers located in the laboratory. More specifically, as Figure 6h illustrates, the participants were asked to replace the various printer cartridges. To perform this activity, the participants were required to open the service panel of the printer and then replace the old cartridge with a new cartridge. Finally, the participant would close the service panel of the printer. No tools were required to open and close the service panel of the printer.

Our analysis focuses on recognising activities that a technical support staff member would perform and how this process can be enhanced by location information. There are, however, other activities that the participants can perform before or after they engage in one of the activities we described above. As the set of these activities depends on the context and the environment in which the system operates, we would expect that inside a computer laboratory, a participant could also be walking, standing still, sitting on a chair, etc. Our system can be adapted in order to address this. One approach we can adopt is to expand our training dataset to include a wider range of activities. This would result in a higher number of classes in our multiclass classification problem. Another approach is the inclusion of the null class, which is formed by activities that have similar patterns, but are irrelevant with the application in question. However, since in theory there is an infinite number of arbitrary activities that can belong to the null class, modelling it is particularly difficult [43].

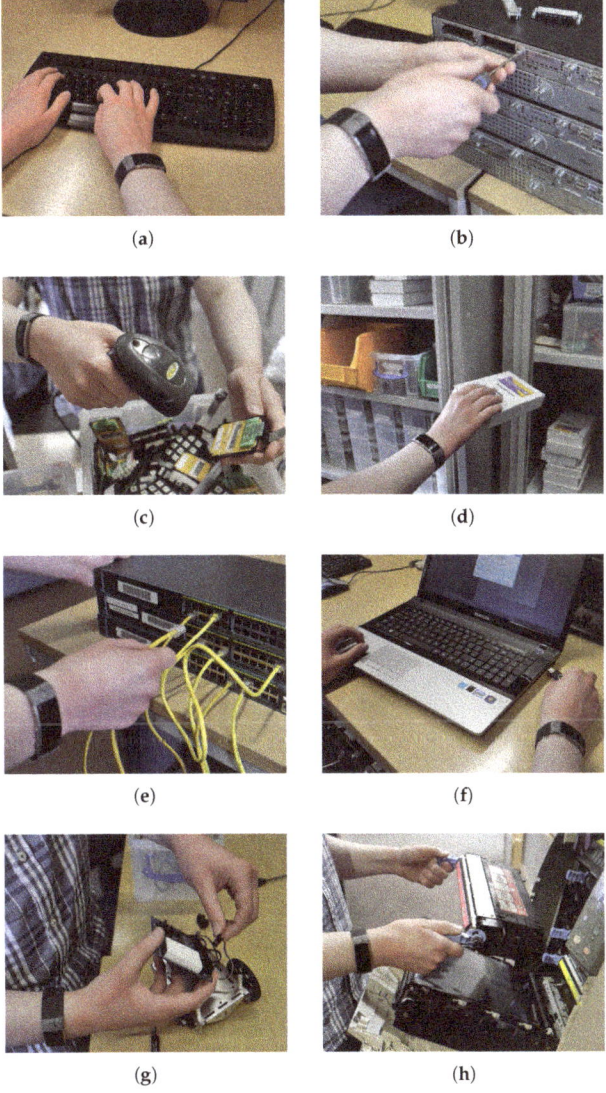

Figure 6. The activities performed by the participants in our laboratory. (**a**) Typing; (**b**) servicing; (**c**) scanning; (**d**) relocating; (**e**) patching; (**f**) installing; (**g**) assembling; (**h**) refilling.

The data collection was carried out by using our mobile application in training mode. Data coming from the smart watch and the BLE beacons were logged by the mobile application. Furthermore, when participants were performing activities, they were only given the required basic information to minimise the amount of external influence on the participant. This allowed us to perform the activities under a more naturalistic setting, closer to real-life conditions.

Each of the aforementioned activities was performed for a time between 170 s and 180 s by three different participants, while two out of three participants repeated the activities one more time. This resulted in a total dataset duration of about 290 min.

6. Results

In this section, we present the results of our activity recognition system. We have evaluated the system in a wide range of window sizes, classification algorithms and feature types, as discussed in Section 4. We first provide an overview of our system's performance for different windows sizes and feature types and continue with an evaluation of individual activities. In order to provide a comparison with the methods that only use COTS or custom wearable devices, as discussed in Section 2, we have also evaluated the performance of our system when only using data generated by the smart watch. As the main focus of this work is to demonstrate that location enhancement significantly benefits activity recognition, these results form the baseline against which we measure the enhancement in system performance when incorporating BLE beacon data.

6.1. Overview of Results

We begin with providing a high level view of our system's performance over the range of different parameter values. A first metric we used for our evaluation is the F_1 score [51], which takes into account both precision and recall and is robust to class imbalance. It is defined as:

$$F_1 = 2 \times \frac{precision \times recall}{precision + recall} \quad (1)$$

where $F_1 \in [0,1]$, $precision = \frac{tp}{tp+fp}$, $recall = \frac{tp}{tp+fn}$, $tp = true\ positives$, $fp = false\ positives$ and $fn = false\ negatives$. A value of F_1 close to one indicates the best classification performance.

Figures 7 and 8 present the F_1 score performance of our system. We must note that we have calculated the weighted average of F_1 score over all activities, weighted by the number of true instances for each class, for different window sizes, feature types and classification models.

More specifically, in Figure 7a, we illustrate our system's performance when using the first feature type without beacon feature fusion. We can observe that LR performs considerably worse compared to the other three classifiers. More specifically, KNN, RF and SVM are all able to achieve a maximum F_1 score of 0.8 for a window size of 4 s, while LR achieves a F_1 score of 0.7 for the same window size. Increasing the window size improves the classification performance; however, exceeding a size of 4 s does not yield further improvement. The same performance pattern can be seen in Figure 7b, where there is a significant performance gap between LR and the rest of the classifiers. Both figures indicate that using a higher dimensional feature space for the smart watch data (Feature Type 2), improves the performance of all classifiers.

Figure 8a,b presents our system's performance when using BLE beacon data in conjunction with smart watch data. It is evident that there is a significant enhancement in the system's performance as illustrated by the improved F_1 scores for all classifiers. We should note that when using location-enhancement, all classifiers, except LR, are able to achieve F_1 scores above 0.9 even for the smallest window size of 1 s. As a small window size improves our system's response time (less time required to recognise the performed activity), this result highlights the benefit of using beacon feature fusion in our activity recognition system. We can also observe a similar performance pattern for the case where no beacon data are used, both with respect to window size and to the gap between

LR and the rest of the classifiers. However, we should note that now there is a more clear distinction among the classifiers in terms of performance. SVM achieves the best F_1 score for all experimental configurations, followed by KNN and RF, respectively.

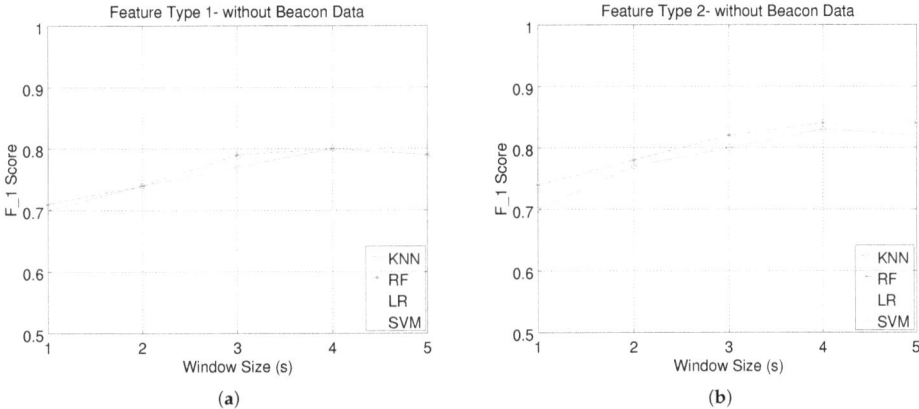

Figure 7. Activity recognition system performance without beacon data: weighted average of $F_1 score$ over all activities, for different window sizes, feature types and classification models. (**a**) Wearable Feature Type 1 (mean, standard deviation); (**b**) Wearable Feature Type 2 (mean, standard deviation, mean crossing rate, maximum and minimum).

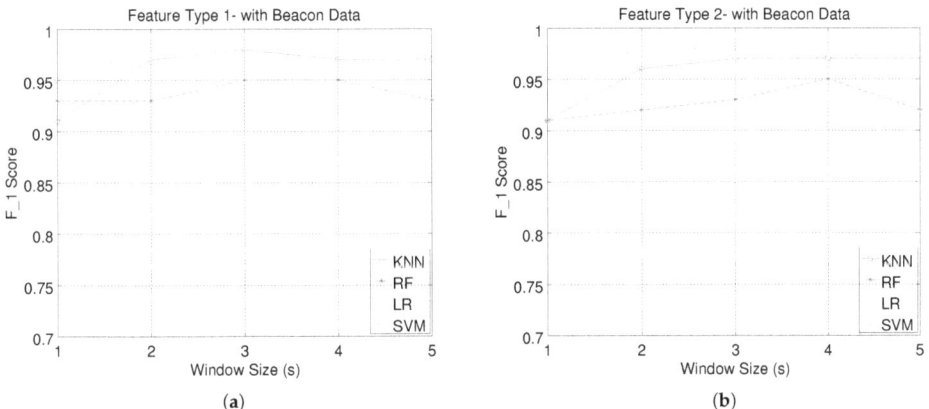

Figure 8. Activity recognition system performance with beacon data: weighted average of $F_1 score$ over all activities, for different window sizes, feature types and classification models. (**a**) Wearable Feature Type 1 (mean, standard deviation); (**b**) Wearable Feature Type 2 (mean, standard deviation, mean crossing rate, maximum and minimum).

An overview of activity-specific classification performance across all experimental configurations is illustrated in Figure 9. We can again confirm that the performance pattern observed in Figures 7 and 8 is present: LR has a consistently worse performance compared to the other classifiers; increasing the smart watch feature dimensionality improves classification performance; and beacon feature fusion significantly enhances classification performance for all activities and classifiers.

Activities	w/oLocation FT1	w/oLocation FT2	with Location FT1	with Location FT2	Activities	w/o Location FT1	w/o Location FT2	with Location FT1	with Location FT2
A1	0.87	0.85	0.97	0.97	A1	0.73	0.76	0.73	0.80
A2	0.79	0.84	0.97	0.96	A2	0.79	0.80	0.79	0.83
A3	0.83	0.92	0.98	0.98	A3	0.73	0.84	0.95	0.99
A4	0.72	0.74	0.98	0.97	A4	0.47	0.61	0.97	0.95
A5	0.66	0.72	0.97	0.96	A5	0.63	0.64	0.76	0.79
A6	0.88	0.87	0.99	0.99	A6	0.81	0.83	0.85	0.87
A7	0.71	0.76	0.96	0.95	A7	0.57	0.64	0.70	0.75
A8	0.67	0.70	0.99	1.00	A8	0.61	0.59	0.99	1.00

(a)   (b)

Activities	w/o Location FT1	w/o Location FT2	with Location FT1	with Location FT2	Activities	w/o Location FT1	w/o Location FT2	with Location FT1	with Location FT2
A1	0.90	0.91	0.94	0.93	A1	0.85	0.89	0.99	1.00
A2	0.81	0.85	0.94	0.90	A2	0.82	0.85	0.98	0.98
A3	0.85	0.93	0.98	0.98	A3	0.88	0.91	1.00	1.00
A4	0.70	0.69	0.98	0.98	A4	0.71	0.75	0.98	0.97
A5	0.69	0.73	0.93	0.90	A5	0.69	0.74	0.97	0.97
A6	0.90	0.90	0.96	0.94	A6	0.87	0.91	0.99	0.99
A7	0.72	0.78	0.91	0.90	A7	0.75	0.80	0.98	0.97
A8	0.62	0.69	0.99	0.98	A8	0.65	0.68	1.00	1.00

(c)   (d)

Figure 9. F_1 Scores for all classifiers and activities, for a window size of 3 s. (**a**) KNN; (**b**) LR; (**c**) RF; (**d**) SVM.

6.2. Evaluation of Individual Activities

The observations of Section 6.1 have informed the choice of system parameters that are investigated here, where we elaborate on our system's performance for individual activities. Based on these observations, window sizes higher than 4 s do not significantly benefit the system's performance. Furthermore, there is a clear performance gain when using the second feature type for the smart watch data. Thus, we analyse individual activity classification for window sizes up to 4 s when using the second smart watch feature type, with and without beacon feature fusion. We will refer to the activities with the codes assigned in Table 2.

To better illustrate our system's performance, we present our results for each classifier using a normalised confusion matrix. A row of the matrix represents the instances in an actual class, while a column represents the instances in a predicted class. The diagonal elements represent the number of instances where the predicted label is equal to the true label. Off-diagonal elements represent instances that are misclassified. Furthermore, we have normalised the confusion matrices by the number of elements in each actual class. In the case of class imbalance, this approach better illustrates which classes are being misclassified. Furthermore, we have colour-coded the matrices by assigning black to 1.0 (100%) and white to 0.0 (0%). Finally, we should emphasise that the evaluation results have been calculated using only the test set data (20% of the original dataset), which the classifiers have never seen before, in order to provide a more reliable estimation of their out of sample error.

As shown in Section 6.1, the LR classifier results in the lowest classification performance in all experimental configurations. Figures 10 and 11 confirm this observation for individual activities. More specifically, for activities A1, A2, A3 and A6, the LR classifier without beacon information is able to achieve a classification accuracy that increases with window size and manages to reach 80%. Adding beacon information does not significantly change the performance of the classifier for activities A1, A2 and A6. However, A3 benefits significantly and reaches 100% accuracy for a window value of 4 s. Looking at Table 2, we can see that A3 takes place in Sector 1, while A1, A2 and A6 do not. This is beneficial for the classification and allows the LR classifier to better distinguish between the activities. We must note that, although A6 can also take place in Sector 1, the actual micro-location within this sector is different (scanning and installing take place in subtly different locations along the bench). This is adequately different for the classifier to improve its performance. Looking at activities A4, A5, A7 and A8, we observe that LR gives poor classification performance without beacon data. For example, A4 is misclassified as A5, with more than 50% of examples classified incorrectly. More specifically, we can note that the activities of patching and relocating both involve translational hand movement while grasping an object (a cable or a piece of equipment). This can be confirmed by Figure 6d,e.

(a)

	A1	A2	A3	A4	A5	A6	A7	A8
A1	0.67	0	0	0	0	0.28	0.04	0
A2	0.01	0.71	0.02	0.01	0.11	0.01	0.08	0.06
A3	0.01	0.01	0.84	0	0.02	0.05	0.08	0
A4	0.01	0.06	0.06	0.23	0.31	0	0.13	0.2
A5	0.02	0.23	0.02	0.02	0.43	0	0.19	0.09
A6	0.08	0	0.01	0	0	0.88	0.03	0
A7	0.17	0.13	0.02	0	0.07	0.05	0.47	0.09
A8	0.04	0.17	0.02	0.03	0.22	0	0.1	0.41

(b)

	A1	A2	A3	A4	A5	A6	A7	A8
A1	0.78	0	0	0	0	0.19	0.03	0
A2	0.01	0.78	0.01	0.01	0.12	0	0.03	0.05
A3	0	0	0.87	0.01	0.01	0.08	0.02	0.01
A4	0.01	0.03	0.03	0.45	0.26	0	0.05	0.17
A5	0.03	0.16	0.02	0.06	0.58	0	0.1	0.05
A6	0.09	0	0.01	0	0	0.88	0.02	0
A7	0.16	0.1	0.03	0	0.06	0.03	0.52	0.09
A8	0.04	0.12	0.01	0.04	0.25	0	0.11	0.42

(c)

	A1	A2	A3	A4	A5	A6	A7	A8
A1	0.79	0	0	0	0	0.19	0.02	0
A2	0.01	0.85	0	0.01	0.04	0	0.05	0.05
A3	0	0	0.87	0	0.02	0.05	0.06	0
A4	0	0	0.03	0.54	0.2	0	0.16	0.07
A5	0.01	0.12	0.01	0.07	0.63	0	0.1	0.07
A6	0.13	0	0.02	0	0	0.84	0.02	0
A7	0.1	0.1	0.02	0	0.07	0.02	0.6	0.08
A8	0.02	0.09	0.02	0.02	0.2	0	0.09	0.57

(d)

	A1	A2	A3	A4	A5	A6	A7	A8
A1	0.81	0	0	0	0	0.14	0.04	0
A2	0	0.88	0	0.01	0.07	0	0.03	0.02
A3	0	0	0.84	0	0	0.03	0.13	0
A4	0	0.02	0.04	0.56	0.22	0	0.1	0.06
A5	0	0.12	0.01	0.02	0.72	0	0.08	0.05
A6	0.09	0	0.01	0.01	0	0.84	0.05	0.01
A7	0.11	0.04	0.02	0	0.06	0.01	0.67	0.09
A8	0.02	0.05	0.01	0.05	0.28	0	0.09	0.5

Figure 10. Normalised confusion matrices for logistic regression, with Wearable Feature Type 2, without beacon data. (**a**) C = 10, w = 1 s; (**b**) C = 100, w = 2 s ; (**c**) C = 10, w = 3 s; (**d**) C = 10, w = 4 s.

To further explain this, we must note that each of the complex activities that we aim to classify can be composed into a set of simpler activities, with varying time durations. For example, patching the routers requires grasping a network cable, moving it towards the respective socket and pushing the cable until it is securely connected to the socket. Similarly, changing the printer cartridges requires pulling the cartridge out of the printer slot and then pushing the new cartridge into the printer slot. During the training phase, this activity structure is taken into account in a straightforward manner, simply by applying the same label to all windowed data collected for one activity. This is done automatically by our data gathering application while the participant performs an activity. In the classification phase, the performance of our system depends on the similarity between the complex activities. This can be expressed in terms of the similarity among the simple activities of which two complex activities are composed.

We can also observe that activity A8 is misclassified as A5. These activities are again similar in nature (hand movements involve inserting an object (cable or cartridge) inside a slot (Ethernet port or printer cartridge bay), as can be observed in Figure 6e,h. Adding beacon information drastically improves results for A4 and A8. Looking at Table 2, we can see that the locations of these activities are distinct compared to the rest of the activities, and beacon information helps the classifier discriminate the relevant data points. For example, A8 is no longer misclassified as A5. Although A5 and A8 can be both performed in Sector 2, the locations of the printers within this sector are, as one would expect, distinct from the locations where patching takes place.

Activities A5 and A7 also benefit from beacon data, but to a lesser degree. For example, A5 is still misclassified as A2 for more than 10% of the data. This is due to the fact that both activities take place in the same sector. Although this does not mean that their locations are exactly the same (in which case there would be no benefit from additional location information), they are not sufficiently different to result in greater classification improvement. We must also highlight the fact that increasing the window size improves by a small degree the performance of the LR classifier. As a small window size results in a more responsive activity recognition system (less waiting time to construct a data point), it is evident that LR suffers in that respect since for a window size of 1 s, the results are poor.

	A1	A2	A3	A4	A5	A6	A7	A8
A1	0.71	0	0	0	0	0.2	0.09	0
A2	0	0.72	0.01	0.01	0.16	0.01	0.09	0.01
A3	0.01	0	0.91	0	0	0.04	0.01	0.03
A4	0.01	0.03	0.03	0.8	0.07	0.01	0.05	0.01
A5	0.01	0.23	0.01	0.03	0.62	0	0.08	0.02
A6	0.08	0	0.01	0	0	0.88	0.02	0.01
A7	0.17	0.1	0.01	0.01	0.1	0.04	0.56	0.01
A8	0.02	0.02	0.03	0.01	0.02	0.01	0.01	0.9

(a)

	A1	A2	A3	A4	A5	A6	A7	A8
A1	0.8	0	0	0	0	0.1	0.1	0
A2	0	0.78	0	0	0.14	0	0.07	0
A3	0	0	0.91	0	0	0.05	0.01	0.03
A4	0.01	0.02	0	0.89	0.04	0	0.04	0
A5	0.01	0.17	0	0.02	0.74	0	0.06	0
A6	0.06	0	0	0	0	0.89	0.05	0
A7	0.09	0.09	0	0	0.1	0.03	0.69	0
A8	0	0	0.01	0	0	0	0	0.99

(b)

	A1	A2	A3	A4	A5	A6	A7	A8
A1	0.81	0	0	0	0	0.12	0.07	0
A2	0.01	0.85	0	0	0.09	0	0.05	0
A3	0	0	0.98	0	0	0	0	0.02
A4	0	0	0	0.93	0.03	0	0.03	0
A5	0.01	0.13	0	0.01	0.77	0	0.08	0
A6	0.1	0	0	0	0	0.87	0.03	0
A7	0.07	0.07	0	0	0.08	0.04	0.74	0
A8	0	0	0	0	0	0	0	1

(c)

	A1	A2	A3	A4	A5	A6	A7	A8
A1	0.82	0	0	0	0	0.09	0.09	0
A2	0	0.83	0.01	0	0.13	0	0.03	0
A3	0	0	1	0	0	0	0	0
A4	0	0	0	0.94	0.02	0	0.04	0
A5	0	0.12	0	0.03	0.82	0	0.02	0
A6	0.08	0.01	0.01	0	0	0.83	0.07	0
A7	0.07	0.04	0	0	0.04	0.03	0.82	0
A8	0	0	0	0	0	0	0	1

(d)

Figure 11. Normalised confusion matrices for logistic regression, with Wearable Feature Type 2, with beacon data. (a) C = 10, w = 1 s; (b) C = 10, w = 2 s ; (c) C = 10, w = 3 s; (d) C = 100, w = 4 s.

Figures 12 and 13 illustrate the performance of the KNN classifier. We can observe that activities A1, A2, A3 and A6 are classified with over 90% accuracy without beacons, an improvement in performance compared to the LR classifier. Adding beacon data further improves performance, as expected. KNN benefits significantly from increasing the window size. This is shown for activities A4, A5 and A7 where for a 1-s window, they are below 60%. However, when the window size increases, they all reach an accuracy close to 75%, without beacon data. Adding beacon data further improves the performance of these activities. We must again note that, although these activities are performed in common sectors, the micro-locations inside each sector are different. For example, activity A7 (assembling the robot) and activity A5 (patching the router) take place on different parts of the workbenches inside the sectors. The KNN classifier can take advantage of this information to improve performance, something that the LR classifier could not achieve to the same degree. Finally, the benefit of location information is clearly shown in the case of activity A8. Without location information, the best accuracy obtained is 62%. With location information, it reaches 99% for the same window size (3 s).

As seen in Figures 14 and 15, the RF classifier exhibits a performance similar to KNN in terms of being able to take advantage of micro-location information. We can again confirm that adding beacon information improves drastically the classifier's performance. Mores specifically, the classification accuracy for activities A4 and A8 (for their optimal window sizes) increases from 76 and 67% without beacon data to 98% for both activities when beacon features are fused with smart watch features. However, the RF classifier cannot fully take advantage of the feature fusion in the case of activities A5 and A7: the RF classifier cannot achieve accuracy above 93% and 91% when we use beacon information, and it only manages this for the maximum window size of 4 s.

	A1	A2	A3	A4	A5	A6	A7	A8
A1	0.86	0	0	0	0	0.13	0.01	0
A2	0.01	0.77	0.02	0.01	0.09	0	0.06	0.03
A3	0	0	0.92	0	0.01	0.01	0.07	0
A4	0.01	0.06	0.02	0.51	0.16	0	0.09	0.14
A5	0.02	0.2	0.02	0.03	0.58	0	0.09	0.07
A6	0.1	0	0.01	0	0	0.86	0.03	0
A7	0.11	0.06	0.04	0.01	0.1	0.07	0.57	0.03
A8	0.02	0.14	0.02	0.05	0.21	0.01	0.12	0.44

(a)

	A1	A2	A3	A4	A5	A6	A7	A8
A1	0.9	0	0	0	0	0.09	0.02	0
A2	0	0.84	0.01	0.01	0.08	0	0.04	0.03
A3	0	0	0.96	0	0	0.03	0.01	0
A4	0	0.04	0	0.53	0.14	0	0.06	0.24
A5	0	0.12	0.01	0.05	0.68	0	0.08	0.06
A6	0.12	0	0	0	0	0.86	0.02	0
A7	0.1	0.04	0.03	0.01	0.06	0.06	0.71	0
A8	0	0.07	0.01	0.03	0.17	0	0.17	0.54

(b)

	A1	A2	A3	A4	A5	A6	A7	A8
A1	0.97	0	0	0	0	0.03	0	0
A2	0.02	0.89	0.01	0	0.05	0	0.01	0.02
A3	0	0	1	0	0	0	0	0
A4	0	0.03	0.02	0.7	0.08	0	0.08	0.08
A5	0	0.12	0	0.05	0.71	0	0.07	0.04
A6	0.14	0	0.01	0	0	0.83	0.01	0
A7	0.09	0.04	0.02	0	0.06	0.07	0.71	0
A8	0.01	0.09	0.02	0.03	0.16	0	0.08	0.62

(c)

	A1	A2	A3	A4	A5	A6	A7	A8
A1	0.94	0	0	0	0	0.05	0.01	0
A2	0	0.92	0	0.01	0.05	0	0.02	0
A3	0	0	1	0	0	0	0	0
A4	0	0	0.02	0.74	0.14	0	0.04	0.06
A5	0.01	0.09	0	0.02	0.78	0	0.05	0.05
A6	0.08	0	0.01	0.01	0	0.85	0.05	0
A7	0.03	0.01	0.04	0	0.03	0.04	0.82	0.05
A8	0	0.12	0	0.05	0.16	0	0.12	0.56

(d)

Figure 12. Normalised confusion matrices for KNN, with Wearable Feature Type 2, without beacon data. (**a**) $n = 9$, w = 1 s; (**b**) $n = 10$, w = 2 s ; (**c**) $n = 8$, w = 3 s; (**d**) $n= 5$, w = 4 s.

	A1	A2	A3	A4	A5	A6	A7	A8
A1	0.97	0	0	0	0	0.02	0.01	0
A2	0.01	0.9	0	0.01	0.05	0	0.02	0
A3	0	0.01	0.97	0	0.01	0.02	0	0
A4	0.01	0.03	0.01	0.91	0.03	0.01	0.01	0.01
A5	0.02	0.09	0	0.02	0.83	0	0.03	0
A6	0.02	0	0	0	0	0.98	0	0
A7	0.05	0.05	0	0.01	0.03	0.02	0.85	0
A8	0.01	0.03	0.03	0.02	0.01	0.01	0.01	0.89

(a)

	A1	A2	A3	A4	A5	A6	A7	A8
A1	1	0	0	0	0	0	0	0
A2	0	0.97	0	0	0.03	0	0	0
A3	0	0.01	0.97	0	0	0.02	0	0
A4	0	0	0	0.96	0.02	0	0	0.01
A5	0	0.06	0	0.01	0.92	0	0.01	0
A6	0.01	0	0	0	0	0.98	0	0
A7	0.05	0.02	0	0.01	0.01	0.01	0.91	0
A8	0	0.01	0.02	0.01	0.01	0	0	0.95

(b)

	A1	A2	A3	A4	A5	A6	A7	A8
A1	0.99	0	0	0	0	0.01	0	0
A2	0.01	0.97	0	0	0.02	0	0.01	0
A3	0	0	1	0	0	0	0	0
A4	0	0	0.02	0.97	0	0	0.02	0
A5	0	0.03	0	0.01	0.95	0	0.02	0
A6	0	0	0	0	0	0.99	0	0
A7	0.04	0.02	0	0	0.01	0.01	0.93	0
A8	0	0	0.01	0	0	0	0	0.99

(c)

	A1	A2	A3	A4	A5	A6	A7	A8
A1	0.99	0	0	0	0	0.01	0	0
A2	0	0.97	0	0	0.02	0	0.01	0
A3	0	0	1	0	0	0	0	0
A4	0	0	0.02	0.96	0.02	0	0	0
A5	0	0.02	0	0.02	0.95	0	0.01	0
A6	0.01	0	0.01	0.01	0	0.97	0.01	0
A7	0.02	0.02	0	0	0	0.02	0.95	0
A8	0	0.01	0.01	0.01	0	0	0.01	0.95

(d)

Figure 13. Normalised confusion matrices for KNN, with Wearable Feature Type 2, with beacon data. (**a**) $n = 3$, w = 1 s; (**b**) $n = 3$, w = 2 s ; (**c**) $n = 3$, w = 3 s; (**d**) $n = 3$, w = 4 s.

Figures 16 and 17 illustrate that SVM has the optimal recognition performance and also benefits the most from beacon information. More specifically, classification accuracy for activities A1, A2, A3 and A6 is above 85% without beacon data. This is further improved, as expected, when beacon information is used and reaches a classification accuracy of over 95%. Correctly classifying activities A4 and A5 proves more challenging since, as we explained above, both activities involve similar translational hand movement. However, SVM is the only classifier that reaches above 60% accuracy without beacon data for window sizes greater than 1 s. Adding beacon data increases the classification performance to near perfect accuracy levels. Furthermore, although SVM has a classification accuracy similar to that of the other classifiers for activity A7 without beacon information, it outperforms them with beacon information and reaches 97% accuracy. Looking more closely at the confusion matrices, we observe that activity A7 proves one of the most challenging activities to classify accurately for the other classifiers, even with beacon data. Although activity A7 takes place in the same set of sectors with activities A2, A5 and A5, the micro-locations inside each sector are different (i.e., location along a workbench). SVM can use this micro-location information, revealed by the beacon data, better than other classifiers, and this results in higher classification accuracy. The same behaviour is observed for activity A8: when using information solely from smart watches, classification accuracy does not reach a level above 65%. Adding beacon information results in perfect accuracy for most window sizes.

	A1	A2	A3	A4	A5	A6	A7	A8		A1	A2	A3	A4	A5	A6	A7	A8
A1	0.87	0	0	0	0	0.1	0.03	0	A1	0.9	0	0	0	0	0.08	0.02	0
A2	0	0.74	0.01	0.01	0.13	0	0.07	0.03	A2	0	0.81	0	0.01	0.09	0	0.05	0.04
A3	0	0	0.93	0	0	0.02	0.04	0.01	A3	0	0.01	0.92	0	0	0.02	0.03	0.01
A4	0	0.05	0.01	0.5	0.17	0	0.12	0.15	A4	0	0.04	0	0.51	0.17	0	0.11	0.16
A5	0.01	0.15	0.01	0.03	0.63	0	0.09	0.08	A5	0	0.11	0	0.04	0.68	0	0.1	0.07
A6	0.07	0	0	0	0	0.87	0.05	0	A6	0.08	0	0	0	0	0.89	0.03	0
A7	0.06	0.04	0.02	0.01	0.09	0.02	0.72	0.03	A7	0.05	0.03	0	0.02	0.06	0.03	0.79	0.01
A8	0.01	0.1	0.01	0.04	0.25	0.01	0.1	0.48	A8	0.01	0.07	0	0.02	0.17	0	0.15	0.57

(a) (b)

	A1	A2	A3	A4	A5	A6	A7	A8		A1	A2	A3	A4	A5	A6	A7	A8
A1	0.95	0	0	0	0	0.04	0.01	0	A1	0.94	0	0	0	0	0.04	0.02	0
A2	0.01	0.88	0	0	0.06	0	0.02	0.03	A2	0	0.88	0	0.01	0.08	0	0.02	0.01
A3	0	0	1	0	0	0	0	0	A3	0	0	0.97	0	0	0	0.03	0
A4	0	0.02	0	0.62	0.18	0	0.1	0.08	A4	0	0	0	0.76	0.06	0	0.08	0.1
A5	0	0.1	0	0.04	0.73	0	0.05	0.07	A5	0	0.1	0	0	0.82	0	0.04	0.04
A6	0.08	0	0.01	0	0	0.88	0.02	0	A6	0.04	0	0	0	0	0.89	0.07	0
A7	0.03	0.04	0.02	0.01	0.05	0.04	0.78	0.02	A7	0.02	0	0.04	0.01	0.06	0.01	0.82	0.04
A8	0	0.06	0.02	0.02	0.12	0	0.11	0.67	A8	0	0.07	0	0.07	0.22	0	0.07	0.57

(c) (d)

Figure 14. Normalised confusion matrices for random forest, with Wearable Feature Type 2, without beacon data. (**a**) 49, w = 1 s; (**b**) 50, w = 2 s ; (**c**) 43, w = 3 s; (**d**) 45, w = 4 s.

	A1	A2	A3	A4	A5	A6	A7	A8		A1	A2	A3	A4	A5	A6	A7	A8
A1	0.95	0	0	0	0	0.03	0.02	0	A1	0.93	0	0	0	0	0.05	0.02	0
A2	0	0.87	0	0	0.07	0	0.05	0	A2	0	0.92	0	0	0.05	0	0.02	0
A3	0	0	0.97	0	0	0.01	0.01	0.01	A3	0	0	0.95	0	0	0.02	0	0.02
A4	0	0.01	0	0.96	0	0	0.03	0	A4	0	0.01	0.01	0.95	0.02	0	0	0
A5	0	0.08	0	0	0.86	0	0.05	0	A5	0	0.07	0	0.01	0.88	0	0.04	0
A6	0.02	0	0	0	0	0.96	0.01	0	A6	0.04	0	0	0	0	0.92	0.04	0
A7	0.05	0.04	0	0	0.06	0.01	0.83	0	A7	0.05	0.03	0	0	0.05	0	0.88	0
A8	0	0.01	0.01	0	0	0	0.01	0.96	A8	0.01	0.01	0.01	0	0	0	0.01	0.97

(a) (b)

	A1	A2	A3	A4	A5	A6	A7	A8		A1	A2	A3	A4	A5	A6	A7	A8
A1	0.97	0	0	0	0	0.02	0.01	0	A1	0.95	0	0	0	0	0.04	0.01	0
A2	0	0.92	0	0	0.05	0	0.02	0.01	A2	0	0.94	0	0	0.05	0	0.02	0
A3	0	0	1	0	0	0	0	0	A3	0	0	1	0	0	0	0	0
A4	0	0	0.02	0.98	0	0	0	0	A4	0	0	0.02	0.98	0	0	0	0
A5	0	0.07	0	0.01	0.88	0	0.04	0	A5	0	0.05	0	0	0.93	0	0.02	0
A6	0.06	0	0	0	0	0.92	0.02	0	A6	0.01	0	0	0.01	0	0.94	0.05	0
A7	0.03	0.04	0	0	0.02	0.01	0.9	0	A7	0.02	0.01	0	0	0.05	0.01	0.91	0
A8	0	0	0.01	0	0	0.01	0.01	0.97	A8	0	0.01	0	0	0.01	0	0	0.98

(c) (d)

Figure 15. Normalised confusion matrices for random forest, with Wearable Feature Type 2, with beacon data. (**a**) n = 48, w = 1 s; (**b**) n = 46, w = 2 s ; (**c**) n = 42, w = 3 s; (**d**) n = 41, w = 4 s.

As a general note, we should highlight the fact that LR is a linear classifier, while KNN, RF and SVM are non-linear classifiers. When adding beacon data and increasing the dimensionality of our feature space, the data become non-linearly separable, and LR is not able to take advantage of the additional information. This results in worse classification performance compared to the other classifiers. We can also confirm this by inspecting Figures 7a and 8a, where the gap in average $F_1 score$ between LR and the other classifiers increases from 0.1 (without beacon data) to 0.15 (with beacon data).

	A1	A2	A3	A4	A5	A6	A7	A8
A1	0.83	0	0	0	0	0.14	0.03	0
A2	0.01	0.74	0.01	0.02	0.14	0	0.07	0.02
A3	0	0	0.96	0.01	0	0.01	0.03	0
A4	0.01	0.05	0.01	0.57	0.15	0.01	0.08	0.12
A5	0.01	0.14	0.01	0.04	0.65	0	0.08	0.06
A6	0.08	0	0	0	0	0.88	0.04	0
A7	0.08	0.05	0.02	0.02	0.09	0.03	0.68	0.03
A8	0.01	0.08	0.01	0.06	0.19	0.01	0.12	0.5

(a)

	A1	A2	A3	A4	A5	A6	A7	A8
A1	0.87	0	0	0	0	0.1	0.03	0
A2	0	0.86	0	0.01	0.08	0	0.03	0.02
A3	0	0	0.92	0	0.01	0.02	0.04	0
A4	0	0.03	0.01	0.6	0.14	0	0.05	0.17
A5	0	0.08	0.01	0.03	0.72	0	0.08	0.07
A6	0.09	0	0.01	0	0	0.88	0.01	0
A7	0.08	0.03	0.01	0.02	0.04	0.01	0.78	0.03
A8	0	0.09	0	0.03	0.17	0.01	0.14	0.57

(b)

	A1	A2	A3	A4	A5	A6	A7	A8
A1	0.94	0	0	0	0	0.05	0.01	0
A2	0.01	0.83	0	0	0.08	0	0.04	0.04
A3	0	0	1	0	0	0	0	0
A4	0	0.03	0.02	0.74	0.1	0	0.03	0.08
A5	0	0.07	0	0.06	0.76	0	0.05	0.05
A6	0.08	0	0.01	0	0	0.88	0.01	0
A7	0.04	0.03	0.04	0.01	0.04	0.03	0.77	0.03
A8	0.01	0.04	0.02	0.02	0.19	0	0.08	0.65

(c)

	A1	A2	A3	A4	A5	A6	A7	A8
A1	0.93	0	0	0	0	0.05	0.02	0
A2	0	0.92	0	0	0.02	0	0.03	0.03
A3	0	0	0.97	0	0	0	0.03	0
A4	0	0	0	0.76	0.12	0	0.04	0.08
A5	0	0.12	0	0.03	0.74	0	0.05	0.06
A6	0.04	0	0	0	0.01	0.92	0.04	0
A7	0.02	0.01	0.02	0	0.04	0.03	0.84	0.04
A8	0	0.08	0	0.08	0.14	0	0.07	0.63

(d)

Figure 16. Normalised confusion matrices for SVM, with Wearable Feature Type 2, without beacon data. (a) C = 10, $\gamma = 0.1$, w = 1 s; (b) C = 10, $\gamma = 0.1$, w = 2 s; (c) C = 10, $\gamma = 0.1$, w = 3 s; (d) C = 10, $\gamma = 0.1$, w = 4 s.

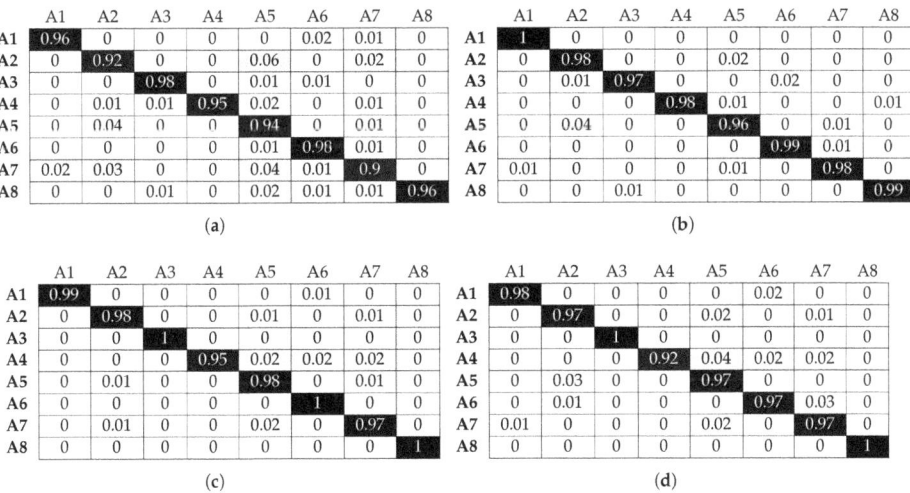

Figure 17. Normalised confusion matrices for SVM, with Wearable Feature Type 2, with beacon data. (a) C = 100, $\gamma = 0.1$, w = 1 s; (b) C = 10, $\gamma = 0.1$, w = 2 s; (c) C = 10, $\gamma = 0.1$, w = 3 s; (d) C = 10, $\gamma = 0.1$, w = 4 s.

7. Conclusions

In this work, we proposed an activity recognition framework for indoor environments, composed of off-the-shelf smart watches and BLE beacons. A mobile phone is responsible for gathering smart watch and beacon data and transmitting them to a server where the processing and classification takes place. Our approach uses location information revealed by the beacon data, to enhance the classification accuracy of the machine learning algorithms we employ. Our experimental results have shown that there is a clear improvement in the performance of our system when beacon data are used. However, the extent to which the location information can be advantageous depends on the type of classifier. LR cannot take full advantage of location information, while KNN and RF benefit more from the fusion of beacon data. SVM exhibits the highest performance gain when using beacon data. Furthermore, we observe that the more unique the location of an activity is with respect to the others, the higher the benefit in activity recognition performance. However, we must highlight that even subtle differences in activity locations are sufficient for a significant improvement in the classification accuracy (e.g., working on different parts of a workbench inside the same sector). Finally, location information can make the system more adaptive, as it allows for smaller window sizes, which results in less time required to collect and classify data.

In future work, we will further investigate human activities that can take place in an indoor setting, such as building emergency management [52,53]. This could prove beneficial for an emergency operation, as it could improve situational awareness with respect to the activities of building occupants in the instances before or after an incident took place. Finally, we will investigate a wider range of machine learning algorithms and consider the use of neural networks and deep learning for further improving our system's performance.

Acknowledgments: This work was supported by the University of Greenwich Research & Enterprise Investment Programme.

Author Contributions: Avgoustinos Filippoupolitis conceived the experiments. Avgoustinos Filippoupolitis and George Loukas designed the experiments. William Oliff and Babak Takand developed the mobile application and performed the experiments. Avgoustinos Filippoupolitis analysed the data. All authors have participated in writing the paper. Avgoustinos Filippoupolitis and George Loukas edited the paper.

Conflicts of Interest: The authors declare no conflict of interest.

Abbreviations

The following abbreviations are used in this manuscript:

ANN	Artificial Neural Networks
AP	Access Point
API	Application Program Interface
BLE	Bluetooth Low Energy
COTS	Commercial-Off-The-Shelf
CRF	Conditional Random Field
DT	Decision Trees
EP	Emerging Pattern
GNSS	Global Navigation Satellite System
HAR	Human Activity Recognition
HMM	Hidden Markov Models
IMU	Inertial Measurement Unit
IPS	Indoor Positioning System
NB	Naive Bayes

KNN	K-Nearest Neighbours
LR	Logistic Regression
MLP	Multi-Layer Perceptron
RF	Random Forests
RSSI	Received Signal Strength Indicator
SNR	Signal-to-Noise Ratio
SVM	Support Vector Machines
UUID	Universally Unique Identifier

References

1. Zhang, Q.; Su, Y.; Yu, P. Assisting an elderly with early dementia using wireless sensors data in smarter safer home. In Proceedings of the International Conference on Informatics and Semiotics in Organisations, Shanghai, China, 23–35 May 2014; pp. 398–404.
2. Suryadevara, N.K.; Mukhopadhyay, S.C.; Wang, R.; Rayudu, R. Forecasting the behavior of an elderly using wireless sensors data in a smart home. *Eng. Appl. Artif. Intell.* **2013**, *26*, 2641–2652.
3. Han, Y.; Han, M.; Lee, S.; Sarkar, A.; Lee, Y.K. A framework for supervising lifestyle diseases using long-term activity monitoring. *Sensors* **2012**, *12*, 5363–5379.
4. Zhu, C.; Sheng, W. Motion-and location-based online human daily activity recognition. *Pervasive Mob. Comput.* **2011**, *7*, 256–269.
5. Kim, S.C.; Jeong, Y.S.; Park, S.O. RFID-based indoor location tracking to ensure the safety of the elderly in smart home environments. *Pers. Ubiquitous Comput.* **2013**, *17*, 1699–1707.
6. Statista. Global Smartwatch Unit Sales 2014–2018 | Statistic. Available online: https://www.statista.com/statistics/538237/global-smartwatch-unit-sales/ (accessed on 22 February 2017).
7. The Hitchhikers Guide to iBeacon Hardware: A Comprehensive Report by Aislelabs. Available online: http://www.aislelabs.com/reports/beacon-guide/ (accessed on 31 March 2017).
8. Filippoupolitis, A.; Takand, B.; Loukas, G. Activity Recognition in a Home Setting Using Off the Shelf Smart Watch Technology. In Proceedings of the 2016 15th International Conference on Ubiquitous Computing and Communications and 2016 International Symposium on Cyberspace and Security (IUCC-CSS), Granada, Spain, 14–16 December 2016; pp. 39–44.
9. Cornacchia, M.; Ozcan, K.; Zheng, Y.; Velipasalar, S. A Survey on Activity Detection and Classification Using Wearable Sensors. *IEEE Sens. J.* **2017**, *17*, 386–403.
10. Lara, O.D.; Labrador, M.A. A survey on human activity recognition using wearable sensors. *IEEE Commun. Surv. Tutor.* **2013**, *15*, 1192–1209.
11. Trost, S.G.; Zheng, Y.; Wong, W.K. Machine learning for activity recognition: Hip versus wrist data. *Physiol. Meas.* **2014**, *35*, 2183.
12. Dieu, O., Mikulovic, J.; Fardy, P.S.; Bui Xuan, G.; Béghin, L.; Vanhelst, J Physical activity using wrist-worn accelerometers: Comparison of dominant and non-dominant wrist. *Clin. Physiol. Funct. Imaging* **2016**, doi:10.1111/cpf.12337.
13. Kefer, K.; Holzmann, C.; Findling, R.D. Comparing the Placement of Two Arm-Worn Devices for Recognizing Dynamic Hand Gestures. In Proceedings of the ACM 14th International Conference on Advances in Mobile Computing and Multi Media, Singapore, 28–30 November 2016; pp. 99–104.
14. Gjoreski, M.; Gjoreski, H.; Luštrek, M.; Gams, M. How accurately can your wrist device recognize daily activities and detect falls? *Sensors* **2016**, *16*, 800.
15. Weiss, G.M.; Timko, J.L.; Gallagher, C.M.; Yoneda, K.; Schreiber, A.J. Smartwatch-based activity recognition: A machine learning approach. In Proceedings of the 2016 IEEE-EMBS International Conference on Biomedical and Health Informatics (BHI), Las Vegas, NV, USA, 24–27 February 2016; pp. 426–429.
16. Sen, S.; Subbaraju, V.; Misra, A.; Balan, R.K.; Lee, Y. The case for smartwatch-based diet monitoring. In Proceedings of the 2015 IEEE International Conference on Pervasive Computing and Communication Workshops (PerCom Workshops), St. Louis, MO, USA, 23–27 March 2015; pp. 585–590.
17. Radhakrishnan, M.; Eswaran, S.; Misra, A.; Chander, D.; Dasgupta, K. Iris: Tapping wearable sensing to capture in-store retail insights on shoppers. In Proceedings of the 2016 IEEE International Conference on Pervasive Computing and Communications (PerCom), Sydney, NSW, Australia, 14–19 March 2016; pp. 1–8.

18. Rawassizadeh, R.; Tomitsch, M.; Nourizadeh, M.; Momeni, E.; Peery, A.; Ulanova, L.; Pazzani, M. Energy-Efficient Integration of Continuous Context Sensing and Prediction into Smartwatches. *Sensors* **2015**, *15*, 22616–22645.
19. Bai, L.; Efstratiou, C.; Ang, C.S. weSport: Utilising wrist-band sensing to detect player activities in basketball games. In Proceedings of the 2016 IEEE International Conference on Pervasive Computing and Communication Workshops, Sydney, NSW, Australia, 14–19 March 2016; pp. 1–6.
20. Garcia-Ceja, E.; Brena, R.F.; Carrasco-Jimenez, J.C.; Garrido, L. Long-term activity recognition from wristwatch accelerometer data. *Sensors* **2014**, *14*, 22500–22524.
21. GENEActiv by Activinsights. Available online: https://www.geneactiv.org/ (accessed on 24 March 2017).
22. Shoaib, M.; Bosch, S.; Incel, O.D.; Scholten, H.; Havinga, P.J. Complex human activity recognition using smartphone and wrist-worn motion sensors. *Sensors* **2016**, *16*, 426.
23. Moschetti, A.; Fiorini, L.; Esposito, D.; Dario, P.; Cavallo, F. Recognition of daily gestures with wearable inertial rings and bracelets. *Sensors* **2016**, *16*, 1341.
24. Parate, A.; Chiu, M.C.; Chadowitz, C.; Ganesan, D.; Kalogerakis, E. Risq: Recognizing smoking gestures with inertial sensors on a wristband. In Proceedings of the ACM 12th annual international conference on Mobile Systems, Applications, and Services, Bretton Woods, NH, USA, June 16–19 2014; pp. 149–161.
25. Nguyen, M.; Fan, L.; Shahabi, C. Activity recognition using wrist-worn sensors for human performance evaluation. In Proceedings of the 2015 IEEE International Conference on. IEEE Data Mining Workshop (ICDMW), Atlantic City, NJ, USA, 14–17 November 2015; pp. 164–169.
26. Sarcevic, P.; Kincses, Z.; Pletl, S. Comparison of different classifiers in movement recognition using WSN-based wrist-mounted sensors. In Proceedings of the 2015 IEEE Sensors Applications Symposium (SAS), Zadar, Croatia, 13–15 April 2015; pp. 1–6.
27. Margarito, J.; Helaoui, R.; Bianchi, A.M.; Sartor, F.; Bonomi, A.G. User-independent recognition of sports activities from a single wrist-worn accelerometer: A template-matching-based approach. *IEEE Trans. Biomed. Eng.* **2016**, *63*, 788–796.
28. Wei, Z.; Bao, T. Research on a novel strategy for automatic activity recognition using wearable device. In Proceedings of the 2016 8th IEEE International Conference on Communication Software and Networks (ICCSN), Beijing, China, 4–6 June 2016; pp. 488–492.
29. Cho, Y.; Cho, H.; Kyung, C.M. Design and Implementation of Practical Step Detection Algorithm for Wrist-Worn Devices. *IEEE Sens. J.* **2016**, *16*, 7720–7730.
30. Ni, Q.; García Hernando, A.B.; de la Cruz, I.P. The elderly's independent living in smart homes: A characterization of activities and sensing infrastructure survey to facilitate services development. *Sensors* **2015**, *15*, 11312–11362.
31. Okeyo, G.; Chen, L.; Wang, H. Combining ontological and temporal formalisms for composite activity modelling and recognition in smart homes. *Future Gener. Comput. Syst.* **2014**, *39*, 29–43.
32. Hardegger, M.; Roggen, D.; Calatroni, A.; Tröster, G. S-SMART: A unified bayesian framework for simultaneous semantic mapping, activity recognition, and tracking. *ACM Trans. Intell. Syst. Technol. TIST* **2016**, *7*, 34.
33. Ni, Q.; García Hernando, A.B.; Pau de la Cruz, I. A Context-Aware System Infrastructure for Monitoring Activities of Daily Living in Smart Home. *J. Sens.* **2016**, *2016*, 9493047.
34. Bouten, C.V.; Koekkoek, K.T.; Verduin, M.; Kodde, R.; Janssen, J.D. A triaxial accelerometer and portable data processing unit for the assessment of daily physical activity. *IEEE Trans. Biomed. Eng.* **1997**, *44*, 136–147.
35. Santoso, F.; Redmond, S.J. Indoor location-aware medical systems for smart homecare and telehealth monitoring: State-Of-The-Art. *Physiol. Meas.* **2015**, *36*, R53.
36. Sugino, K.; Katayama, S.; Niwa, Y.; Shiramatsu, S.; Ozono, T.; Shintani, T. A Bluetooth-based Device-Free Motion Detector for a Remote Elder Care Support System. In Proceedings of the 2015 IIAI 4th International Congress on Advanced Applied Informatics (IIAI-AAI), Okayama, Japan, 12–16 July 2015; pp. 91–96.
37. Fujihara, A.; Yanagizawa, T. Proposing an extended iBeacon system for indoor route guidance. In Proceedings of the 2015 IEEE International Conference on Intelligent Networking and Collaborative Systems (INCOS), Taipei, Taiwan, 2–4 September 2015; pp. 31–37.
38. He, Z.; Cui, B.; Zhou, W.; Yokoi, S. A proposal of interaction system between visitor and collection in museum hall by iBeacon. In Proceedings of the 2015 10th International Conference on Computer Science Education (ICCSE), Cambridge, UK, 22–24 July 2015; pp. 427–430.

39. Volam, P.K.; Kamath, A.R.; Bagi, S.S. A system and method for transmission of traffic sign board information to vehicles and relevance determination. In Proceedings of the 2014 IEEE International Conference on Advances in Electronics, Computers and Communications (ICAECC), Bangalore, India, 10–11 October 2014; pp. 1–6.
40. Corna, A.; Fontana, L.; Nacci, A.; Sciuto, D. Occupancy detection via iBeacon on Android devices for smart building management. In Proceedings of the 2015 Design, Automation & Test in Europe Conference & Exhibition, Grenoble, France, 9–13 March 2015; pp. 629–632.
41. Filippoupolitis, A.; Oliff, W.; Loukas, G. Occupancy Detection for Building Emergency Management Using BLE Beacons. In Proceedings of the Computer and Information Sciences: 31st International Symposium, ISCIS 2016, Kraków, Poland, 27–28 October 2016; Czachórski, T., Gelenbe, E., Grochla, K., Lent, R., Eds.; Springer: Cham, Switzerland, 2016; pp. 233–240.
42. Filippoupolitis, A.; Oliff, W.; Loukas, G. Bluetooth Low Energy Based Occupancy Detection for Emergency Management. In Proceedings of the 2016 15th International Conference on Ubiquitous Computing and Communications and 2016 International Symposium on Cyberspace and Security (IUCC-CSS), Granada, Spain, 14–16 December 2016; pp. 31–38.
43. Bulling, A.; Blanke, U.; Schiele, B. A tutorial on human activity recognition using body-worn inertial sensors. *ACM Comput. Surv.* **2014**, *46*, 33.
44. Banos, O.; Galvez, J.M.; Damas, M.; Pomares, H.; Rojas, I. Window size impact in human activity recognition. *Sensors* **2014**, *14*, 6474–6499.
45. Faragher, R.; Harle, R. An analysis of the accuracy of bluetooth low energy for indoor positioning applications. In Proceedings of the 27th International Technical Meeting of The Satellite Division of the Institute of Navigation (ION GNSS+ 2014), Tampa, FL, USA, 8–12 September 2014; Volume 812, p. 2.
46. Bao, L.; Intille, S.S. Activity recognition from user-annotated acceleration data. In *Pervasive Computing*; Springer: Berlin, Heidelberg, 2004; pp. 1–17.
47. Preece, S.J.; Goulermas, J.Y.; Kenney, L.P.; Howard, D. A comparison of feature extraction methods for the classification of dynamic activities from accelerometer data. *IEEE Trans. Biomed. Eng.* **2009**, *56*, 871–879.
48. Zhu, C.; Sheng, W. Human daily activity recognition in robot-assisted living using multi-sensor fusion. In Proceedings of the 2009 IEEE International Conference on Robotics and Automation (ICRA'09), Kobe, Japan, 12–17 May 2009; pp. 2154–2159.
49. Pansiot, J.; Stoyanov, D.; McIlwraith, D.; Lo, B.P.; Yang, G.Z. Ambient and wearable sensor fusion for activity recognition in healthcare monitoring systems. In Proceedings of the 4th international workshop on wearable and implantable body sensor networks (BSN 2007), Aachen, Germany, 26–28 March 2007; pp. 208–212.
50. Hsu, C.W.; Chang, C.C.; Lin, C.J. A practical guide to support vector classification. 2003. Available online: http://www.csie.ntu.edu.tw/~cjlin/papers/guide/guide.pdf (accessed on 24 March 2017).
51. Sokolova, M.; Lapalme, G. A systematic analysis of performance measures for classification tasks. *Inf. Process. Manag.* **2009**, *45*, 427–437.
52. Filippoupolitis, A.; Gorbil, G.; Gelenbe, E. Spatial computers for emergency support. *Comput. J.* **2012**, *56*, 1399–1416.
53. Filippoupolitis, A.; Loukas, G.; Timotheou, S.; Dimakis, N.; Gelenbe, E. Emergency response systems for disaster management in buildings. In Proceedings of the NATO Symposium on C3I for Crisis, Emergency and Consequence Management (NATO), Bucharest, Romania, 11–12 May 2009.

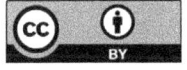

© 2017 by the authors. Licensee MDPI, Basel, Switzerland. This article is an open access article distributed under the terms and conditions of the Creative Commons Attribution (CC BY) license (http://creativecommons.org/licenses/by/4.0/).

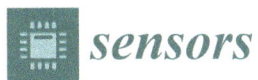

Article

Context Mining of Sedentary Behaviour for Promoting Self-Awareness Using a Smartphone [†]

Muhammad Fahim [1,*], Thar Baker [2], Asad Masood Khattak [3], Babar Shah [3], Saiqa Aleem [3] and Francis Chow [4]

1. Institute of Information Systems, Innopolis University, Innopolis 420500, Russia
2. Department of Computer Science, Faculty of Engineering and Technology, Liverpool John Moores University, Liverpool L3 3AF, UK; t.baker@ljmu.ac.uk
3. College of Technological Innovation, Zayed University, Abu Dhabi Campus, Abu Dhabi 144534, UAE; asad.khattak@zu.ac.ae (A.M.K.); Babar.Shah@zu.ac.ae (B.S.); Saiqa.Aleem@zu.ac.ae (S.A.)
4. University College, Zayed University, Dubai 144534, UAE; Francis.Chow@zu.ac.ae
* Correspondence: m.fahim@innopolis.ru; Tel.: +7-917-225-0915
† This paper is an extended version of our paper published in Fahim, M.; Khattak, A.M.; Baker, T.; Chow, F.; Shah, B. Micro-context recognition of sedentary behaviour using smartphone. In Proceedings of the Sixth International Conference on Digital Information and Communication Technology and Its Applications (DICTAP), Konya, Turkey, 21–23 July 2016.

Received: 29 October 2017; Accepted: 13 March 2018; Published: 15 March 2018

Abstract: Sedentary behaviour is increasing due to societal changes and is related to prolonged periods of sitting. There is sufficient evidence proving that sedentary behaviour has a negative impact on people's health and wellness. This paper presents our research findings on how to mine the temporal contexts of sedentary behaviour by utilizing the on-board sensors of a smartphone. We use the accelerometer sensor of the smartphone to recognize user situations (i.e., still or active). If our model confirms that the user context is still, then there is a high probability of being sedentary. Then, we process the environmental sound to recognize the micro-context, such as working on a computer or watching television during leisure time. Our goal is to reduce sedentary behaviour by suggesting preventive interventions to take short breaks during prolonged sitting to be more active. We achieve this goal by providing the visualization to the user, who wants to monitor his/her sedentary behaviour to reduce unhealthy routines for self-management purposes. The main contribution of this paper is two-fold: (i) an initial implementation of the proposed framework supporting real-time context identification; (ii) testing and evaluation of the framework, which suggest that our application is capable of substantially reducing sedentary behaviour and assisting users to be active.

Keywords: context recognition; self-management; unhealthy sitting habits

1. Introduction

In past decades, sedentary behaviour has appropriately received considerable attention in both developed and developing countries due to societal changes. People spend most of their time in sedentary activities, and their metabolic health is compromised due to low levels of energy expenditure (e.g., while sitting watching television, working on a computer in the workplace, using a cellphone, driving automobiles, playing video/board games, reading books and lying on the couch [1]). To address sedentary behaviour, some initial clarification is required about the terminology. We refer to all sitting activities in different contexts with an energy expenditure of $\leq$1.5 resting metabolic equivalents (METs) as sedentary behaviours [2]. Hence, a person is considered sedentary if s/he spends a large amount of the day in such activities. Sedentary behaviours are associated with chronic disease [3], physiological and psychological problems [4], cardiovascular disease, diabetes [5] and poor sleep [6]. The most noticeable one is the high risk of being overweight and obesity, which have become serious public health threats worldwide and comprise the second leading cause of preventable death, trailing only tobacco [7]. Therefore, a self-management approach is required to support self-awareness and promote healthy behaviour to reduce the health risks caused by sedentary behaviour. The research community has suggested that new technologies like smartphone alerts of elapsed sedentary time and short breaks during prolonged sitting could be adopted in our daily routines [1,8].

Recently, activity trackers such as Fitbit [9], smartphone apps such as Google Fit [10] and smartwatch activity apps [11] can recognize many user activities. However, these trackers generate a time-series of user activities, but do not make the user aware of the detected unhealthy behaviour. This paper presents our model to detect the sedentary behaviour patterns and create a personal behaviour profile to store collected information. In the future, these profiles may assist practitioners to counsel the users or predict the future based on everyday rhythms of sedentary activity and past sedentary habits. Integrating smartphone technology has great potential to promote healthy behaviours [12]. Users do not have to wear/carry extra gear to monitor and track their daily routine behaviour. The smartphone has various embedded sensors (e.g., accelerometer, audio, WiFi, Global Positioning System (GPS), Bluetooth, gyroscope, magnetometer), high computational power and storage and programmable capabilities, along with wireless communication technologies [13]. Furthermore, it has become an integral part of our daily routines; and one of the best devices to recognize the user's context.

In order to mine the contexts of sedentary behaviour, there is a need to develop a ubiquitous system that can track the sedentary elapsed time accurately with all its minor routines ranging from office work to watching television during leisure time. Previously, we conducted a pilot study on micro-context recognition [14] and visualizing the user behaviour over the web through the Internet. In this paper, we propose a user-centric smartphone-based approach to recognize the context of sedentary behaviour based on the onboard accelerometers and audio sensors of the smartphone. We compute the acceleration and acoustic features over the collected sensory data streams and mine the contexts by applying the non-parametric nearest neighbour classification algorithm [15]. The main contribution of this paper is two-fold: (i) an initial implementation of the proposed framework supporting real-time context identification; (ii) testing and evaluation of the framework, which prove that our application is capable of substantially reducing sedentary behaviour and assisting humans to be active. The aim of the proposed framework is to monitor human sedentary behaviour in a proactive way. Based on the tracked behaviour, users will be able to monitor and manage their daily routines, which may help them to adopt active lifestyle.

The rest of the paper is structured as follows: Related work and the limitations of existing systems are discussed in Section 2. In Section 3, we provide the proposed architecture and its implementation inside the smartphone environment to track sedentary behaviour. In Section 4, we explain our experimental setup and present the obtained results. We provide a detailed discussion in Section 5 and interventions for our experimental study. Finally, the paper concludes with our findings and proposes future work in Section 6.

2. Related Work

Large proportions of the population report insufficient physical activity, high volumes of sedentary behaviour and poor sleep [16–21]. The most common methods to capture sedentary behaviour are self-reporting diaries, direct observations, smartphone applications and wearable devices [22]. Self-reporting diaries and direct observation mechanisms are difficult with respect to recording daily routines of a long duration and are time consuming to manage on a daily basis. On the other hand, wearable devices and smartphone applications represent a comprehensive way to monitor sedentary behaviour continuously. We report the efforts of the research community in monitoring sedentary behaviour in the following section.

2.1. Wearable Devices

Globally-accepted wearable devices to monitor sedentary behaviour are ActiGraph and actiPAL [23]. Matthews et al. [24] used the ActiGraph device to record the acceleration information and estimate the body movement. The wearable device was set to provide information in 1-min epochs. Participants wear this on their right hip attached with an elastic belt. After the collection of the data, the device was attached to computer, and data were analysed using specially-developed software. This mechanism is intrusive, and the user needs to attach the device to his/her body. Chelsea et al. [25] explored how the DigMem system is used to successfully recognize activity and create temporal memory boxes of human experience, which can be used to monitor sedentary behaviour. Users can track where they exactly were, what they were doing and how their bodies were reacting. Their solution is comprised of multimodal sensors including GPS, camera, ECG monitor, environmental sensor, sound and accelerometer. This notwithstanding, such a system is still not a handy solution to embrace in daily routines in order to promote self-awareness.

Stratton et al. [26] created an intelligent environment to monitor and manipulate the physical activity and sedentary behaviour. They also discussed the broad range of approaches already designed to increase physical activity among different populations. Their proposed solution is obtrusive due to the need to wear an additional sensor to monitor the sedentary behaviour. Such methods are intrusive and unable to process the sensor data inside the devices. Furthermore, they provide limited information about the sedentary behaviour in everyday routines. One of the drawbacks of wearable devices is the inability to detect the contextual information.

2.2. Smartphone Applications

Qian et al. [1] explored smartphone usage to predict sedentary behaviours. They were able to classify user contexts such as location, time and application usage to predict if the user would be sedentary in the coming hours. Their methodology is still unable to distinguish between different types of sedentary behaviour. Dantzig et al. [27] developed the SitCoach mobile application to monitor the physical activity and sedentary behaviour of office workers. The objective of their research was to avoid prolonged sitting by providing timely information to the user in terms of alert messages. They concluded that mobile applications can motivate people to take regular breaks from long sitting. Shin et al. [28] developed a mobile application to recognize user sedentary activity using a mobile device. Their method was based on rotated acceleration using quaternions, which classified sedentary behaviour with higher accuracy. However, their application required server-side processing to classify user activities patterns. It is seen that many systems and models were therefore proposed to track sedentary behaviour; however, they had limitations.

Our proposed approach is to expand upon the lessons learned from existing research work and to enable the detection of the contextual information by utilizing the embedded sensors of the smartphone and processing data in real time inside the smartphone environment.

3. Methodology

The contextual mining of sedentary behaviour consists of: (a) the smartphone environment to mine the sensory data streams; (b) cloud computing infrastructure to make it an acceptable and usable solution; and (c) sedentary behaviour analysis. The proposed model is illustrated in Figure 1, and the details of the sub-components are as follows.

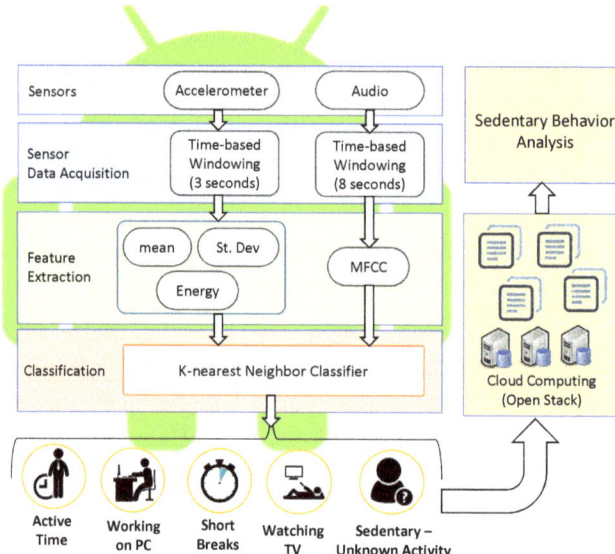

Figure 1. The proposed architecture of context mining. MFCC, Mel-Frequency Cepstral Coefficient.

3.1. The Smartphone Environment

We implement our proposed model using the most competitive open source Google Android platform (Ice Cream Sandwich) [29]. The developed system's components are detailed as follows.

3.1.1. Sensor Data Acquisition

We collect the temporal sensory data stream of the onboard tri-axial accelerometer and audio sensor of the smartphone. The accelerometer sensor is capable of measuring the acceleration in three orthogonal directions (i.e., x, y and z axis). These raw signals need to be pre-processed to segment the continuous temporal data before extracting the feature set. Therefore, we apply the time-based windowing method to divide it into fixed time segments (i.e., 3 s) [30]. The selection of time-based windowing is based on the its good handling of continuous data [15,28,31]. The audio data stream is an important source to know the user contexts by processing the environmental sound. We collected the audio data stream and applied signal segmentation by dividing it into fixed time segments (i.e., 8 s). The duration of fixed time segments is based on the analysis of audio data, and it will be enough to process for mining contexts. In order to maintain the user privacy, we did not store the audio signal, nor accelerometer signal, but rather, we processed it immediately in real time.

3.1.2. Feature Extraction

Feature extraction is the most important part of mining contexts, since the selected features play a crucial role in determining the user's situation. In the past, many complex features extraction techniques such as Principal Component Analysis (PCA) followed by Linear Discriminant Analysis (LDA) [32] and wavelet features [33] were used; however, they are computationally expensive and difficult to implement inside the smartphone environment, as they require a strong statistical background. Many researchers reported that simple and low cost computational features, such as mean, median and standard deviation, and low and high pass filters are able to achieve high accuracy [33,34]. First, we solve the orientation issue of acceleration data suggested by Mizell [35] and then reduce the complexity of feature computation for mobile devices by extracting the time and frequency domain features, which are the mean, standard deviation and energy feature. We extract the mean to measure the central tendency, the standard deviation to measure the data spread for different activities and the energy feature to find the quantitative characteristics of the data over a defined time period. In order to capture the characteristics of environmental sound, we extract the Mel-Frequency Cepstral Coefficients (MFCC) feature vector. It is calculated on the basis of Fast Fourier Transformation (FFT), which is closest to the human auditory system due to the utilized Mel-scale filter bank and represented as the short-term power spectrum of a sound [36]. The calculation of MFCC can be structured into several steps. Figure 2 shows the block diagram for calculating the MFCC feature.

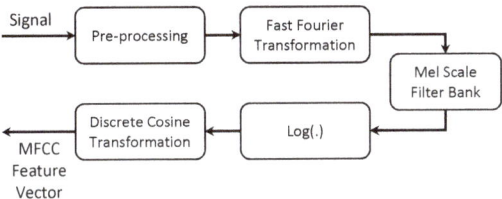

Figure 2. Block diagram of MFCC feature vector calculation.

After the feature extraction step, the feature vector is supplied to the classifier to know the current context of the user.

3.2. Classifier

The classifier has the ability to learn the concept during the training phase, mine the situations and assign the context label during the recognition phase in real time. The extracted feature vectors (i.e., Section 3.1.2) are provided to the classifier for the classification. In the first stage, accelerometer data are classified into "active" or "still". In the second stage, audio data are classified by the classifier. In the audio data classifier, we take into consideration only two contexts, while the rest of the contexts are recognized as "sedentary-unknown context". The following sections explain the training and testing of the classifier.

3.2.1. Training Phase

We trained our model over three participants and asked them to annotate the daily routines' context by miming short duration trials and keeping a note on a piece of paper of the start and end time. We employ non-overlapping time-based windows to cut the signal into equal-length frames. After windowing, feature vectors were extracted (i.e., explained in the feature extraction section) from signal frames and fed into a classifier trainer function to construct a training model. Figure 3 illustrates a block diagram of the training module.

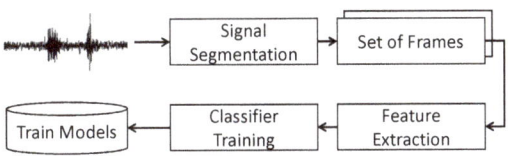

Figure 3. Training of contextual models.

We implement a simple, yet robust non-parametric *k*-nearest neighbour algorithm in our proposed model [37]. It features two stages: the first is the determination of the nearest neighbours, and the second is assigning the context label using those neighbours. In the proposed method, the Euclidean distance metric is applied to find the neighbours, and three neighbours (i.e., k = 3) are taken into account. The value of k = 3 has been proven to provide good results in some related work and for different settings [30,38,39]. Assume "C_{fv}" is the current feature vector that wants to discover the most relevant instances in the context miner "CM".

$$C_{fv} \leftarrow CM(X_n) \qquad (1)$$

where X_n is the number of stored training examples to classify the contexts. In order to find the optimal similarities between the current feature vector and selected classifier module, we calculate the Euclidean distance of "C_{fv}" with all instances of selected "CM" as follows:

$$\text{Euclidean distance}: d(x_i, x_j) = \sqrt{\sum_{k=1}^{n}(C_{fv}(x_{ik}) - CM(x_{jk}))^2} \qquad (2)$$

In Equation (2), the Euclidean distance between two instances "x_i" and "x_j" is denoted by "d_{ij}". The distance is calculated for the k-th attribute of instance x; where, $C_{fv}(x_{ik})$ is the feature vector that wants to associate itself with the instances of $CM(x_{jk})$. Based on this structure, most relevant instances are filtered out, and context class labels are assigned by considering the three nearest neighbours. The selection of the k-nearest neighbour algorithm is based on one of the most useful and lightweight algorithms for various applications. It is also ranked among the top 10 data-mining algorithms [15].

3.2.2. Recognition Phase

Once we train the model, the trained application will be installed on all participants' smartphones. Our application is capable of running in the background so that users can use their smartphone for other tasks. Our model is a two-step process, where we process the accelerometer data stream and know the contexts either "still" or "active". If the classifier labels the context as "still", we process the environmental sound to recognize the micro-context: working on a PC, watching television, "sedentary-unknown context". We consider every context as sedentary-unknown if the user is "still" and it does not lie in the defined micro-contexts. Unknown context includes for example sleeping, reading books and attending classes or seminars. In order to preserve privacy, we do not store the environmental sound. We extract the features in real time from the sensory data and fed to the classifier to recognize the micro-contexts. The time scale for inference is set to one-minute epochs, which is sufficient to distinguish among the micro-contexts. If a user is found to be sedentary, then we activate the audio sensor for 8 s to analyse the environmental sound and recognize the micro-context. Furthermore, if we found the micro-context and the user is still in the sedentary state, we check the environment after fifteen minutes to distinguish between the different micro-contexts while staying sedentary. In this way, we save the battery consumption of the smartphone by only checking the environment when the user is in a sedentary state. The training models were used to classify the contexts in real time, as is shown in Figure 4.

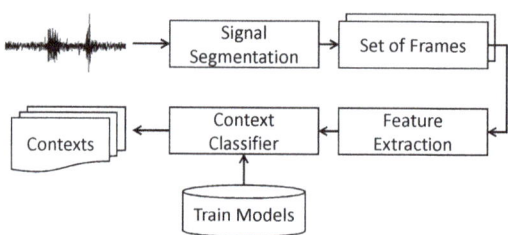

Figure 4. Real-time mining of users' contexts.

We processed all these data inside our smartphone application, and furthermore, it requires a ubiquitous service to transfer this contextual information to our private cloud. We deployed the software as a service model, which will automatically scale the services with dynamic provisioning of resources. This approach will reduce the chances of denial of service to the users even at peak usage. It will also enable the user's phone to be independent in case of any issue with the smartphone. We also present the flowchart of the proposed model in Figure 5.

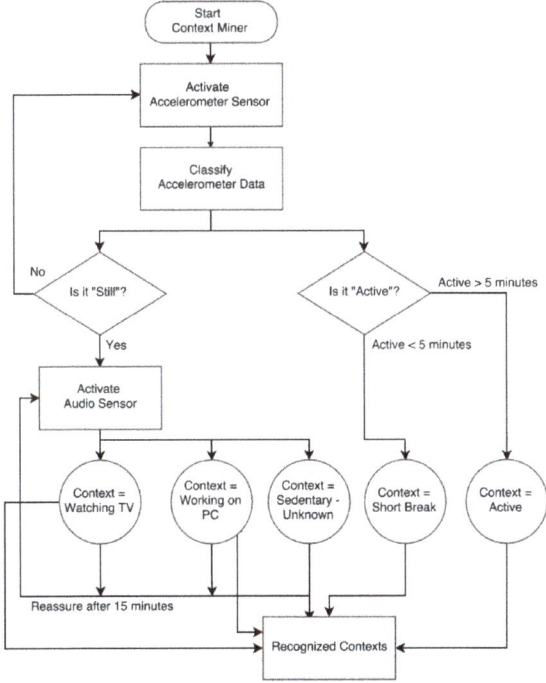

Figure 5. Flowchart of the context miner model.

3.3. Cloud Computing

Cloud computing provides scalable and flexible computing model, where resources, such as computing power, storage, network and software, are abstracted and provided as services over the Internet [40] based on a pay-per-use utility model. Cloud computing has been widely used for data hosting and analysis including healthcare/patients' data storing [41]. It also helps in solving numerous problems in the domain of ambient assisted living. Therefore, we have developed and deployed an open source OpenStack cloud environment in our machine learning research laboratory [42] to provide the user's profile storage, computing and access services from anywhere at anytime. Our smartphone application recognizes the user's context in real time inside the smartphone environment and sends the sedentary behaviour profile to our deployed cloud through the Internet. Furthermore, recognized behaviour is analysed to infer the useful information.

3.4. Sedentary Behaviour Analysis

Our behaviour analytics provide information about the user daily patterns in terms of sedentary time, active time, short breaks, watching television during leisure time and working in the office while using a computer. These contexts of sedentary behaviour provide better understanding of user's daily routines and may help users to minimize the amount of prolonged sitting. We are using MPAndroidChart [43] to present information over the smartphone. We create a limited number of credentials that is equal to the number of participants to interact with the system and able to visualize the sedentary behaviour patterns in daily routines.

4. Results

In this section, we evaluate the proposed contextual mining of sedentary behaviour model and present the results of the performed experiments. Our approach belongs to the family of instance-based learning (i.e., *k*-nearest neighbour). Such approaches do not require optimizing the classifier parameters. It stores the training instances and classifies the new data by calculating the similarities of the stored instances. In order to get these training instances, we asked the participants to annotate the daily routines by miming short duration trials and keeping a note of the start and end time of each context. The training dataset is labelled over the time intervals' information. To assess the performance of our approach, we split the dataset into a ratio of 60:10:30 (i.e., training:validation:test) of the annotated dataset. Our dataset is balanced by considering the equal instances of each considered context. In this experimental setting, the simple performance metric "accuracy" is able to provide correct information about the ability of the model. Initially, we get an overall accuracy of 93% over the collected dataset. We analysed the dataset and performed the data pre-processing. In this step, we discard the first and last few instances of the recorded context. Our analysis showed that start and end instances do not present the true representation of the class. Such a setting enhanced the quality of the training instances in terms of better context representation. In the same experimental setting with the same dataset, we get an accuracy of 98%. The real test setup consists of six volunteer graduate students. The participants installed our developed application on their smartphone for two weeks in order to have enough time to analyse the significance and to perform a comparative analysis of sedentary behaviour. Examples of the scenes of context mining are shown in Figure 6.

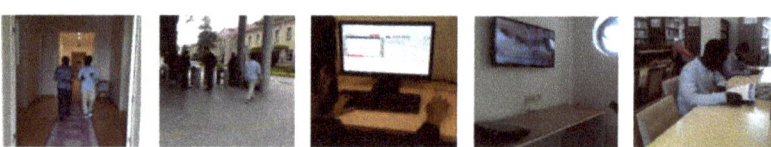

Figure 6. Example photos for "short break", "active", "working on a PC", "watching TV" and "sedentary-context unknown".

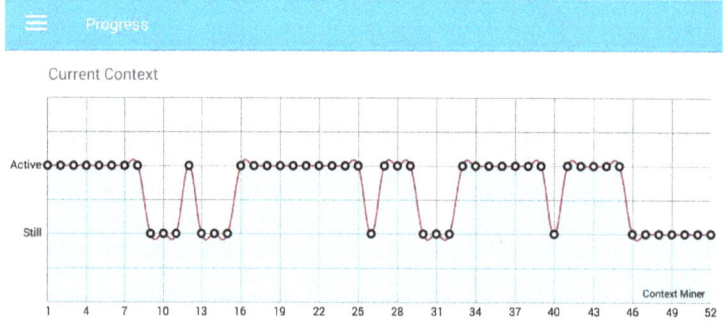

Figure 7. Current progress of the user in the last hour.

In Figure 7, we can observe the progress of the last hour in real time by identifying the context, either active or still. We can see in the "progress graph" (i.e., Figure 7) that the *x*-axis presents the recognized context, the while *y*-axis provides the time stamp in minutes. Furthermore, each point presents each minute of the human behaviour and reports the information about the last 52 min. The annotation of the recognized context shows that the participant was waling from the dormitory to the campus. A user can also visualize the hourly status of the sedentary behaviour of the day. We presented the hourly status of the behaviour, which is the "today context", as shown in Figure 8.

In Figure 8, each bubble presents the number of minutes, and the size of each bubble increases or decreases with the recognized context. For example, at 11:00, the person is in sedentary activity for the whole 60 min. We can also observe that 0.00 means that person is not active even for a single minute.

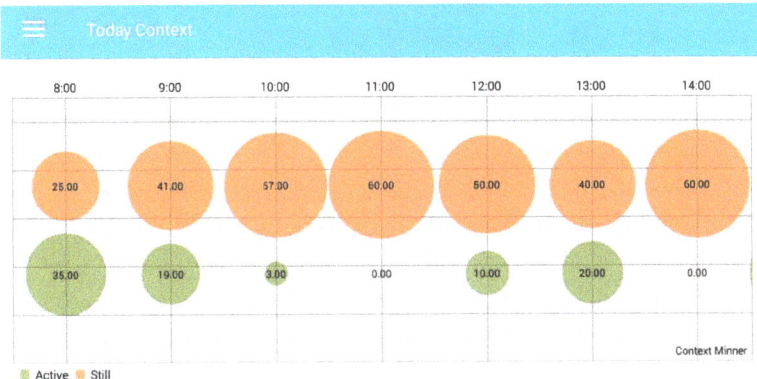

Figure 8. Hourly sedentary behaviour recognition.

In order to provide rich contextual information, we facilitate the user awareness about the micro-contexts of sedentary behaviour, which explains how much time the user spent watching TV, working on a PC or sedentary-context unknown. As we discussed earlier, our micro-context recognition list is very limited due to limited processing of environmental sound. Figure 9 shows the details of micro-contexts that our model identifies by processing the environmental sound.

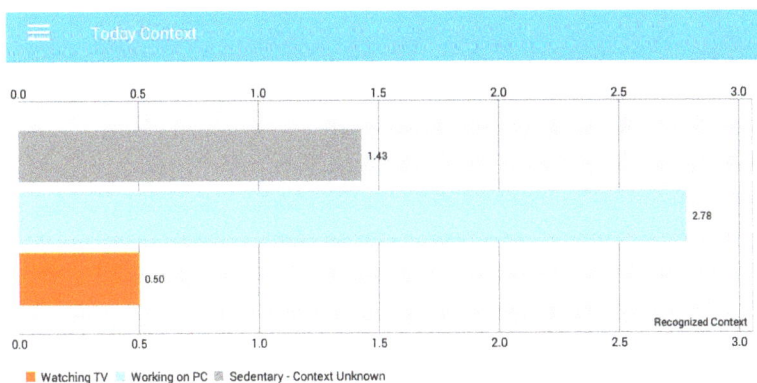

Figure 9. Micro-context recognition.

In Figure 9, the *x*-axis represents the time in hours, while *y*-axis presents the recognized micro-context. All the sedentary contexts other than watching TV and working on a PC are considered as sedentary-context unknown. In the unknown context, a user can be located on a public bus, in a library, in a cafeteria, sleeping or any other situation. We also present the entire week of behaviour in terms of recognized context and visualize it through our developed application. The user can query any specific context from the recognized context to get the information about the time spent. Figure 10 shows the total active hours of the user each day throughout the week.

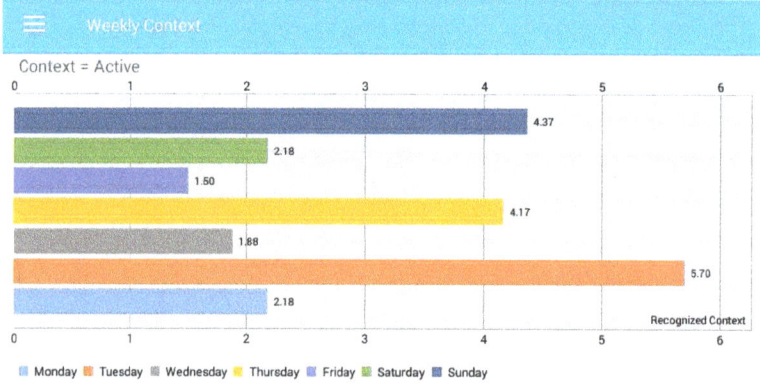

Figure 10. Total time spent during a week while being "active".

It is obvious in Figure 10 that very limited activity is observed during Friday and Wednesday against the context "active", while the user is very active on Tuesday and Sunday. Figure 11 presents the total duration spent in short breaks for each day. Our model recognized the short breaks between the sedentary hours of a user. Along the *x*-axis, we placed the time in hours, and the *y*-axis presents the days.

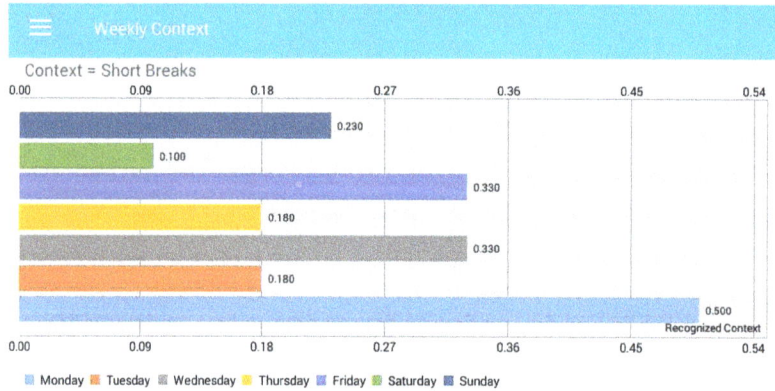

Figure 11. Total time spent during a week for "short breaks".

In Figure 11, the user took a small number of short breaks during Saturday, while a large number of short breaks can be seen on Monday. This information about the number of short breaks may help the subject to avoid longer sedentary activity, as well as provide an abstraction to compare different days. In Figure 12, we present the recognized context information while the user is working on a PC. During the wee, the user spent a maximum of 7 h on a PC, while zero hours were recognized on Wednesday.

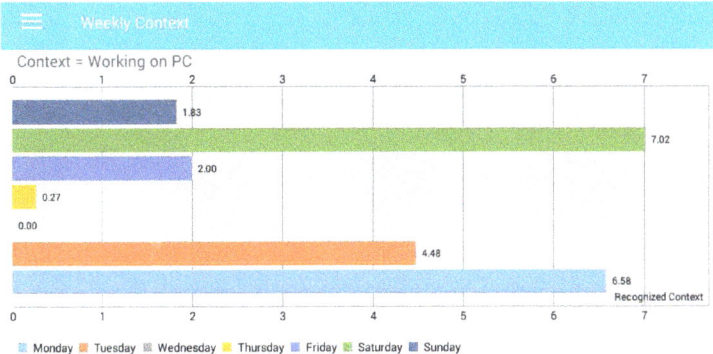

Figure 12. Total time spent during a week for "working on a PC".

In Figure 13, we can observe the total time spent while watching TV during leisure time. In the presented "weekly context", the x-axis presents the context of watching TV, while the y-axis presents the time spent in hours. Furthermore, zero means that the user did not watch the television on Monday, Tuesday, Wednesday and Thursday.

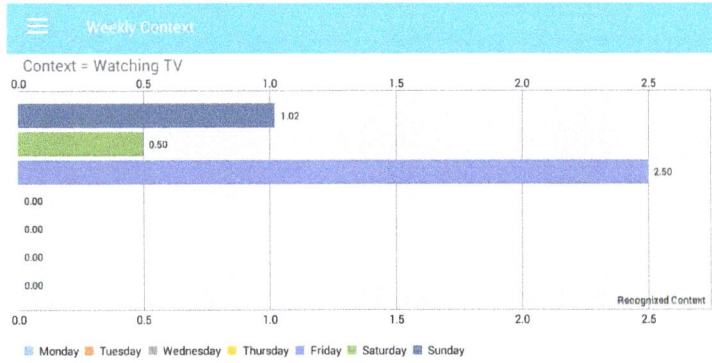

Figure 13. Total time spent during a week for "watching TV".

In Figure 14, we present the sedentary behaviour when the context is unknown. In unknown context sleeping time is also included and sedentary behaviour that is other than watching TV or working on a PC. The y-axis presents the context for the whole week, and each bar presents the number of hours spent during the sedentary activity. We found that the SitCoach [27] application is aligned in the same direction of our research. The SitCoach application monitors office workers' prolonged sitting routines and generates alerts. The alerts may help to reduce sedentary behaviour, and their intervention successfully helps office workers. Their application is restricted in terms of visualization of the user behaviour, as well as mining the micro-contexts. In our proposed research, we are providing rich information to the user about the recognized contexts. We found that self-awareness helps to reduce the sedentary behaviour and motivate the user to avoid prolonging sitting. The following section provides more details about this.

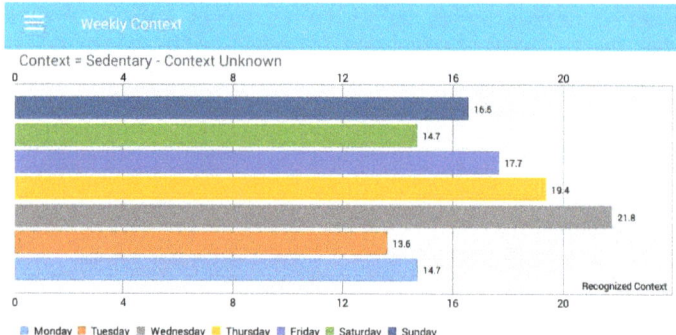

Figure 14. Total time spent during a week for "sedentary-context unknown".

5. Discussion

Context mining of sedentary behaviour and visualization of individual patterns may promote self-awareness to reduce it. In this regard, technology and hand-held smart devices can play a significant role. Whether a person spends much time in sedentary activities is somewhat dependent on the age group, health status, environmental conditions and life roles [12]. Our research goal is to promote self-awareness to reduce sedentary behaviours. Our approach identifies sedentary behaviour based on daily, weekly and monthly patterns. This information can be used to intervene in sedentary behaviour across the working hours, as well as leisure time. Furthermore, it can be used to predict the subject alarming condition while being sedentary in the future. In order to provide rationales for our study, we provide the comparison of one subjects' two-week comparison of recognized sedentary behaviour. The visualization of recognized contexts is presented in Figure 15.

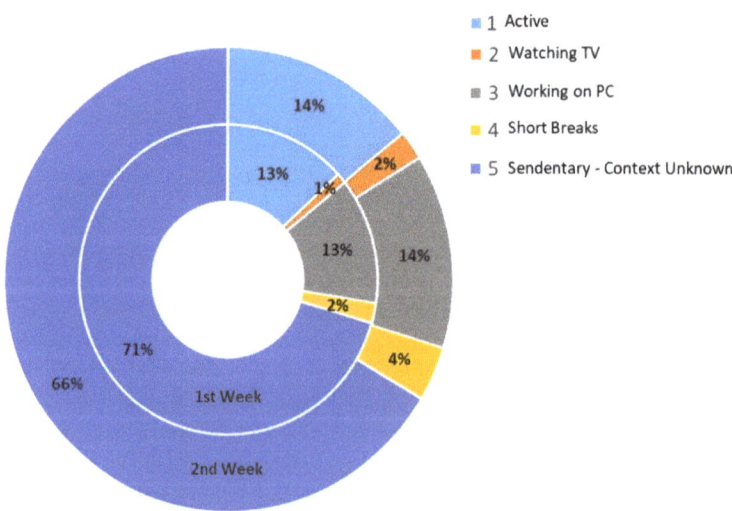

Figure 15. Two-week comparison of the mining contexts.

In Figure 15, the inner circle presents the first week recognized context in percentage, while the outer circle presents the second week contextual information. We can observe quite subtle differences in the recognized sedentary behaviour. For instance, after knowing the sedentary routines, the user took more short breaks during prolonged sitting. In Figure 15, we can observe a 50% increase in short breaks, and sedentary time is reduced from 71% to 66%. The participant also reported that after knowing his/her sedentary behaviour patterns, he/she started making small changes in his/her daily routines. For instance, he/she preferred to use stairs instead of elevators and took short breaks during prolonged sitting.

In Figure 16, we also present the accumulated results of active or still contexts in terms of hours to get abstract information about the sedentary behaviour.

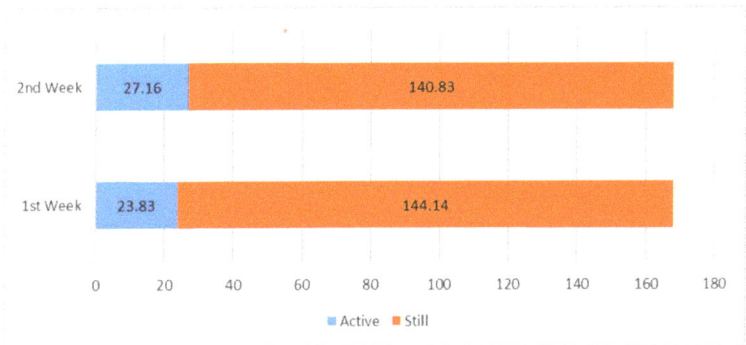

Figure 16. Time spent active or still during two weeks.

It is obvious from Figure 16 that the participants are becoming more active after knowing the sedentary patterns. Several issues with the study approach were noted throughout. In particular, our trained classifier module classifies the context "sedentary-context unknown" in certain situations where the user is working on a PC and listening to music in the background or using a PC in public places. However, we consider both situations as a sedentary context. It can be seen in Figure 17 that we presented the 57-min contextual data while participants were working on a PC and listening to music. On the other hand, the subject may not have carried his/her smartphone all the time, which may introduce errors in context recognition.

We also collected the participant feedback to find out more about the UX (i.e., user experience). The participants commented that the information they received about the sedentary behaviour is more helpful than they had expected. They found themselves checking the progress and daily status of sedentary behaviour frequently and adjusting their activity accordingly.

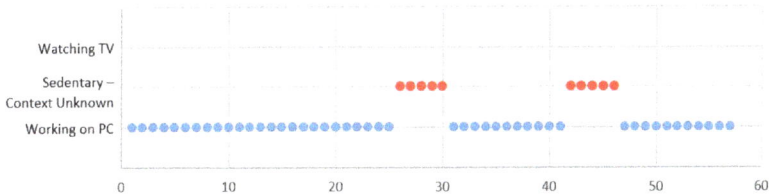

Figure 17. Misrecognized context while working on a PC.

6. Conclusions

Quantifying sedentary behaviour can provide valuable information about individuals' daily life patterns. In this research, we proposed a context-mining model to promote self-awareness by monitoring sedentary behaviour and providing a proactive platform for self-management. Participants reported a high level of satisfaction with active or sedentary behaviour, while moderate satisfaction while recognizing the micro-contexts. Micro-context recognition is a complex process that can take place in a wide variety of settings and is influenced by various environmental factors. Furthermore, our model processes the collected sensory data in real time and inside the smartphone environment, which prove the ubiquity of our solution and demonstrate how it does not require any server-side processing, which can obviously undermine privacy. Ultimately, it relaxes the assumption of a strong reliable communication channel to transfer the bulk amount of collected sensory data. The work is ongoing, and we are applying a deep learning model on environmental sound to learn more concrete contexts and situations. We are also working on a dashboard in our application, which will be able to demonstrate the visual representation of users' progress toward achieving a predetermined standard level of each behaviour for different age groups.

Acknowledgments: This research was supported by Zayed University RIF funding # R17063.

Author Contributions: Muhammad Fahim, Thar Baker and Asad Masood Khattak are the principal researchers of this research. Babar Shah, Saiqa Aleem and Fracis Chow contributed to the design of the framework. Muhammad Fahim implemented the idea in the Android platform. Asad Masood Khattak contributed to the development of the experimental protocol. All authors contributed equally to finalizing the manuscript.

Conflicts of Interest: The authors declare no conflict of interest.

References

1. He, Q.; Agu, E.O. Smartphone usage contexts and sensable patterns as predictors of future sedentary behaviours. In Proceedings of the IEEE Healthcare Innovation Point-Of-Care Technologies Conference (HI-POCT), Cancun, Mexico, 9–11 November 2016; pp. 54–57.
2. Biswas, A.; Oh, P.I.; Faulkner, G.E.; Bonsignore, A.; Pakosh, M.T.; Alter, D.A. The energy expenditure benefits of reallocating sedentary time with physical activity: A systematic review and meta-analysis. *J. Public Health* **2017**, 1–9, doi:10.1093/pubmed/fdx062.
3. Atkin, A.J.; Gorely, T.; Clemes, S.A.; Yates, T.; Edwardson, C.; Brage, S.; Salmon, J.; Marshall, S.J.; Biddle, S.J. Methods of measurement in epidemiology: Sedentary behaviour. *Int. J. Epidemiol.* **2012**, *41*, 1460–1471.
4. Park, S.; Thøgersen-Ntoumani, C.; Ntoumanis, N.; Stenling, A.; Fenton, S.A.; Veldhuijzen van Zanten, J.J. Profiles of Physical Function, Physical Activity, and Sedentary Behavior and their Associations with Mental Health in Residents of Assisted Living Facilities. *Appl. Psychol. Health Well-Being* **2017**, *9*, 60–80.
5. Vandelanotte, C.; Duncan, M.J.; Short, C.; Rockloff, M.; Ronan, K.; Happell, B.; Di Milia, L. Associations between occupational indicators and total, work-based and leisure-time sitting: A cross-sectional study. *BMC Public Health* **2013**, *13*, 1110.
6. Duncan, M.J.; Vandelanotte, C.; Trost, S.G.; Rebar, A.L.; Rogers, N.; Burton, N.W.; Murawski, B.; Rayward, A.; Fenton, S.; Brown, W.J. Balanced: A randomised trial examining the efficacy of two self-monitoring methods for an app-based multi-behaviour intervention to improve physical activity, sitting and sleep in adults. *BMC Public Health* **2016**, *16*, 670.
7. Jia, P.; Cheng, X.; Xue, H.; Wang, Y. Applications of geographic information systems (GIS) data and methods in obesity-related research. *Obes. Rev.* **2017**, *18*, 400–411.
8. Synnott, J.; Rafferty, J.; Nugent, C.D. Detection of workplace sedentary behaviour using thermal sensors. In Proceedings of the IEEE 38th Annual International Conference of the Engineering in Medicine and Biology Society (EMBC), Orlando, FL, USA, 16–20 August 2016; pp. 5413–5416.
9. Fit Bit. Available online: https://www.fitbit.com/ (accessed on 23 October 2017).
10. Google Fit. Available online: https://www.google.com/fit/ (accessed on 23 October 2017).

11. He, Q.; Agu, E.O. A frequency domain algorithm to identify recurrent sedentary behaviours from activity time-series data. In Proceedings of the IEEE-EMBS International Conference on Biomedical and Health Informatics (BHI), Las Vegas, NV, USA, 24–27 February 2016; pp. 45–48.
12. Manini, T.M.; Carr, L.J.; King, A.C.; Marshall, S.; Robinson, T.N.; Rejeski, W.J. Interventions to reduce sedentary behaviour. *Med. Sci. Sports Exerc.* **2015**, *47*, 1306.
13. Fahim, M.; Lee, S.; Yoon, Y. SUPAR: Smartphone as a ubiquitous physical activity recognizer for u-healthcare services. In Proceedings of the 36th IEEE Annual International Conference of the Engineering in Medicine and Biology Society (EMBC), Chicago, IL, USA, 26–30 August 2014; pp. 3666–3669.
14. Fahim, M.; Khattak, A.M.; Baker, T.; Chow, F.; Shah, B. Micro-context recognition of sedentary behaviour using smartphone. In Proceedings of the Sixth IEEE International Conference on Digital Information and Communication Technology and Its Applications (DICTAP), Konya, Turkey, 21–23 July 2016; pp. 30–34.
15. Wu, X.; Kumar, V.; Quinlan, J.R.; Ghosh, J.; Yang, Q.; Motoda, H.; McLachlan, G.J.; Ng, A.; Liu, B.; Philip, S.Y.; et al. Top 10 algorithms in data mining. *Knowl. Inf. Syst.* **2008**, *14*, 1–37.
16. Bonke, J. Trends in short and long sleep in Denmark from 1964 to 2009, and the associations with employment, SES (socioeconomic status) and BMI. *Sleep Med.* **2015**, *16*, 385–390.
17. Jean-Louis, G.; Williams, N.J.; Sarpong, D.; Pandey, A.; Youngstedt, S.; Zizi, F.; Ogedegbe, G. Associations between inadequate sleep and obesity in the US adult population: Analysis of the national health interview survey (1977–2009). *BMC Public Health* **2014**, *14*, 290.
18. Bauman, A.; Ainsworth, B.E.; Sallis, J.F.; Hagströmer, M.; Craig, C.L.; Bull, F.C.; Pratt, M.; Venugopal, K.; Chau, J.; Sjöström, M.; et al. The descriptive epidemiology of sitting: A 20-country comparison using the International Physical Activity Questionnaire (IPAQ). *Am. J. Prev. Med.* **2011**, *41*, 228–235.
19. Ng, S.W.; Popkin, B. Time use and physical activity: a shift away from movement across the globe. *Obes. Rev.* **2012**, *13*, 659–680.
20. Duncan, M.J.; Kline, C.E.; Rebar, A.L.; Vandelanotte, C.; Short, C.E. Greater bed-and wake-time variability is associated with less healthy lifestyle behaviours: A cross-sectional study. *J. Public Health* **2016**, *24*, 31–40.
21. Rezende, L.F.M.; Sá, T.H.; Mielke, G.I.; Viscondi, J.Y.K.; Rey-López, J.P.; Garcia, L.M.T. All-cause mortality attributable to sitting time: Analysis of 54 countries worldwide. *Am. J. Prev. Med.* **2016**, *51*, 253–263.
22. Biddle, S.; Cavill, N.; Ekelund, U.; Gorely, T.; Griffiths, M.; Jago, R.; Oppert, J.; Raats, M.; Salmon, J.; Stratton, G.; et al. Sedentary behaviour and obesity: Review of the current scientific evidence. Available online: http://epubs.surrey.ac.uk/763180/ (accessed on 14 March 2018).
23. Sasai, H. Assessing sedentary behaviour using wearable devices: An overview and future directions. *J. Phys. Fit. Sports Med.* **2017**, *6*, 135–143.
24. Matthews, C.E.; Chen, K.Y.; Freedson, P.S.; Buchowski, M.S.; Beech, B.M.; Pate, R.R.; Troiano, R.P. Amount of time spent in sedentary behaviours in the United States, 2003–2004. *Am. J. Epidemiol.* **2008**, *167*, 875–881.
25. Dobbins, C.; Merabti, M.; Fergus, P.; Llewellyn-Jones, D. A user-centred approach to reducing sedentary behaviour. In Proceedings of the IEEE 11th Consumer Communications and Networking Conference (CCNC), Las Vegas, NV, USA, 10–13 January 2014; pp. 1–6.
26. Stratton, G.; Murphy, R.; Rosenberg, M.; Fergus, P.; Attwood, A. Creating intelligent environments to monitor and manipulate physical activity and sedentary behaviour in public health and clinical settings. In Proceedings of the IEEE International Conference on Communications (ICC), Ottawa, ON, Canada, 10–15 June 2012; pp. 6111–6115.
27. Van Dantzig, S.; Geleijnse, G.; van Halteren, A.T. Toward a persuasive mobile application to reduce sedentary behaviour. *Pers. Ubiquitous Comput.* **2013**, *17*, 1237–1246.
28. Shin, Y.; Choi, W.; Shin, T. Physical activity recognition based on rotated acceleration data using quaternion in sedentary behaviour: A preliminary study. In Proceedings of the 2014 36th Annual International Conference of the Engineering in Medicine and Biology Society (EMBC), Chicago, IL, USA, 26–30 August 2014; pp. 4976–4978.
29. Butler, M. Android: Changing the mobile landscape. *IEEE Pervasive Comput.* **2011**, *10*, 4–7.
30. Fahim, M.; Fatima, I.; Lee, S.; Park, Y.T. EFM: Evolutionary fuzzy model for dynamic activities recognition using a smartphone accelerometer. *Appl. Intell.* **2013**, *39*, 475–488.
31. Banos, O.; Galvez, J.M.; Damas, M.; Pomares, H.; Rojas, I. Window size impact in human activity recognition. *Sensors* **2014**, *14*, 6474–6499.

32. Kao, T.P.; Lin, C.W.; Wang, J.S. Development of a portable activity detector for daily activity recognition. In Proceedings of the ISIE IEEE International Symposium on Industrial Electronics, Seoul, Korea, 5–8 July 2009; pp. 115–120.
33. Preece, S.J.; Goulermas, J.Y.; Kenney, L.P.; Howard, D. A comparison of feature extraction methods for the classification of dynamic activities from accelerometer data. *IEEE Trans. Biomed. Eng.* **2009**, *56*, 871–879.
34. Helmi, M.; AlModarresi, S.M.T. Human activity recognition using a fuzzy inference system. In Proceedings of the FUZZ-IEEE 2009 IEEE International Conference on Fuzzy Systems, Jeju Island, Korea, 20–24 August 2009; pp. 1897–1902.
35. Mizell, D. Using Gravity to Estimate Accelerometer Orientation. Available online: http://citeseerx.ist.psu.edu/viewdoc/download?doi=10.1.1.108.332&rep=rep1&type=pdf (accessed on 14 March 2018).
36. Lu, L.; Ge, F.; Zhao, Q.; Yan, Y. A svm-based audio event detection system. In Proceedings of the IEEE International Conference on Electrical and Control Engineering (ICECE), Wuhan, China, 25–27 June 2010; pp. 292–295.
37. Cover, T.; Hart, P. Nearest neighbour pattern classification. *IEEE Trans. Inf. Theory* **1967**, *13*, 21–27.
38. Banos, O.; Damas, M.; Pomares, H.; Prieto, A.; Rojas, I. Daily living activity recognition based on statistical feature quality group selection. *Expert Syst. Appl.* **2012**, *39*, 8013–8021.
39. Banos, O.; Damas, M.; Pomares, H.; Rojas, I. On the use of sensor fusion to reduce the impact of rotational and additive noise in human activity recognition. *Sensors* **2012**, *12*, 8039–8054.
40. Atul, J.; Johnson, D.; Kiran, M.; Murthy, R.; Vivek, C. OpenStack Beginner's Guide (for Ubuntu–Precise). CSS CORP, May 2012. Available online: https://cssoss.files.wordpress.com/2012/05/openstackbookv3-0_csscorp2.pdf (accessed on 14 March 2018).
41. Fahim, M.; Idris, M.; Ali, R.; Nugent, C.; Kang, B.; Huh, E.N.; Lee, S. ATHENA: A personalized platform to promote an active lifestyle and wellbeing based on physical, mental and social health primitives. *Sensors* **2014**, *14*, 9313–9329.
42. Machine Learning Research Laboratory. Available online: http://ml.ce.izu.edu.tr/ (accessed on 23 October 2017).
43. MPAndroidChart. Available online: https://github.com/PhilJay/MPAndroidChart/ (accessed on 23 October 2017).

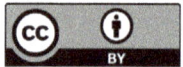

© 2018 by the authors. Licensee MDPI, Basel, Switzerland. This article is an open access article distributed under the terms and conditions of the Creative Commons Attribution (CC BY) license (http://creativecommons.org/licenses/by/4.0/).

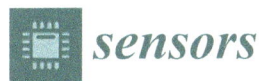

Article

Increasing the Intensity over Time of an Electric-Assist Bike Based on the User and Route: The Bike Becomes the Gym

Daniel H. De La Iglesia [1,*], Juan F. De Paz [1], Gabriel Villarrubia González [1], Alberto L. Barriuso [1], Javier Bajo [2] and Juan M. Corchado [1]

1 Computer and Automation Department, University of Salamanca, 37002 Salamanca, Spain; fcofds@usal.es (J.F.D.P.); gvg@usal.es (G.V.G.); albarriuso@usal.es (A.L.B.); corchado@usal.es (J.M.C.)
2 Artificial Intelligence Department, Polytechnic University of Madrid, 28660 Madrid, Spain; jbajo@fi.upm.es
* Correspondence: danihiglesias@usal.es; Tel.: +34-923-294-500 (ext. 5476)

Received: 27 October 2017; Accepted: 12 January 2018; Published: 14 January 2018

Abstract: Nowadays, many citizens have busy days that make finding time for physical activity difficult. Thus, it is important to provide citizens with tools that allow them to introduce physical activity into their lives as part of the day's routine. This article proposes an app for an electric pedal-assist-system (PAS) bicycle that increases the pedaling intensity so the bicyclist can achieve higher and higher levels of physical activity. The app includes personalized assist levels that have been adapted to the user's strength/ability and a profile of the route, segmented according to its slopes. Additionally, a social component motivates interaction and competition between users based on a scoring system that shows the level of their performances. To test the training module, a case study in three different European countries lasted four months and included nine people who traveled 551 routes. The electric PAS bicycle with the app that increases intensity of physical activity shows promise for increasing levels of physical activity as a regular part of the day.

Keywords: personalized assistance level; coaching; physical activity; electric bicycles

1. Introduction

Advances in the field of technology and developments in common transport systems have greatly reduced people's physical activity [1]. In developed countries, the majority of people travel to and from work using motor transport systems, e.g., statistics from 2011 show that, in England and Wales, 85% of the population used motorized transport as their usual commute mode [2]. Nowadays, citizens spend much more time at sedentary activities, such as working in front of the computer. In 2012, data from 66 high and low income countries show that the percentage of adults who spent four or more hours sitting each day was 41.5% [1]. Due to these changes in our lifestyle, the risk of suffering health problems as a result of physical activity is increasingly high [3]. Experts from diverse entities, such as WHO (World Health Organization), recommend an average of 150 min of exercise per week or 30 min daily [4]. Physical activity provides a well-known set of health benefits [5]. Exercise has been proven to reduce the risk of suffering from high blood pressure, stroke and others [4]. It increases cardiorespiratory and muscular fitness, bone health or increased functional health. Moreover, it can help prevent depression [4]. In 2010, the Global Health Observatory (GHO) estimated that the daily physical activity of more than 20% of adults is insufficient [6]. The low exercise, combined with the daily ingestion of fat and calorie rich foods, is leading our society to an obesity epidemic [7].

Nowadays, people who wish to make exercise a part of their daily routine usually go to gyms or sign up for different sports. This commitment implies an economic cost of registration and sports equipment, travel to sports centers, as well as the necessary free time to carry out the activity and a willingness to attend regularly. Performing a team sport (e.g., basketball, football or volleyball) also requires adequate sports facilities, a group of people to carry out the activity and a skill in that sport. For these reasons, many people do not perform physical activity regularly [8,9]. As a result, the daily use of a bicycle in routine trips is an important alternative to the gym or other sports [10].

One of the most widespread ways of fostering active transport among users is by promoting the use of bicycles in the city [11,12]. Biking will not only help people to get fit but will also reduce traffic congestion, environmental contamination, climate change and energetic sustainability [13,14]. The upgrading of infrastructures for cyclists helps provide a positive experience and as a result increases the use of bicycles in the city [15,16]. In recent years, cities have been promoting the use of bicycles through the implementation of bicycle-sharing systems (BSS), in order to allow users to travel short distances by bike [17]. Recent studies have shown that the use of BSS has a positive impact on health [18] and reduces the use of motor vehicles [19,20].

A decisive factor for encouraging the use of bicycles is the development of electric bicycles or e-bikes. An electric bicycle consists of three main elements: Engine, battery and control system. These elements are installed in a conventional pedal assist bicycle, which combines the power exerted by the user with the power supplied by the electric set. In comparison to conventional bicycles, these are power assisted bicycles which can travel greater distances, providing greater mobility and reducing barriers (such as age, physical limitations, steep slopes, and lack of time) [21].

Some people have barriers that make the use of a traditional bike challenging or impossible, however electric bicycles may give them an opportunity to start cycling [22]. Bicycles of this type are essential if an increase in the number of bikers in the city is to be achieved [23]. Electric bicycles can help users get active, especially those who have a sedentary work, can at least do exercise by cycling between home and work [24]. The bicycle industry esteems that the e-bike market will continue to grow. It is estimated that, in the last decade, more than 150 million electric bicycles have been sold worldwide [25]. In 2015, 1.2 million were sold in Europe, and it is estimated that this number will triple in 2022 [25]. The increase of sales is a result of the relatively low cost of these vehicles (generally, less than 1000 euros) and they are increasing in popularity over scooters [26,27]. In addition, the new e-bike BSS systems are increasingly popular among users in comparison to traditional bicycles because they make travel easier and more comfortable when factors such as long travel distance, high temperatures or poor air quality are involved [28]. On the current market, it is possible to find two types of electric bicycles [26]: Throttle electric bikes and Pedal Assist Systems (PAS) e-bikes.

Of these electric bikes, the throttle e-bike [29], offer an acceleration device to the users, similar to the one used on the handlebar of mopeds. With this system, the users can activate and deactivate the assistance of the engine, as well as regulate its intensity. Thus, the user is in total control of the assistance provided by the engine, making the use of bicycles much simpler. The use of pedals and the user's physical implication is optional, given that the user does not have to put any physical effort into activating the accelerator. Generally, these bicycles are used by expert users who wish to have precise control of the level of power supplied by the engine. In many countries, such as Spain, Finland or the UK, there are strict rules that regulate the users of these bicycles. In Spain, the use of these bicycles on public roads is prohibited and, to be able to use them, the user needs to have liability insurance.

Assist level electric bicycles or bicycles with a PAS, function differently. Unlike in throttle electric bicycles where, thanks to the acceleration system, the user does not have to exert any physical pressure on the pedals, in PAS bicycles, it is necessary [29]. These e-bikes incorporate a sensor that registers the pedaling velocity of the user and activate the electric engine when pedaling starts. As to the control of the power supplied by the engine, a set of assist levels is employed which will progressively increase or decrease the power provided. A remote control installed on the bike's handlebar is used to manage assistance levels, it can also be used to interact with any app for smartphones. In this way, the user can freely perform all the operations without removing his hands from the handlebar. The use of these bicycles is also regulated by the law in many European countries. In countries such as Spain and the UK, engine assistance cannot exceed 25 km/h and the electric power of the engine cannot be greater than 250 W [30]. Moreover, the engine has to remain in a resting state when the user stops pedaling. The proposed system is designed for PAS bicycles. Almost all the commercial electric bicycles that we find on the current market are pedal assist.

While electric-bikes lower the levels of physical activity compared with pedaling a regular bike, pedaling a regular bike on flat land for a very short distance is beneficial but not necessarily highly health-inducing. Individuals could go to the gym or engage in sports but that takes time and money. The goal of this work is to increase the levels of physical activity while riding an electric bike, thus allowing the bike to become the gym through an activity that is a routine part of the day. A secondary goal is to achieve an increase in the number of bicyclists, either riding regular bikes or electric-assist bikes. To this end, a personalized pedaling intensity level system for power assisted electric bicycle users has been developed. With this system, users will be able to gradually progress their physical activity, as they travel different routes on their e-bikes. Many studies have shown that riding on a bicycle with constant or incremental velocity in time has significant health benefits [31,32] and contributes to the user's fitness [33].

2. Background

In the current literature, it is possible to find numerous studies that address the use of mobile devices as a means of encouraging physical activity. The authors studied the influence of apps that send motivational messages or messages that provide information on performing an exercise to the users' mobiles [34–39]. The results of these studies show that users' physical activity improves significantly, e.g., out of the 149 users in the case study [37], the group that used a mobile phone lost per month an average of 0.5 kg more than the control group. In a review, the authors analyze the effectiveness of using a Smartphone for the promotion of daily activity [40]. However, only 6 out of the 13 articles have recorded a change in the behavior of users. Recent studies conducted with patients in medical centers, measured the progress of patients in rehabilitation by counting the number of steps they walked daily, the doctor could then evaluate their progress by comparing these numbers [41,42]. These studies have demonstrated that with the use of a Smartphone and with the supervision of a medical professional, the patients' daily physical activity could be increased.

Moreover, social environments can also be very effective in encouraging exercise. In other study, the authors questioned whether it would be more effective to encourage physical activity through support among users as opposed to competition [43]. The authors demonstrated that social competition had a greater influence over users than the social support of their friends. Other authors describes a combination of an augmented reality game, such as Pokémon Go [44] with social interaction among users, which succeeded at increasing users' physical activity [45].

The use of video games or active video games (AVGs) as a means of promoting physical activity, has also been widely studied. Authors reviewed 52 articles which were focused on AVG systems in [46]. After the analysis of these studies, the authors pointed to an increased interest in light and moderate activities. However, these systems are not likely to produce any significant changes in sedentary behavior. Only the youngest part of our population could benefit from using AVGs but they are not considered to be an effective tool for increasing daily activity.

Recent studies, looked for solutions that promote active forms of transport, such as walking or cycling, with the use of Smartphone applications that monitor physical activity [47]. These authors' goal was to improve active transport and increase daily physical activity when commuting in the city [48]. Electric bicycles were viewed as a new method for promoting daily physical activity [49]. Authors looked at electric bicycles as tools that can benefit the health of elderly people and be a fun and practical way of incorporating exercise into their daily commute [50]. Moreover, authors studied the health benefits of swapping the car for an electric bicycle, especially when used for daily commuting [51]. Other studies analyzed security mechanisms for electric bicycle users, where the user's heart rate determined the level of assistance that was provided to them [52–54]. These mechanisms make it possible for people with health problems to use e-bikes safely.

After a careful analysis of the current literature, no studies were found on the increase of pedaling intensity over time in e-bikes. No relevant research has been conducted in this area. Thus, the proposal made in this study is novel as it is focused specifically on the area of e-bikes and on using them as tools for encouraging physical activity and increasing the intensity of exercise. Therefore, this work proposes a novelty among studies focused on promoting and increasing the intensity of physical activities, specifically for e-bikes. Consequently, this work makes the first reference to this field of study, with the aim of encouraging other researchers to address this problem.

3. System Overview

This section describes the different elements that make up the final system proposed in this work. It is a personalized system whose purpose is to adjust the intensity of exercise for electric bicycle users, in this way facilitating their progress which is marked by the different ability levels. The objective of the system is to promote physical activity among users, with training that is constant and incremental in its intensity. Figure 1 shows the different components that make up the designed system. First, a user of an electric bicycle that is registered in the mobile application, activates the "training" mode and selects the route that they wish to travel. The selected route can be a mountain route or a simple ride, such as the usual route from home to work. Optionally, users can have a Heart Rate sensor which takes their pulse, it allows to measure progress, estimate effort and prevent fatigue. Once the user selects the route they want to travel, it is sent to the remote server which is in charge of managing the data of the platform. When obtained, the server divides the route into segments in order to calculate the power required to travel the route. This is done by establishing the assist level for each of the segments; this level is calculated by considering the user's physical characteristics (height and weight), his ability level (beginner, intermediate, advanced), the characteristics of the electric bicycle (power, battery, weight) and the profile of the route (slope and distance). The objective of calculating assist levels is to prevent excessive variations in velocity over the whole route, by combining the power supplied by the engine with the power provided by the user. The power provided by the user will increase gradually, with each of the exercises that he completes on the platform. Time will not be the only factor taken into account when calculating the difficulty of the travelled route, the slopes found on that route will also be considered. In this way, it will be possible to compare the different routes more effectively.

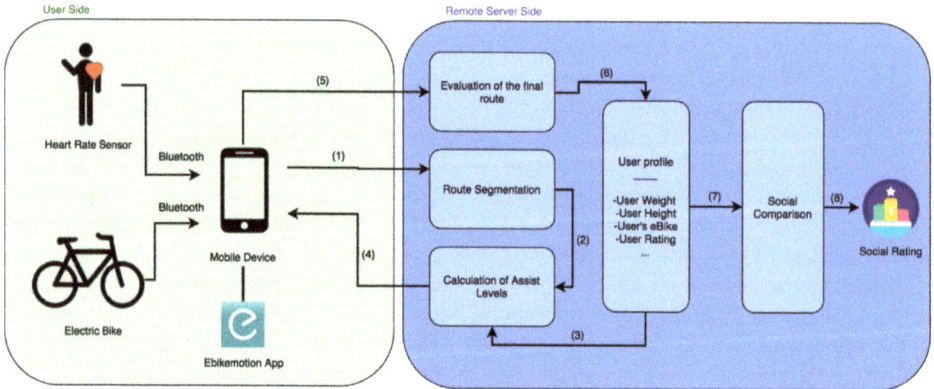

Figure 1. Overall architecture of the system: (**1**) the route selected by the user; (**2**) segmented route; (**3**) user profile data; (**4**) calculated assist levels; (**5**) data collected over the course of the route; (**6**) score obtained on the route; (**7**) comparison of the scores of other users; and (**8**) final social rating.

The resulting assist levels are sent to the user's mobile application, together with the waypoints indicating the beginning of each segment. Over the course of the ride, the assist levels will change automatically when the user reaches the different waypoints. Once the route is completed, the application will send the data registered over the course of the route to the server, which will proceed with their analysis. After the evaluation of the results, the system moves on to calculating the score obtained by the user in the route he completed. The scores obtained in different routes accumulate to a total and the general rating of the user is obtained. These data are necessary for evaluating the user's progress and for calculating the assist levels of future routes.

Finally, the system has an interactive component based on the development social competition. This element allows users to view their progress in comparison to others, to suggest improvements and routes based on their profile. It also allows motivating them through a series of general ratings and the ratings made by friends who use the application.

3.1. Electric Bike and Sensor Data

3.1.1. Assist Levels

As described in the previous paragraph, PAS bicycles increase or decrease the power supplied by the engine with a set of assist levels. Not all electric bicycle manufacturers configure assist levels in the same way. However, in the majority of cases, assist levels oscillate between 5 and 10 levels. There are also bicycles that have a lower power engine which only has a total of three assist levels. However, independently of the assist levels available in bicycles, their functioning is similar in the majority of cases. Each of the assist levels provides an incremental percentage of power. Higher levels provide greater power than lower levels.

Figure 2 shows a graph of the power supplied by an electric bicycle with an engine of 750 W and a total of five assist levels. As it can be observed, the first assist levels provide less power, what means lower velocity, while the highest level provides the maximum power of the engine. In some bicycle models, it is possible to configure engine settings associated with assist levels. In this way, an advanced user could configure the established power profile, so that it suits his needs. The relation between watts and assist levels is obtained directly from the mobile application, since it is possible to monitor the intensity of the battery current at the different levels. Thanks to this possibility, the system is suitable for different types of batteries and engines with no previous configurations.

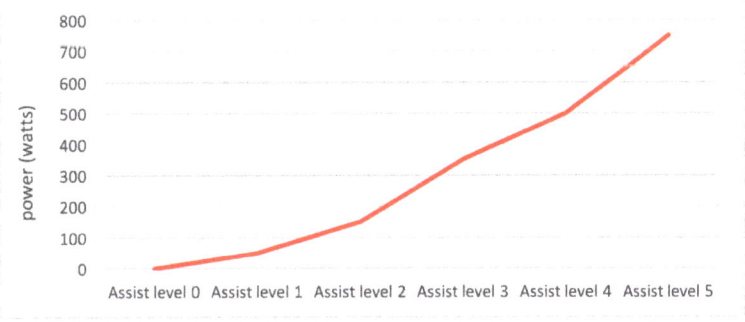

Figure 2. Assist levels and power in an e-bike of 750 w.

When controlling assistance, it is necessary to have a device connected to the bicycle's control system, capable of increasing and decreasing the power. Commercial bicycles have a remote control installed on their handlebar, through which the user can control the behavior of the electric system. Figure 3 shows three different models of remote controls for electric bicycles. Generally, these remote controls, besides an on/off button, also have two additional buttons: one for increasing the assist level and another for decreasing it. They also incorporate Bluetooth wireless communication technology. Some models, such as the iwok model (Figure 3b), incorporate auxiliary buttons, which make it possible to interact with the *ebikemotion* mobile application.

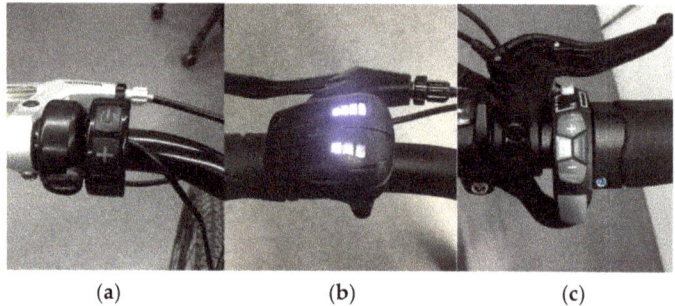

Figure 3. Example of three assist level commercial controllers: (**a**) Bafang controller; (**b**) *ebikemotion* controller; and (**c**) BionX controller.

The remote control is not the only control interface for the assist levels of an electric bicycle. Manufacturers incorporate a control interface in their communication protocols through commands sent by a third party, such as a mobile application. Thanks to this interface, the assistance of an electric bicycle can change automatically and it is not necessary for a user to intervene. This is a fundamental element in this work; as the user travels a route in the "training" mode, the system will change the assist levels in the e-bike in a dynamic and independent manner, by means of the application.

3.1.2. Heart Rate Sensor

The system measures the heart rate by means of an external wireless heart rate sensor connected to the app by Bluetooth. Any of the current commercial sensors with Bluetooth 4.0 is compatible and can be used in the system. There are two reasons for which in the proposed system the user's heart rate is measured by an external sensor. On the one hand, to register the user's improvement along the different exercises he does, which is key for establishing the level of progress and physical development. Users who are not physically fit have a greater number of ppm (pulsations per minute) than users who are used to exercise. The continuous evaluation of changes in the heart rate, while the user performs physical activities, is an important indicator of the user's progress, as reported previously in different works [55].

Similarly, the heart rate registered during a physical activity, such as cycling, provides a measure of the athlete's effort. When calculating the training thresholds, the time the user spent exercising at each of the training zones has to be considered together with the maximum heart rate. This value is calculated based on Equation (1), which has been previously described in the literature [56]. This is the most accepted way of calculating the heart rate even though it has a significant margin of error, so it should be considered as an approximate value and in no case as a precise value.

$$HR_{max} = 205.8 - 0.685 \cdot (age) \tag{1}$$

Table 1, is a general list of the four main training zones for an athlete during physical exercise, as described in [57]. The designed system can calculate the percentage of time that a user spent training in each of these zones, for each of the routes he travelled; this measures the quality of exercise. Zone 1 is considered as exercise that is safe for the heart and is recommended to users who are only beginning to introduce physical activity into their daily routine and who are not physically fit. Zone

3 is considered the anaerobic threshold and it is a turning point in the improvement of capabilities, from here a decrease in performance can be observed. Lastly, training zone 4, can only be maintained during a few seconds and can only be achieved by users with a high level of physical training.

Table 1. Heart Rate training zones.

Target Zone	Intensity% of HR_{max} (bpm)	Training Benefit
Zone 1: Light	50–60%	Increases overall health and metabolism
Zone 2: Moderate	70–80%	Improves aerobic fitness
Zone 3: Hard	80–90%	Increases maximum performance capacity
Zone 4: Maximum	90–100%	Increases maximum sprint race speed

The use of a heart rate sensor is not only important for measuring physical progress. In the designed system, the monitoring of the user's pulse is also seen as a security measure that helps to avoid and prevent fatigue. When the system detects the user's pulse to be very high, over the maximum threshold, the assistance system increases the power of the engine automatically. In this way, the user is helped in his exercise and their heart rate is reduced. This threshold can be established manually by the user on the mobile application or it can be calculated automatically with Equation (1).

3.1.3. *ebikemotion* App

The *ebikemotion* project has been co-developed by the University of Salamanca and the company StageMotion [58]. The *ebikemotion* application for mobile devices [59] is central to the system developed in this article. This application, is compatible with more than 20 electric bicycle brands on the market and it has more than 5000 users from all over the world. This application visualizes all the values of the electric bicycle in real-time (battery level, assist level, velocity, altitude etc.) as can be seen in Figure 4. This application is free and is available in the two main mobile operating systems, Android and iOS. The application was launched in the middle of 2016 and it is possible to use it with electric bicycles as well as with traditional bicycles for recording routes via GPS.

As part of this work, a "training" module has been designed for this application. This application will be in charge of registering the values of the different routes travelled by the user in the "training" mode and of automatically changing the assist levels on the basis of the parameters calculated by the server. The application is linked to the e-bike by Bluetooth wireless technology. Some e-bike models obtain their Bluetooth connection through the remote control while in other models this technology is incorporated in the casing of the battery of the e-bike.

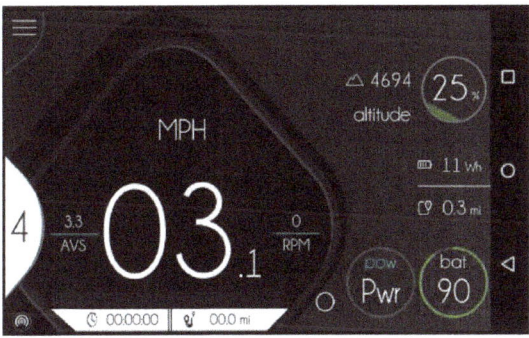

Figure 4. Screenshot of *ebikemotion* app.

3.2. Route Segmentation

The routes travelled by the users through the exercise plan have a high number of GPS localizations. First, it is necessary to identify each of the segments that make up a given route. To this end, the route is segmented into independent sections of different lengths that are connected to each other. The aim of performing this segmentation is to be able to make an individual analysis of each section; reducing its complexity and establishing the assist level required for that route. As described previously, electric bicycles are operated through a series of assist levels, where each one corresponds to a particular amount of power that is provided by the engine. The higher the assist level, the greater the power generated by the engine. Thus, the higher is the assist level, the lesser is the effort of the user.

The second criterion for making this division is based on the difference of slopes at the different points of the route. Slopes are obtained for each of the GPS points p, therefore it is possible to group the adjacent route points which have similar magnitude of slope g_i, in the same segment S_i. The segments obtained can have different lengths l_i. Thus, a route with origin **O** and destination **D** is divided into a series of $i = 1, \ldots, N$ segments S_i, which are connected one to another, as shown in Figure 5.

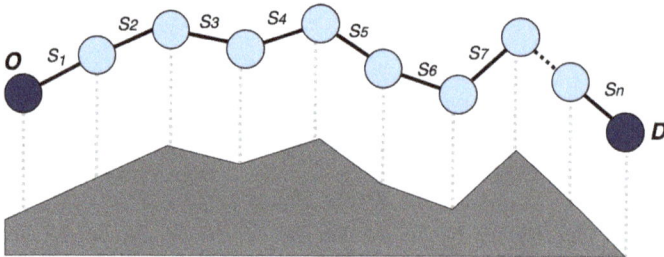

Figure 5. Example of route segmentation. The bottom side and the upper side of the route is segmented according to its profile.

By grouping the points p according to the magnitude of the slope, the profile of the route is reconstructed with the set of segments S_i, as can be seen in Figure 5. Thanks to this grouping, it is possible to establish a single assist level for each segment; this level will be adapted to its slope. When calculating the starting and ending waypoints of a segment, not only the magnitudes of these points should be considered but also the magnitudes of the adjacent points.

The algorithm used to perform this segmentation is based on the previous work of the same authors [60]. In the segmentation algorithm, does not only consider whether the slope is positive or negative, its magnitude is also considered. In this way, within segments with slopes of the same signs, different segments can be grouped according to their magnitude. As for segments of 0% slope, they are considered to be positive or negative, according to the adjacent slopes.

3.3. Calculation of Assist Level

When the system calculates the assist level for each segment, two elements are taken into account. On the one hand, the user's ability level (calculated with the scores obtained on the routes they travelled previously in the "training" mode). On the other hand, the average slope of the segment within the route. The objective is to apportion the power required, according to the level of assist for each of the segments. The power provided by the engine must be complemented with the power derived from the user's physical effort. Thus, the sum of the power to be supplied by the engine and the power that is to be provided by the user in each of the segments, is the total power required to travel the route, as shown in Equation (2).

$$\sum_{i=0}^{n}(p_g + p_u) = \text{Total power to travel a route} \qquad (2)$$

where p_g represents the power supplied by the engine and p_u the power supplied by the user, in each segment n of a route.

To calculate the power required to cycle a bike route, it is necessary to apply Equation (3) as described in [61].

$$P = k_r M s + k_a A s v^2 d + g i M s \qquad (3)$$

where

- P: Represents the total power required to cycle a route, in watts.
- k_r: Rolling resistance coefficient, is a constant (0.005).
- M: Mass of the bike and the cyclist.
- s: Speed of the bike on the road.
- k_a: Wind resistance coefficient, is a constant (0.5).
- A: The frontal area of the bike and cyclist.
- v: Speed of the bike through the air (bike speed +headwind or −tailwind).
- d: Air density, is a constant (1.226 kg/m^3).
- g: Gravitational constant (9.8 m/s^2).
- i: Gradient (slope).

Equation (3) can be divided into three different parts. In the first part ($k_r M s$) calculates the power necessary to overcome the resistance produced by the friction between the wheel and the ground. For this part, it is necessary to add the power required to overcome wind resistance ($k_a A s v^2 d$) and finally the power required to overcome the resistance of the slope of the road ($g i M s$).

To calculate the total mass (sum of the mass of the user and the mass of the bicycle), the user's profile with their data is accessed. The weight of the bicycle is also known since the system registers the bicycle that the user is using to cycle a route. Likewise, knowing the user's height and the size of the bicycle, makes it possible to obtain the user's frontal area.

For the system designed in this work, speed is considered to be a key factor. From the user's overall score (which is the sum of the points obtained at previous routes), the average speed that is to be maintained constant by the user during the completion of a new route is determined. The goal of the "training" mode is to maintain a constant average speed throughout the route, regardless of its profile, and to increase that speed progressively at new routes. In this way, the user gradually observes progress in his training, as the average speed at the routes they cycle is increased and the power supplied by the engine is reduced. Table 2 shows the ability levels established in the system and the score necessary to reach each one of them. The table also indicates the average speed at each of the levels which is used to calculate the power. These power estimates are defined, in ideal conditions, for a person of 75 kg and a bicycle of 8 kg (a total of 83 kg).

Each route is divided into a set of segments, as shown in Figure 5 and Equation (4).

$$r = \{S_1, \ldots, S_n\} \qquad (4)$$

The slope of each segment within a route is calculated, thus obtaining a set of values for each of the segments (Equation (5)).

$$I = \{h_1, \ldots, h_n\} \qquad (5)$$

For each segment S_i, the automatic assist level is calculated. First, the power that is to be generated by the user is established. The power p is kept constant for each of the intervals and the speed of the user is determined using the formula indicated in Equation (3). The speed calculated for each interval is shown in Equation (6).

$$V = \{v_1, \ldots, v_n\} \tag{6}$$

At this point, the tentative speed v' that is to be maintained is considered and the power that should be generated to maintain that speed v' is calculated for each interval (Equation (7)).

$$P = \{p_1, \ldots, p_n\} \tag{7}$$

The power supplied by the battery will be the difference between the power required to maintain the speed constant at each interval and the p value maintained by the user (Equation (8)).

$$P\prime = \{p'_1 = p_1 - p, \ldots, p'_n = p_n - p\} \tag{8}$$

Once the p'_i values are obtained, the level of assist is calculated. Each assist level r is associated with a power p^l_r, whereby the possible power values are as given in Equation (9).

$$p^l = \left\{0, p^l_1, \ldots, p^l_r\right\} \tag{9}$$

Based on the power values defined in Equation (9), the power intervals are established Equation (10).

$$I = \left\{ \left[0, \frac{0 + p^l_1}{2}\right), \left[\frac{p^l_1 + p^l_2}{2}, \frac{p^l_2 + p^l_3}{2}\right), \ldots, \left[\frac{p^l_{r-1} + p^l_r}{2}, p^l_r\right] \right\} \tag{10}$$

Therefore, the assistance for segment q defined as p^e_q, is represented by Equation (11).

$$p^e_q = p^l_j / \left[\frac{p^l_{j-1} + p^l_j}{2}, \frac{p^l_j + p^l_{j+1}}{2}\right) \tag{11}$$

As shown in Figure 6, after establishing the assist levels for each segment, the amount of power that the user must provide and the power that the bicycle must supply is determined. The total sum of the powers must be equal to the power required to travel the segment at a constant speed.

Table 2. Ability levels, average speed and the score required for each level.

Level	Average Speed	Total Points	Power in 0% Slope
Level 1	15 km/h	[0, 50]	33.19 Watts
Level 2	17 km/h	[51, 100]	42.35 Watts
Level 3	18 km/h	[101, 150]	4757 Watts
Level 4	19 km/h	[151, 200]	53.27 Watts
Level 5	20 km/h	[201, 250]	59.46 Watts
Level 6	21 km/h	[251, 300]	66.17 Watts
Level 7	23 km/h	[301, 350]	81.27 Watts
Level 8	25 km/h	[351, 400]	98.76 Watts
Level 9	26 km/h	[401, 500]	108.47 Watts
Level 10	28 km/h	[501, 600]	129.95 Watts

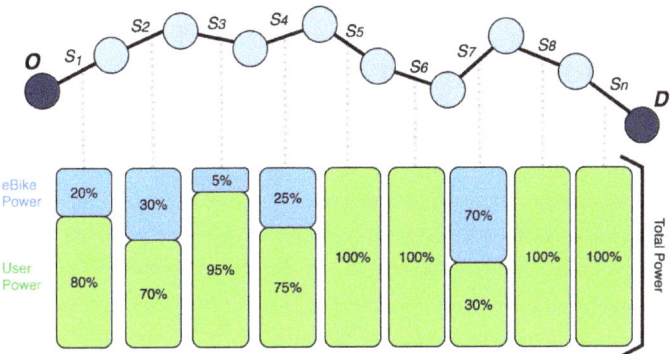

Figure 6. Example of how power is distributed for each of the segments of a route.

3.4. Evaluation of the Final Route

An important aspect is the evaluation of the user's performance on the routes cycled. However, to be able to make a fair evaluation of these routes it must be taken into account that the profile of each route is different. Thus, a procedure has been designed to make a fair comparison. The power generated by the user over the course of the route is the aspect that is considered in the evaluation; as it can be seen in Equation (3), the calculation of this power depends on a number of factors. The power generated by the user is defined in Equation (12).

$$p_u = \sum_{i=1}^{n}(p_i - p_i^e) \quad (12)$$

Once the power generated by the user has been calculated, the system determines the final score that is to be awarded for the route represented by s_r. This score will accrue to the one already obtained by the user. The score is therefore calculated as Equation (13):

$$s_r = \begin{cases} p_u & p_u < 600 \\ 600 & eoc \end{cases} \quad (13)$$

The value of 600 W is considered as the energy required to maintain an average speed of 50 km/h for one hour on a flat surface, considering a user of 75 kg and a bicycle of 8 kg and with average parameters for the coefficients of friction, resistance etc. Considering the records registered by International Cyclist Union [62], the 600 W value is the maximum limit for a person.

3.5. Social Competition for the Promotion of Physical Activity

The objective of the proposed system is to promote users' physical activity through the cycling of routes on electric bicycles. Thanks to social interaction through the application, users are motivated to compete with each other by increasing their physical activity. As described previously, the application implements a social component in order to provide users with a comparative of their progress. The system generates three different rankings on the application; general ranking by area (includes the scores of users in the same location) which shows 10 users with higher scoring. Another ranking with users who have similar profiles (age, gender, routes cycled, the number of routes cycled per week). Finally, a ranking with the user's friends on Facebook. The *ebikemotion* application has native support for Facebook, making it simple for users to find friends on the social network through the application. Eighty-six percent of current *ebikemotion* users have their Facebook account linked to the application, this shows that social interaction among users is high.

4. Case Study

To validate the proposed system, a case study was carried out with real participants using the platform and the application for mobile devices called *ebikemotion*. The testing took place over four months between March and June of 2017 and included nine participants who travelled a total of 551 routes. Out of the nine case study participants, seven were located in Spain (five in Salamanca and two in Palencia), one in Italy (Volverra) and another in Switzerland (Corseaux). All of them are members of the team that worked on developing the software and hardware of the *ebikemotion* platform and on its testing. None of the participants presented any notable health problems and they were not remunerated for their collaboration in the study. All participants wore a heart rate sensor that was compatible with the app. After completing the study, the users made a personal evaluation of their experience in the study.

Before starting the study, the participants' physical fitness was determined to make two groups of users: Users with high physical activity and users with low physical activity. Users with high physical activity are those who practice sports for more than 6 h a week, including cycling. Users who have low physical activity are those who do exercise for less than 3 h a week and do not use the bicycle. The objective of distinguishing these two groups is to be able to compare the progress of the most active users with that of less active users. Table 3 defines the characteristics of the nine users participating in the study. As can be seen, Users 1, 2, 3, 5, 8 have a high activity during the week, exceeding 9 h of exercise per week, while Users 6, 7, 4, 9 have very little physical activity during the week.

Table 3. Set of users for the case of study.

User	Sex	Age	Hours of Activity/Week
User 1	Male	33	13 h
User 2	Male	29	10 h
User 3	Male	32	9 h
User 4	Female	26	1 h
User 5	Male	42	10.5 h
User 6	Female	31	1 h
User 7	Male	28	0 h
User 8	Male	30	0 h
User 9	Female	27	1 h

For the purposes of this case study, all participants had an electric bicycle at their disposal. All bicycles were equipped with the PAS system and were compatible with the *ebikemotion* application. The bicycle of User 1 was road type while the rest of the users' bikes were MTB type or city bikes. The power of the engines of the different bicycles oscillated depending on their model, ranging in their maximum power from 250 W to 750 W.

5. Results and Discussion

5.1. Route Analysis

To illustrate how the route analysis system described in the work functions, a detailed analysis of one of the routes cycled by one of the users was carried out. It is a 14.5 km route in the city of Corseaux (Switzerland) whose altitude profile is shown in Figure 7. The route was made with a 750 W electric bike with a configuration of six levels of assist, as shown in Figure 2. First, the route was processed using the previously described algorithm to divide it into segments. After this analysis, the system determined that the route was composed of a total of 200 segments. Next, the system calculated the power that the user must provide and the power that the engine must supply to perform the exercise. As detailed in Section 3.3, in this calculation, it is necessary to consider the slope of each segment and the user's ability level in the system. In this case, the user had ability level 4, so the system determined their average speed to be 19 km/h over the course of the route. Based on these data, levels of assist are established for each of the segments. The resulting set of assist levels is shown in Figure 8. Finally, these assist levels are sent to the mobile application and the user begins the route.

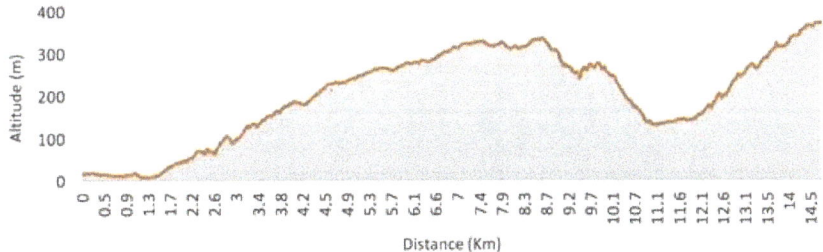

Figure 7. Profile (in altitude) of the analyzed route.

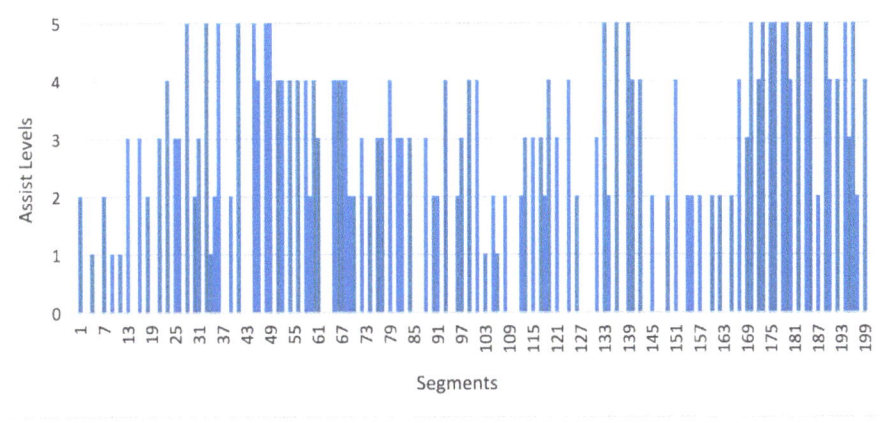

Figure 8. Levels of assistance calculated for each segment.

Once the route is completed, the data collected over the course of the route are sent to the central server for analysis. In Figure 9, we can see the actual power that was provided by the engine (in blue) and the power provided by the user (in green). First, Figure 8 shows how the amount of power is adjusted to the slopes of the route. A greater amount of power has been provided in the segment from 2 to 4 km, due to the inclination of that part of the route. The same happened in the segment from 9 to 10 km and in the final segment of the route, from 12 to 14.5 km. On the contrary, at the segment starting at 10 km and finishing at 12 km, the power provided is lower since the slope of this part of the route is descending. It is also possible to observe how the user's speed is kept as constant as possible on the slopes, although if the selected speed is very high, the power of the engine does not allow the speed to be maintained. With this system, the user's physical effort is not affected by the profile of the route. Regardless of the profile of the route, speed is kept as constant as possible; this helps prevent fatigue and makes exercise healthier. In addition, a heart rate monitor is employed as a safety measure which allows to increase the level of assistance automatically when the threshold of pulsations per minute is exceeded, as indicated in Section 3.1.2.

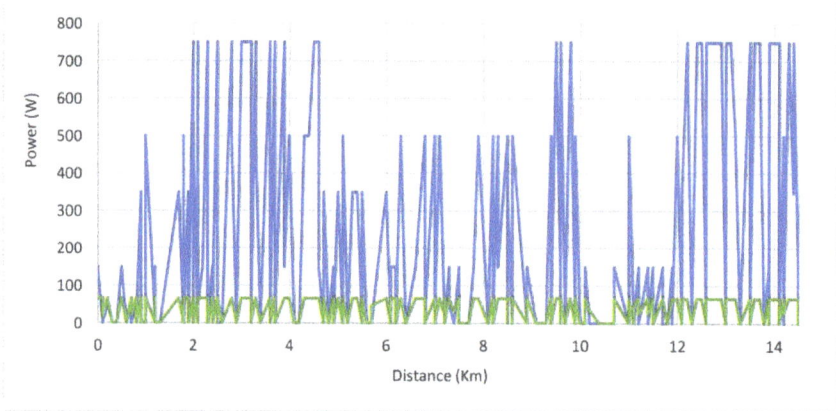

Figure 9. Power apportioned to each of the segments of the analyzed route. The power provided by the user (in blue) and the power provided by the electric engine (in green).

The total watt hours consumed when the route was completed were 240 Wh: 210 Wh were provided by the electric assistance system and 30 Wh were provided by the user. Therefore, the user was awarded a final score of 30 points upon the completion of the route.

5.2. Results Overview

The results obtained at the end of the four-month case study are discussed below to show the progress of the participants. Figure 10 shows the results obtained by the participants and it illustrates the powers each of the users reached to, over the 16 weeks (four months).

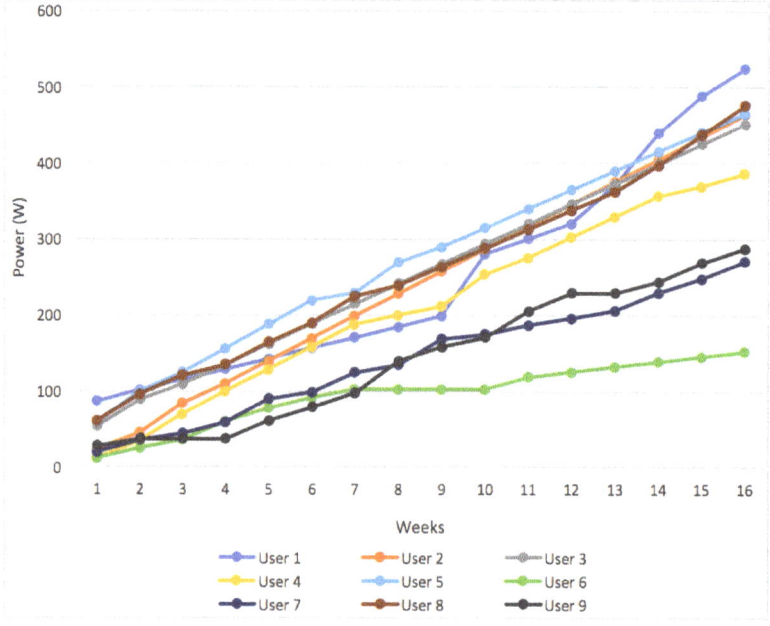

Figure 10. Results obtained by the nine case study participants.

As can be seen, most users have exceeded 300 W, which means that they reached ability level 7 in the system. These users could cycle flat routes with an average speed of 23 km/h, which implies a high level of physical activity. Only three users (6, 7, and 9) were below level 7 in the system, since they did not exceed the 300 Wh. Considering the data analyzed in Table 3, these users do the least amount of exercise per week. After participating in this case study, the three least active users, have managed to do an average of between 4 and 6 h of physical activity a week. The most active users, such as Users 1 and 8, have increased their activity exponentially, surpassing the number of hours that they normally spent cycling.

After analyzing the data provided by the heart rate sensor, it was found that the progress of users who exercised regularly throughout the week was less evident than the progress of those who did little exercise. These data are influenced by factors such as the fitness of the user, the duration of the routes and their difficulty. Users who traveled longer routes with higher slopes, made a greater physical effort and therefore their average heart rate had been affected. However, we can look at the data of the two most representative users of the two groups, users who spent a considerable amount of hours exercising each week and those who did little exercise over the week. Figure 11 compares the mean evolution of the heart rate of these two users over the 16 weeks during which the study had been conducted. In the less active group, User 6 did an average of 1 h of exercise each week. In the first weeks, the user's heart rate was high, however it gradually lowered over the next weeks. On the other hand, the progress of User 1 who did 13 h of physical activity weekly, is not as pronounced. This is because active users' heart rate value tends to stabilize once they have reached a stable level of fitness.

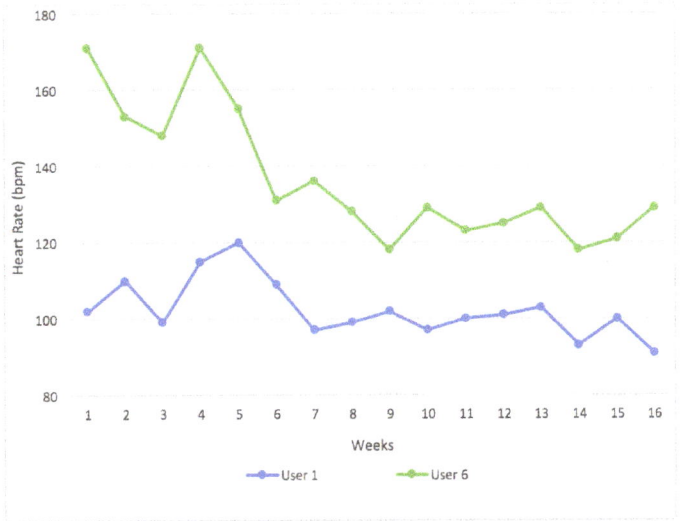

Figure 11. The evolution of the user's heart rate during exercise, over the course of the case study.

If we look closely at the percentage of routes performed according to the days of the week, we can clearly see that there are two groups. On the one hand, users whose cycling activity is high and constant on the weekends. In Figure 12, it can be read that users in this first group did their activities between 30% and 65% on Saturday and Sunday. While the activities carried out between Monday and Friday do not exceed 15% on average. This kind of users (Users 1, 2, 3, 5 and 8) have improved their average speed significantly over the 16 weeks.

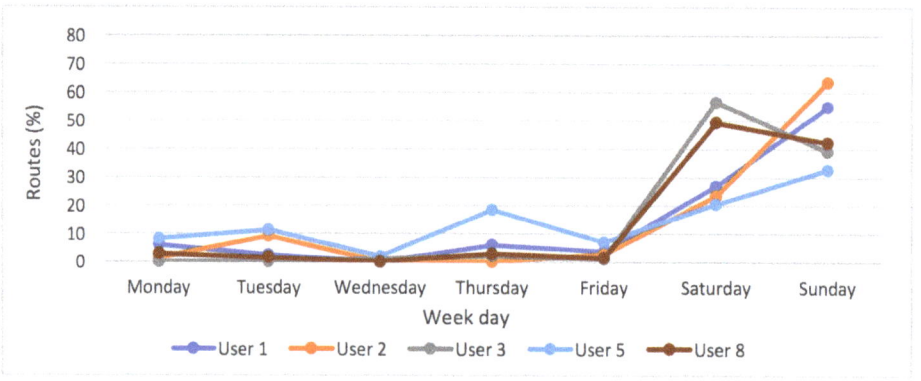

Figure 12. Distribution of the routes cycled by users from the first group over the week.

Figure 13 shows the data of the rest of users, the second user group. These users perform a greater amount of activities over the week than during weekends. In this case, on average, 85% of activities were done between Monday and Friday. This is because the users used their bicycles to commute daily in the city. Cyclists such as User 6 progressed in the number of hours they cycled over the week, from 1 h of exercise a week to an average of 5 h per week, thanks to the support offered by the electrical assistance system.

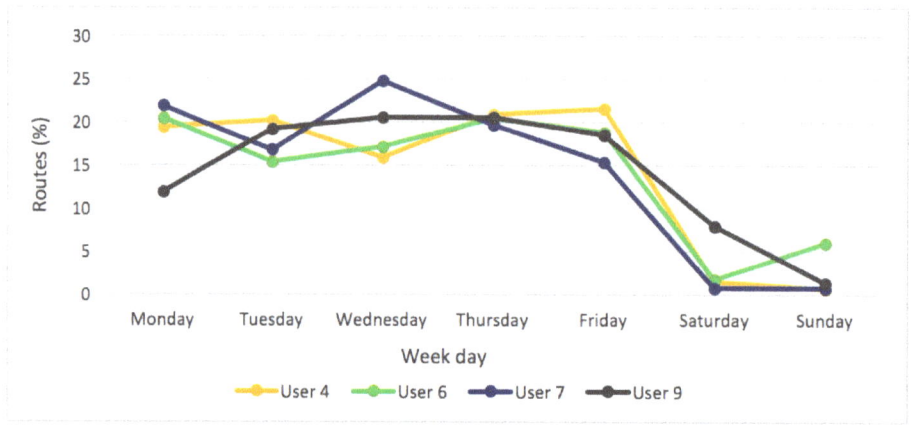

Figure 13. Distribution of the routes cycled by users from the second group over the week.

The web application took record of the days that users checked social statistics on their accounts. The statistics provided by the web application can be seen in Figure 14. In general, all users monitored their performance on the platform. The number of times users accessed these statistics was low in the beginning of the study, however it started increasing with time, especially in the final weeks. Specifically, the activity of Users 1, 2, 3, 4, 8 and 9 increased significantly towards the end of the study and Users 3, 4, 7 and 8 were increasing the number of their cycling activities because they were competing with other users for a higher score. This increase in activity can be seen in Figure 10 in the last weeks of the study.

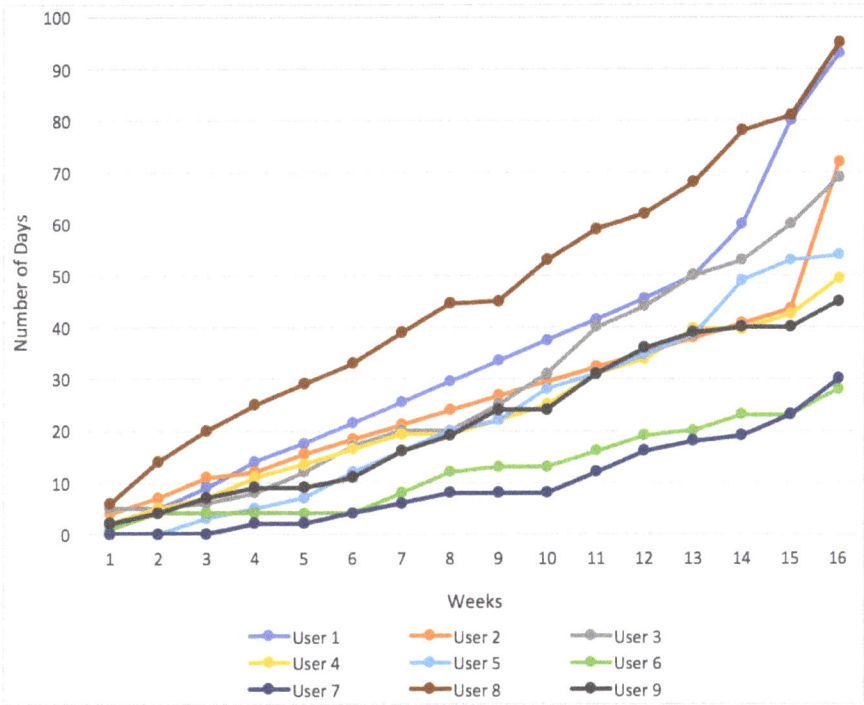

Figure 14. Number of days over the duration of the study in which users consulted social statistics.

Finally, Figure 15 shows a screenshot of the *ebikemotion* web application, where the results of the system can be visualized. On the bottom right-hand side, the rankings of friends who are also users can be viewed. In addition, it is possible to visualize other parameters such as the routes cycled, the calories burned or the scores obtained and the user's ability level.

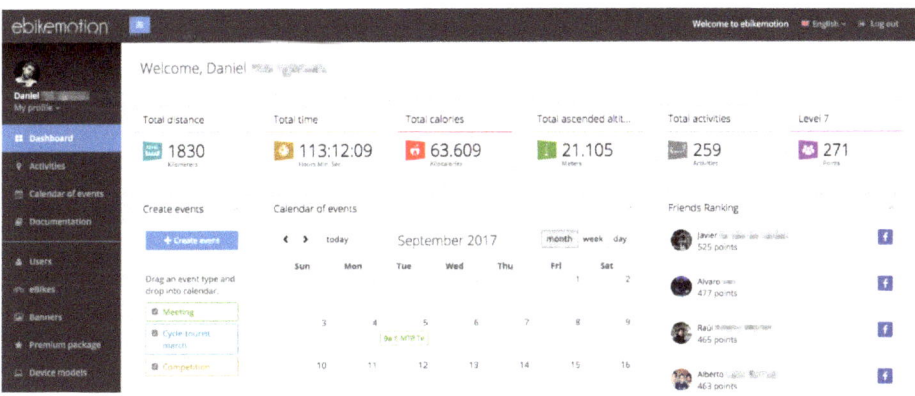

Figure 15. Screenshot of the visualization of results on the *ebikemotion* web application. The names of the users have been erased for privacy reasons.

5.3. Case Study Limitations

It should be noted that the case study participants were located in four different cities, in three different European countries. In this study, it is not possible to see concrete behavior patterns in the evolution of the users from different countries, however it should be kept in mind that the cycling culture varies from country to country. Factors such as climate, infrastructures or terrain orography have an influence on the mode of transport chosen by citizens. It is also important to note that users have not travelled the same routes. Each user travelled different routes with different characteristics. For this reason, it is not possible to directly compare routes with others. The value of the heart rate sensor depends on the physical activities performed by the users. Those users who have performed activities that demand more physical activity, have higher HR values than users with simpler routes.

6. Conclusions

In this work, a personalized intensity level system for the users of assisted electric bicycles has been designed and implemented. The designed system establishes different assist levels in a personalized way, considering the profile of the route, the power required and the user's ability level. As the user travels new routes, the system awards them with higher scores. The higher the score, the greater the average speed on the routes cycled by the user and the greater the amount of power that the user needs to generate. Thanks to the progressive increase in speed, the user gradually does more physical exercise, improving and increasing their fitness. Therefore, it is possible to replace the gym with the use of the electric bicycle for daily commutes saving economic and time costs. This is an important finding of this work.

The innovative component presented in this work is the personalized calculation of exercise for electric bicycle users. Thanks to this system, the user will be able to cycle the routes according to their physical state and ability level. As the user moves up the designed ability levels, the cycling difficulty increases. As demonstrated in Section 5.1, where a route cycled by one of the users has been analyzed, the performance of the designed system is satisfactory. It can segment the route according to its slopes and establish the power that is to be provided by the user, according to its characteristics. The proposed system also evaluates the data collected along the route that had been cycled. This study also demonstrated that the amount of hours the nine case study participants spent on physical activities in a week increased over the four months. This improvement was achieved for both users who were physically fit and those that were not. In general, all users said they were satisfied with their results upon the completion of the 16 weeks of testing. The users whose previous average activity was low (between 0 and 2 h a week) reported that the combination of the e-bike and the training module had helped them increase the amount if exercise they did weekly. The users who were used to regular exercise said that the scoring system and social competition had motivated them to further increase the number of hours they dedicated to exercise weekly.

Thanks to the novel system with assist levels, the more advanced users could progress quickly while the users who were less prepared made a gradual and constant improvement over the four months. The case study participants were located in four different cities, in three different European countries. In future work, a case study will be conducted with users from different parts of the world, whose areas will be more heterogeneous. In the future, we would also like to validate the feasibility of the system in terms of its suitability for people of different ages. To this end, we will conduct a case study that will divide participants into different age groups, such as young people, adults and the elderly.

Acknowledgments: This work has been supported by project GatEBike: Arquitectura basada en Computación Social para el control Inteligente e Interacción en Bicicletas Eléctricas. RTC-2015-4171-4. Project co-financed with Ministerio de Economía y Competitividad and Fondo Europeo de Desarrollo Regional (FEDER) funds (RETOS-COLABORACIÓN 2015). The research of Alberto López Barriuso has been co-financed by the European Social Fund and Junta de Castilla y León (Operational Programme 2014–2020 for Castilla y León, EDU/128/2015 BOCYL).

Author Contributions: Daniel Hernández de la Iglesia and Juan F. De Paz developed the system, performed the test and elaborated the review of the state of the art. Javier Bajo, Alberto López Barriuso, Juan M. Corchado and Gabriel Villarrubia formalized the problem, wrote the algorithms and reviewed the work. All authors contributed to the revision of the paper.

Conflicts of Interest: The authors declare no conflict of interest.

References

1. Hallal, P.C.; Andersen, L.B.; Bull, F.C.; Guthold, R.; Haskell, W.; Ekelund, U.; Alkandari, J.R.; Bauman, A.E.; Blair, S.N.; Brownson, R.C.; et al. Global physical activity levels: Surveillance progress, pitfalls, and prospects. *Lancet* **2012**, *380*, 247–257. [CrossRef]
2. Goodman, A. Walking, Cycling and Driving to Work in the English and Welsh 2011 Census: Trends, Socio-Economic Patterning and Relevance to Travel Behaviour in General. *PLoS ONE* **2013**, *8*, e71790. [CrossRef] [PubMed]
3. Booth, F.W.; Roberts, C.K.; Laye, M.J. Lack of exercise is a major cause of chronic diseases. *Compr. Physiol.* **2012**, *2*, 1143–1211. [PubMed]
4. Health Economic Assessment Tool (HEAT) for Cycling and Walking. Available online: http://www.euro.who.int/HEAT (accessed on 20 October 2017).
5. Lee, I.-M.; Shiroma, E.J.; Lobelo, F.; Puska, P.; Blair, S.N.; Katzmarzyk, P.T. Lancet Physical Activity Series Working Group Effect of physical inactivity on major non-communicable diseases worldwide: An analysis of burden of disease and life expectancy. *Lancet* **2012**, *380*, 219–229. [CrossRef]
6. WHO. *Prevalence of Insufficient Physical Activity*; WHO: Geneva, Switzerland, 2015.
7. Ng, M.; Fleming, T.; Robinson, M.; Thomson, B.; Graetz, N.; Margono, C. Global, regional, and national prevalence of overweight and obesity in children and adults during 1980–2013: A systematic analysis for the Global Burden of Disease Study 2013. *Lancet* **2014**, *384*, 766–781. [CrossRef]
8. Zapata-Diomedi, B.; Gunn, L.; Giles-Corti, B.; Shiell, A.; Lennert Veerman, J. A method for the inclusion of physical activity-related health benefits in cost-benefit analysis of built environment initiatives. *Prev. Med. (Baltim)* **2017**. [CrossRef] [PubMed]
9. Withall, J.; Jago, R.; Fox, K.R. Why some do but most don't. Barriers and enablers to engaging low-income groups in physical activity programmes: A mixed methods study. *BMC Public Health* **2011**, *11*, 507. [CrossRef] [PubMed]
10. Donaire-Gonzalez, D.; de Nazelle, A.; Cole-Hunter, T.; Curto, A.; Rodriguez, D.A.; Mendez, M.A.; Garcia-Aymerich, J.; Basagaña, X.; Ambros, A.; Jerrett, M.; et al. The Added Benefit of Bicycle Commuting on the Regular Amount of Physical Activity Performed. *Am. J. Prev. Med.* **2015**, *49*, 842–849. [CrossRef] [PubMed]
11. Maibach, E.; Steg, L.; Anable, J. Promoting physical activity and reducing climate change: Opportunities to replace short car trips with active transportation. *Prev. Med. (Baltim)* **2009**, *49*, 326–327. [CrossRef] [PubMed]
12. Médard de Chardon, C.; Caruso, G.; Thomas, I. Bicycle sharing system "success" determinants. *Transp. Res. Part A Policy Pract.* **2017**, *100*, 202–214. [CrossRef]
13. Johan de Hartog, J.; Boogaard, H.; Nijland, H.; Hoek, G. Do the health benefits of cycling outweigh the risks? *Environ. Health Perspect.* **2010**, *118*, 1109–1116. [CrossRef] [PubMed]
14. Lindsay, G.; Macmillan, A.; Woodward, A. Moving urban trips from cars to bicycles: Impact on health and emissions. *Aust. N. Z. J. Public Health* **2011**, *35*, 54–60. [CrossRef] [PubMed]
15. Heinen, E.; van Wee, B.; Maat, K. Commuting by Bicycle: An Overview of the Literature. *Transp. Rev.* **2010**, *30*, 59–96. [CrossRef]
16. Pucher, J.; Dill, J.; Handy, S. Infrastructure, programs, and policies to increase bicycling: An international review. *Prev. Med. (Baltim)* **2010**, *50*, S106–S125. [CrossRef] [PubMed]
17. Woodcock, J.; Tainio, M.; Cheshire, J.; O'Brien, O.; Goodman, A. Health effects of the London bicycle sharing system: Health impact modelling study. *BMJ* **2014**, *348*, g425. [CrossRef] [PubMed]
18. Rojas-Rueda, D.; de Nazelle, A.; Tainio, M.; Nieuwenhuijsen, M.J. The health risks and benefits of cycling in urban environments compared with car use: Health impact assessment study. *BMJ* **2011**, *343*, d4521. [CrossRef] [PubMed]

19. Bike share's impact on car use: Evidence from the United States, Great Britain, and Australia. *Transp. Res. Part D Transp. Environ.* **2014**, *31*, 13–20.
20. Sun, Y.; Mobasheri, A.; Hu, X.; Wang, W. Investigating Impacts of Environmental Factors on the Cycling Behavior of Bicycle-Sharing Users. *Sustainability* **2017**, *9*, 1060. [CrossRef]
21. Ling, Z.; Cherry, C.; MacArthur, J.; Weinert, J. Differences of Cycling Experiences and Perceptions between E-Bike and Bicycle Users in the United States. *Sustainability* **2017**, *9*, 1662. [CrossRef]
22. Jones, T.; Harms, L.; Heinen, E. Motives, perceptions and experiences of electric bicycle owners and implications for health, wellbeing and mobility. *J. Transp. Geogr.* **2016**, *53*, 41–49. [CrossRef]
23. Cairns, S.; Behrendt, F.; Raffo, D.; Beaumont, C.; Kiefer, C. Electrically-assisted bikes: Potential impacts on travel behaviour. *Transp. Res. Part A Policy Pract.* **2017**, *103*, 327–342. [CrossRef]
24. Langford, B.C.; Cherry, C.R.; Bassett, D.R.; Fitzhugh, E.C.; Dhakal, N. Comparing physical activity of pedal-assist electric bikes with walking and conventional bicycles. *J. Transp. Heal.* **2017**, *6*, 463–473. [CrossRef]
25. Citron, R. *Executive Summary: Electric Bicycles Li-Ion and SLA E-Bikes: Drivetrain, Motor, and Battery Technology Trends, Competitive Landscape, and Global Market Forecasts Section 1*; The Navigant research: Washington, DC, USA, 2016.
26. Fishman, E.; Cherry, C. E-bikes in the Mainstream: Reviewing a Decade of Research. *Transp. Rev.* **2016**, *36*, 72–91. [CrossRef]
27. Cherry, C.R.; Yang, H.; Jones, L.R.; He, M. Dynamics of electric bike ownership and use in Kunming, China. *Transp. Policy* **2016**, *45*, 127–135. [CrossRef]
28. Campbell, A.A.; Cherry, C.R.; Ryerson, M.S.; Yang, X. Factors influencing the choice of shared bicycles and shared electric bikes in Beijing. *Transp. Res. Part C Emerg. Technol.* **2016**, *67*, 399–414. [CrossRef]
29. Rose, G. E-bikes and urban transportation: Emerging issues and unresolved questions. *Transportation (Amst)* **2012**, *39*, 81–96. [CrossRef]
30. Electric Bikes: Licensing, Tax and Insurance—GOV.UK. Available online: https://www.gov.uk/electric-bike-rules (accessed on 15 October 2017).
31. Götschi, T.; Garrard, J.; Giles-Corti, B. Cycling as a Part of Daily Life: A Review of Health Perspectives. *Transp. Rev.* **2016**, *36*, 45–71. [CrossRef]
32. Aguiló, A.; Tauler, P.; Pilar Guix, M.; Villa, G.; Córdova, A.; Tur, J.A.; Pons, A. Effect of exercise intensity and training on antioxidants and cholesterol profile in cyclists. *J. Nutr. Biochem.* **2003**, *14*, 319–325. [CrossRef]
33. Rønnestad, B.R.; Hansen, J.; Hollan, I.; Ellefsen, S. Strength training improves performance and pedaling characteristics in elite cyclists. *Scand. J. Med. Sci. Sports* **2015**, *25*, e89–e98. [CrossRef] [PubMed]
34. Fjeldsoe, B.S.; Miller, Y.D.; Marshall, A.L. MobileMums: A Randomized Controlled Trial of an SMS-Based Physical Activity Intervention. *Ann. Behav. Med.* **2010**, *39*, 101–111. [CrossRef] [PubMed]
35. Kim, B.H.; Glanz, K. Text Messaging to Motivate Walking in Older African Americans. *Am. J. Prev. Med.* **2013**, *44*, 71–75. [CrossRef] [PubMed]
36. Prestwich, A.; Perugini, M.; Hurling, R. Can the effects of implementation intentions on exercise be enhanced using text messages? *Psychol. Health* **2009**, *24*, 677–687. [CrossRef] [PubMed]
37. Prestwich, A.; Perugini, M.; Hurling, R. Can implementation intentions and text messages promote brisk walking? A randomized trial. *Heal. Psychol.* **2010**, *29*, 40–49. [CrossRef] [PubMed]
38. Shaw, R.; Bosworth, H. Short message service (SMS) text messaging as an intervention medium for weight loss: A literature review. *Health Inform. J.* **2012**, *18*, 235–250. [CrossRef] [PubMed]
39. Sirriyeh, R.; Lawton, R.; Ward, J. Physical activity and adolescents: An exploratory randomized controlled trial investigating the influence of affective and instrumental text messages. *Br. J. Health Psychol.* **2010**, *15*, 825–840. [CrossRef] [PubMed]
40. Bort-Roig, J.; Gilson, N.D.; Puig-Ribera, A.; Contreras, R.S.; Trost, S.G. Measuring and Influencing Physical Activity with Smartphone Technology: A Systematic Review. *Sport. Med.* **2014**, *44*, 671–686. [CrossRef] [PubMed]
41. Casey, M.; Hayes, P.S.; Glynn, F.; OLaighin, G.; Heaney, D.; Murphy, A.W.; Glynn, L.G. Patients' experiences of using a smartphone application to increase physical activity: The SMART MOVE qualitative study in primary care. *Br. J. Gen. Pract.* **2014**, *64*, e500–e508. [CrossRef] [PubMed]
42. Bravata, D.M.; Smith-Spangler, C.; Sundaram, V.; Gienger, A.L.; Lin, N.; Lewis, R.; Stave, C.D.; Olkin, I.; Sirard, J.R. Using Pedometers to Increase Physical Activity and Improve Health. *JAMA* **2007**, *298*, 2296–2304. [CrossRef] [PubMed]

43. Zhang, J.; Brackbill, D.; Yang, S.; Becker, J.; Herbert, N.; Centola, D. Support or competition? How online social networks increase physical activity: A randomized controlled trial. *Prev. Med. Rep.* **2016**, *4*, 453–458. [CrossRef] [PubMed]
44. Wong, F.Y. Influence of Pokémon Go on physical activity levels of university players: A cross-sectional study. *Int. J. Health Geogr.* **2017**, *16*, 8. [CrossRef] [PubMed]
45. Wang, D.; Wu, T.; Wen, S.; Liu, D.; Xiang, Y.; Zhou, W.; Hassan, H.; Alelaiwi, A. Pokémon GO in Melbourne CBD: A case study of the cyber-physical symbiotic social networks. *J. Comput. Sci.* **2017**. [CrossRef]
46. LeBlanc, A.G.; Chaput, J.-P.; McFarlane, A.; Colley, R.C.; Thivel, D.; Biddle, S.J.H.; Maddison, R.; Leatherdale, S.T.; Tremblay, M.S. Active Video Games and Health Indicators in Children and Youth: A Systematic Review. *PLoS ONE* **2013**, *8*, e65351. [CrossRef] [PubMed]
47. Zhao, J.; Baird, T. "Nudging" Active Travel: A Framework for Behavioral Interventions Using Mobile Technology. In Proceedings of the Transportation Research Board 93rd Annual Meeting, Washington, DC, USA, 12–16 January 2014.
48. Development of a Technological Platform for Implementing VTBC Programs. *Transp. Res. Procedia* **2014**, *3*, 129–138.
49. Louis, J.; Brisswalter, J.; Morio, C.; Barla, C.; Temprado, J.-J. The Electrically Assisted Bicycle. *Am. J. Phys. Med. Rehabil.* **2012**, *91*, 931–940. [CrossRef] [PubMed]
50. Extending life on the bike: Electric bike use by older Australians. *J. Transp. Heal.* **2015**, *2*, 276–283.
51. Berntsen, S.; Malnes, L.; Langåker, A.; Bere, E. Physical activity when riding an electric assisted bicycle. *Int. J. Behav. Nutr. Phys. Act.* **2017**, *14*, 55. [CrossRef] [PubMed]
52. Cyclist Heart Rate Control via a Continuously Varying Transmission. *IFAC Proc. Vol.* **2014**, *47*, 912–917.
53. Shibahara, D.; Ueno, A. Fuzzy Rule Introduction to Mode Change Algorithm of a Health Assisting Bicycle. *Trans. Jpn. Soc. Med. Biol. Eng.* **2013**, *51*, U-19. [CrossRef]
54. Corno, M.; Giani, P.; Tanelli, M.; Savaresi, S.M. Human-in-the-Loop Bicycle Control via Active Heart Rate Regulation. *IEEE Trans. Control Syst. Technol.* **2015**, *23*, 1029–1040. [CrossRef]
55. Fletcher, G.F.; Ades, P.A.; Kligfield, P.; Arena, R.; Balady, G.J.; Bittner, V.A.; Coke, L.A.; Fleg, J.L.; Forman, D.E.; Gerber, T.C.; et al. Exercise standards for testing and training: A scientific statement from the American heart association. *Circulation* **2013**, *128*, 873–934. [CrossRef] [PubMed]
56. Inbar, O.; Oren, A.; Scheinowitz, M.; Rotstein, A.; Dlin, R.; Casaburi, R. Normal cardiopulmonary responses during incremental exercise in 20- to 70-year-old men. *Med. Sci. Sports Exerc.* **1994**, *26*, 538–546. [PubMed]
57. Carey, D.G. Quantifying Differences in the "Fat Burning" Zone and the Aerobic Zone: Implications for Training. *J. Strength Cond. Res.* **2009**, *23*, 2090–2095. [CrossRef] [PubMed]
58. Stagemotion. Available online: http://stagemotion.com/stagemotion/ (accessed on 15 October 2017).
59. Ebikemotion®—Ebikes Platform. Available online: https://www.ebikemotion.com/web/es/ (accessed on 15 October 2017).
60. De La Iglesia, D.; Villarubia, G.; De Paz, J.; Bajo, J. Multi-Sensor Information Fusion for Optimizing Electric Bicycle Routes Using a Swarm Intelligence Algorithm. *Sensors* **2017**, *17*, 2501. [CrossRef] [PubMed]
61. Swain, D.P. Cycling Uphill and Downhill. Available online: http://www.sportsci.org/jour/9804/dps.html (accessed on 13 January 2018).
62. Union Cycliste Internationale. Available online: http://www.uci.ch/ (accessed on 20 October 2017).

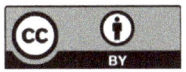
© 2018 by the authors. Licensee MDPI, Basel, Switzerland. This article is an open access article distributed under the terms and conditions of the Creative Commons Attribution (CC BY) license (http://creativecommons.org/licenses/by/4.0/).

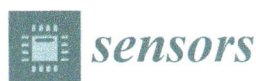

Article

Design and Evaluation of a Pervasive Coaching and Gamification Platform for Young Diabetes Patients [†]

Randy Klaassen [1,*], Kim C. M. Bul [2], Rieks op den Akker [1], Gert Jan van der Burg [3], Pamela M. Kato [4] and Pierpaolo Di Bitonto [5]

1. Human Media Interaction, Faculty of Electrical Engineering, Mathematics and Computer Science, University of Twente, P.O. Box 217, 7500 AE Enschede, The Netherlands; h.j.a.opdenakker@utwente.nl
2. Centre for Innovative Research across the Life Course, Faculty of Health and Life Sciences, Coventry University, CV1 5FB Coventry, UK; ac2658@coventry.ac.uk
3. Gelderse Vallei Hospital, P.O. Box 9025, 6710 HN Ede, The Netherlands; burgg@zgv.nl
4. School of Computing, Electronics and Mathematics, Faculty of Engineering, Environment and Computing, Coventry University, CV1 5FB Coventry, UK; pam@pamkato.com
5. Grifo multimedia Srl, Via Bruno Zaccaro, 19-70126 Bari, Italy; p.dibitonto@grifomultimedia.it
* Correspondence: r.klaassen@utwente.nl; Tel.: +31-53-489-3811
† This paper is an extended version of our paper published in Op den Akker, R.; Klaassen, R.; Kim C.M. Bul, Kato, P.; van der Berg, G.J.; Di Bitonto, P. Let them play: Experiences in the wild with a gamification and coaching system for young diabetes patients. In Proceedings of the Health-i-Coach 2017, Barcelona, Spain, 23–26 May 2017.

Received: 29 October 2017; Accepted: 17 January 2018; Published: 30 January 2018

Abstract: Self monitoring, personal goal-setting and coaching, education and social support are strategies to help patients with chronic conditions in their daily care. Various tools have been developed, e.g., mobile digital coaching systems connected with wearable sensors, serious games and patient web portals to personal health records, that aim to support patients with chronic conditions and their caregivers in realizing the ideal of self-management. We describe a platform that integrates these tools to support young patients in diabetes self-management through educational game playing, monitoring and motivational feedback. We describe the design of the platform referring to principles from healthcare, persuasive system design and serious game design. The virtual coach is a game guide that can also provide personalized feedback about the user's daily care related activities which have value for making progress in the game world. User evaluations with patients under pediatric supervision revealed that the use of mobile technology in combination with web-based elements is feasible but some assumptions made about how users would connect to the platform were not satisfied in reality, resulting in less than optimal user experiences. We discuss challenges with suggestions for further development of integrated pervasive coaching and gamification platforms in medical practice.

Keywords: digital coaching; diabetes education; serious gaming; self-management; user evaluations

1. Introduction

Self-management [1] is of key importance in the successful treatment of patients with chronic conditions, such as Type 1 diabetes (T1D), a condition in which the patient needs daily insulin treatment because their body fails to produce this hormone. In contrast to Type 2 diabetes, T1D is typically diagnosed at a young age when patients are still dependent on their parents who are responsible for managing their child's health condition [2]. Children are supposed to gain more responsibility for their T1D care when they become adolescents. Goals for the management of T1D include achieving optimal glycemic control, avoiding acute complications, and minimizing the risk of long-term microvascular and macrovascular complications. Self-monitoring of blood glucose (BGM), either by using a blood glucose meter or using a system for continuous blood glucose monitoring [3] is one of the most important activities in managing diabetes. Research repeatedly shows that adherence to BGM is linked to glycemic control in pediatric T1D [4–7]. That is, the more frequently the patient measures their blood glucose (BG) using reliable, certified blood glucose meters [8], the more their BG will be within acceptable and appropriate levels. International studies show that metabolic control is unsatisfactory in many adolescents with T1D [7,9]. Despite advances in technologies that support BGM, frequent measuring is still a burden for many children and adolescents [10–12]. Adherence, i.e., the degree to which the person's behavior corresponds with the agreed recommendations from a health-care provider, is a key factor in the successful treatment of chronic conditions. Even when patients have good knowledge about treatment adherence, their actual practice of adherence is often less than ideal [13]. One of the factors that is often underestimated in T1D management is the burden of the disease in everyday life. The patient is constantly required to perform actions and make decisions in their daily diabetes routine. Examples are: finger pricks for glucose measurements, insulin injections, replacing needles for insulin pumps or subcutaneous glucose sensors, carbohydrate counting, and regime adjustments for physical activities or sports, for sick days, for parties, etc. These requirements interfere with normal life, especially for adolescents who want to be perceived as "normal". Aversion to these compelling actions often means that children and adolescents do not achieve a good metabolic control. Research on the motivations for and causes of non-adherence to diabetes care regimens among adolescent diabetes patients points to the contrasting views on adherence between patients and providers. Where providers typically view adherence in pursuing optimal glycemic control and health outcomes, patients have other perspectives [11]. Hence, one of the adherence challenges with T1D is motivating and helping these patients measure their BG at regular times every day in such a way that it is least invasive using methods and tools popular among this target group. Digital coaching systems that monitor the users' BGM send reminders and motivating messages to support the patient adhere to a personalized and clinically appropriate medical regimen. However, to function properly these systems need regular data from the user, which often requires additional actions on the part of the user; e.g., upload glucose data. The challenge is then to motivate the patient to keep using these tools on an ongoing regular basis. How can technology help these patients to make it a bit easier to learn to live with their condition and to adhere to a medical regimen as long as there is no cure?

The pervasive gamification and coaching platform presented here is the product of the EU Horizon 2020 PERGAMON project (No. 644385) in which a number of developments came together that exploit opportunities offered by the availability and acceptance of new technologies in e/m-health: reliable wearable sensors, mobile apps that support self-management and lifestyle behaviour change, digital coaching, serious games and gamification to enhance healthcare education, and Patient Web Portals connected to Personal Health Records, that allow patients to upload personal data and receive personalised guidance from caregivers. The platform integrates the complementary potential offered by the widespread use of wearable sensors and mobile devices and the popularity of games and social networks delivered on a secure and authorized portal that supports patients and their caregivers in self-management of their chronic condition. Reviews of studies in the development and evaluation of the use of each of the above mentioned component technologies show besides (potential) positive impact on diabetes care and opportunities, that there are also challenges that demand a more integrated solution [14].

The management of diabetes is complex and patients need personalized advice and medical control by a pediatrician or diabetes nurse. The growing number of diabetes patients worldwide place a heavy burden on medical budgets. Patient web portals are increasingly set up and maintained by hospitals to support self-management and improve communication between patients and their medical caregivers, as one of the most important predictors of adherence [13]. A review by Osborne et al. showed that they have a positive impact on management for diabetes care [15]. The communication between health provider and patient could benefit from integration of these web portals with the mobile technology and "real-time" sensoring available on smartphones.

What can we say about quality, engagement and effect in terms of adherence when treatment is supported by mobile diabetes apps? While a wide selection of mobile apps is available for self-management of diabetes, some specifically designed for patients with T1D [12], some with a virtual coach [16,17], current research suggests that most do not meet basic requirements for medical applications [18]. From a medical perspective a main finding from a review by Chomutare et al. [19] is that a critical feature strongly recommended by clinical guidelines, namely, personalized education, is not present in current applications. Although mobile health apps have great potential for improving chronic disease care, they face a number of challenges including lack of evidence of clinical effectiveness and lack of integration with the healthcare delivery system. There is a clear need for formal evaluation and review of potential threats to safety and privacy [20]. Brzan et al. [18] reviewed 65 apps for diabetes and concluded that 56 of these apps "did not meet even minimal requirements or did not work properly". They report on a qualitative study in young adults with the objective to explore their experiences with apps that aim at health behavior change and their willingness to use these apps. Many participants in their study "were not motivated enough to regularly and precisely use the apps in making healthy lifestyle changes", a recurring issue in many studies. Boyle et al. [21], reporting on a survey of patients seen at a hospital diabetes clinic in New Zealand found so many concerning issues that they concluded that there is a need for an app assessment process to raise confidence in the quality and safety of diabetes management apps in diabetes patients as well as in healthcare providers.

Although short term user studies often show promising results in terms of adherence to medical treatment there is no evidence of maintenance of high adherence in the long run. According to self-determination theory, it may take many months before external motivation becomes internalized into daily routine behaviours [22]. Hence there is a need for ways to motivate patients with T1D to manage and adhere to their treatments on an ongoing basis.

Gamification techniques have been introduced as possible means to motivate patients to sustain adherence to medical treatment [23]. Gamification is using elements of game design [24], i.e., points, leader boards, levels, competitions, rewards, achievements, mini games, goals, experience points, rules, narrative, graphics, imagination, role identification, or setting step-wise challenges in pursuit of a goal. Use of games or gamification in health behaviour change programs might thus be a way to intrinsically motivate users to expose themselves to and continually engage with these programs (Baranowski et al. [25], Thompson et al. [26], Cugelman [27]). In serious games, elements of game design [28,29] are used to help the user learn to reach non-game goals. The ultimate goal is to foster intrinsic motivation for learning and maintaining desired behaviours [30].

Educational games in diabetes care dates back to the 90s. Lieberman [31] describes 14 diabetes self-management video games. The games typically involve players in problem-solving and decision-making in simulations of diabetes self-management, usually by asking players to balance food intake and insulin injections to keep a game character's blood glucose within a normal range. An important feature of these games is that they provide practice through rehearsal and show cause and effect, while also providing basic information about diabetes self-management. There are many games that teach the relationship between food (carbohydrates), plasma glucose level, exercise, and insulin dose [32,33], or that focus on learning the number of carbohydrates in drinks, snacks and meals [34]. Several studies using randomized controlled trial designs, e.g., Brown et al. [35] and Fuchslocher et al. [36], showed that diabetes related content explicitly presented in games improves diabetes self-management in T1D. In a study by Lieberman [37] a diabetes game reduced diabetes-related urgent and emergency visits by 77% after young patients had the game at home for six months, compared to no reduction in clinical utilization in a control group of young patients who took home an entertainment video game that had no health content.

In a special issue on Games for Diabetes, Theng et al. [38] provide a review of evidence on the efficacy of video games and gamification in diabetes self-management (not specifically targeting, but including T1D). The duration of most of the ten studies was short with small sample sizes of those that studied patients aged between 8 and 16 years old. All the interventions targeted behavioural changes to promote healthy behaviours among the study participants. Video games were found to be effective tools for education while gamification and virtual environments increased intrinsic motivation and positive reinforcement. Remarkably, their study did not find any research specifically targeting medication adherence as part of the behavioral change process.

Charlier et al. [39] reports a review of randomized controlled trials (RCTs) assessing efficacy of serious games in improving knowledge and self-management in young people with chronic conditions. From 9 studies the general conclusion is that educational video games improve knowledge and self-management. Johnson et al. [40] identify potential advantages of gamification from existing research and conducted a systematic literature review of empirical studies on gamification for health and well-being, assessing quality of evidence, effect type, and application domain. They conclude that due to the relatively small number of studies and a lack of studies that compare gamified interventions to non-gamified versions of the intervention, it is hard to draw general conclusions about the efficacy of gamification in digital health interventions. Deacon and O'Farrell [41] and Sardi et al. [42] come to a similar conclusion: there is still a lack of valid empirical evidence that support the use of gamification strategies employed in e-Health.

Some studies indicate that gamification of BGM has positive effects on BGM in adolescents with T1D [43,44]. In the mobile game, DIAL, a group of children (8–18) were given a mobile device with an integrated motivational game in which the participants could guess a BG level following collection of three earlier readings. In a 4 week experiment, the game group sent significantly more glucose values to the platform than the control group that did not have the game. Use of a motivational game appears to increase the frequency of monitoring, reduce the frequency of hyperglycemia, improve diabetes knowledge and may help to optimize glycemic control. Follow-up research in a RCT among adolescent T1D patients over 12 months showed that app usage diminished over the trial. On average, 35% (16/46) of the participants were classified as moderately or highly engaged (uploaded glucose data 3 or more days a week) over the 12 months. S. et al. [14] suggest exploring the utility of integrating mobile applications for T1D support into routine clinical care to facilitate more frequent feedback.

Does access to video games or the possibility of making progress in a video game work as a reward for regular glucose measuring and control? In a study by Klingensmith et al. [45] acceptance of a system that connects a blood glucose meter with a Nintendo game was assessed in a sample of children, adolescents, and young adults with T1D. Users receive reward points that can be transferred from the meter to the video game, allowing access to new levels of play and mini games. Rewards are based on frequency, timing and results of blood glucose testing. Healthcare providers can also set personalized target ranges in the meter to help patients reach glucose goals. The majority of healthcare providers agreed that the coupled system would solve a problem in diabetes management, and that it would motivate patients to test their blood sugar. They observed an increase of use in the home situation compared to the lab situation because users wanted to have more advanced games [45].

Besides monitoring and feedback, personal coaching and goal-setting and learning how to cope with situations that impact blood glucose level, social support is an important strategy to help young diabetes patients to adopt healthier habits. A rationale for using games for serious purposes like health is their ability to motivate and facilitate social encounters [28]. Children like to play together even when playing single player games. The effect of social support on users' motivation to use mobile apps appears to be mixed. Some are motivated by competition among peers, where others feel that sharing data and results introduces too much competition [46]. The gaming framework of Chomutare et al. [30] focuses on completing self-management tasks, rather than rewards or penalties. They emphasize the value of cooperation, social comparison and a focus on positive achievements as core game elements, limiting the extent of competition. Social media in combination with serious games are suggested as a beneficial platform for self-management of T1D by the younger age groups [47]. Social media are popular among adolescents. They can interact and build communities dedicated to specific games.

Social media allow T1D patients to share their game experience with everyone; not only with other patients with diabetes. A disadvantage of such an open community is the lack of a quality control of the content which is mostly provided by the community itself [47]. This is one of the reasons we chose an environment with authorized users where content is moderated by the care institute.

The above review presents a state of the art of existing applications. The PERGAMON platform (introduced in Section 1.1) integrates techniques and design decisions that we find in the applications discussed above. A system that integrates all the diabetes educators by integrating gaming and coaching in a clinical setting through a principled design would overcome many of the shortcomings of the partial solutions in reviewed systems (e.g., no personalization, not specifically focused on medical adherence).

1.1. The PERGAMON Platform

The PERGAMON platform that we present here is a gamification platform that integrates educational gaming and coaching. It gamifies self-care-related activities so users are rewarded for making progress in the game world. The virtual coach can keep track of users' daily BGM, physical activity, food intake and send reminders and motivational messages when the user forgets to follow recommendations agreed upon with their healthcare professional. The coaching system can reward behaviours that correspond to personalized goals. The platform provides a secure way for message exchange and data sharing between patients, their peers and their caregivers.

The platform integrates game elements and virtual coaching with a well designed system of main game and mini games based on an ontology of tasks, sub-goals and goals. Moreover, contrary to many systems medical content and coaching messages are tailored and personalized.

The aim is to see how gamification and digital coaching can be integrated into the continuous care of patients with chronic conditions, with the aim to integrate the findings in existing Patient Web Portals that support care of patients with T1D. Involving young patients with T1D and their caregivers in the development process was part of the development and research process. Young people and adolescents in particular have different requirements for medical devices than adults [48]. They also have different preferences for types of games and gamification methods [49].

In this research we investigate if the PERGAMON framework does support the specification and implementation of a pervasive serious gaming and coaching system for specific target groups. We demonstrated the answer by developing the system for young children with diabetes in a clinical setting. Next to this question, this research tries to investigate if patients do like the PERGAMON platform, how they use the different functions and the games of the platform, and if the integration of the components motivate educative game play as well as self-management of diabetes (in particular adherence to blood glucose monitor use).

After we discuss design principles and the design of the PERGAMON gamification platform, we present preliminary pilot study results obtained with experiences with the platform "in the wild", that is, with young patients with T1D under supervision of paediatricians and diabetes nurses in a Dutch hospital. The aim of the evaluation was to see whether patients had problems using the system and how they assessed the games and the coaching. Such usability and experience evaluations are a prerequisite for future evaluations that measure the impact of the platform in terms of medical outcomes.

2. Design Principles for the Gamification Platform

The design of the gamification and coaching platform adheres to basic principles of healthcare, design principles for serious gaming as well as design principles for behaviour change support systems. Care values were considered in determining design, especially regarding what techniques and content the system implements, how the system communicates with the user, and how the system treats personal information, regarding security and privacy issues. The gamified platform involved introducing intelligent systems to users that could to some extent take over the role of human caregivers. This raised issues of responsibility for protecting care values [50]. In our view, a system can never take away the responsibility from the human user (e.g., the care provider, or the patient). On the contrary, the design should aim at supporting the patient in becoming a responsible person in their self-care by providing the patient the means, along with supportive motivation, to make a well-informed decision. Tailoring to the individual user and his or her social and intellectual abilities was therefore an important requirement for the design. The aim of technology for self-management in healthcare is not to completely replace the human care system but to support and enhance it. The PERGAMON system was designed to be integrated in the care and treatment of young patients by the medical caregivers, e.g., pediatricians, diabetes nurses, and informal carers. Patient's credibility rating of the system depends on how trustworthy the medical experts are that provide input into the design of the system. Educational goals and targets of diabetes self-management formulated by diabetes care organizations were used to drive the content and design of the system as a whole as well as for the specific themes of the games in the system. Specifically, these goals (diabetes educators) were balancing energy through medication intake, healthy eating, being physically active, learning how to monitor blood sugar levels, coping with high and lows of BG and how to reduce risks associated with BGM. The system guides the individual and establishes together with the user specific, measurable, attainable, realistic, and timely (SMART) goals [51].

The design of a behaviour change support system for health interventions [52] involves the implementation of several behaviour change techniques, such as feedback and monitoring, reward and threat, and social support. A behaviour change technique is a component of an intervention designed to alter or redirect causal processes that regulate behaviour [53]. They are based on socio–psychological behaviour theories, e.g., Goal-Setting [54], Self-Determination Theory [55]. Behavior change techniques (BCTs) were integrated into the Persuasive System Design Model (PSD) for behaviour change support systems [52] that we use to describe the system's design. The PSD model has four categories: primary task support, dialogue support, system credibility support and social support, each with a number of design principles (to be distinguished from the moral principles of health care). Key aspects of BCTs were integrated, e.g., self-monitoring, rewards or provide information about others approval. Although Abraham et al. [53] presents 26 BCTs, the principles in the category of System Credibility Support in the PSD model do not occur in the BCTs listed. This is understandable because the PSD is intended for the design and evaluation of a technical system, not human beings per se. These systems function as more or less autonomous entities in situations where the medical care giver is not immediately present for the user. Also, by their very nature, technical systems have —seen from a design perspective— abstract users so that for the system designer tailoring and personalisation become a concern (partly solved by explicit user models and use of persona in the design process) where treatments by human caregivers and coaches (different from rule following machines) are tacitly assumed to tailor their treatment to the individual patient.

Some of the design principles of the PSD model are implemented in our system by means of specific game elements (which encompass game mechanics, themes, game characters, challenges, rewards) from game design [28]. For example, the principles of reduction and tunneling in the PSD model are materialized by dedicated learning tasks in different mini games and by distinguishing different reachable goal levels. Other principles are implemented in actions of the virtual coach: praise, rewards, reminders, suggestions as well as by various game elements. Similarity and social role are materialized by game elements that aim at identification with the main character in the game as well as by the use of a similar character for the virtual coach.

The educational goals for diabetes care (e.g., the BCT provide information on consequences [53]) are implemented in the adventure game, called the Tako Game, in particular in a number of integrated educational mini games and by educational elements such as videos. The Tako Game is a "pervasive" game in the sense that it expands the "magic circle" of play [24,28]: the border between game world and reality is blurred by making daily self-management activities relevant in the game.

3. PERGAMON: A Framework for Gamification, Real-Time Sensoring and Virtual Coaching

The TIKI TAKO system for young T1D patients is an instantiation of the general PERGAMON framework. The PERGAMON framework allows the creation of behaviour change support systems [56] that combine serious gaming (a main game and mini games), virtual coaching and real-time monitoring of activities in daily life via sensors.

The architecture of the PERGAMON framework is a Service Architecture. The system is not a set of isolated applications communicating based on the integration of the different parts of the application. The framework is organized in a collection of services that can published on a communication infrastructure. These services can be used by multiple applications. The main services in the PERGAMON framework are; (1) Saving and sharing data from the sensor network (Glucometer data; Pedometer data; Insulin Pen data), (2) Saving and sharing user state (e.g., achieved goals, badges), (3) Analysis of the data coming from sensors (i.e., Pedometer, Glucometer, Insulin Pen) and (4) Virtual Coach services. The infrastructure enables the various "consumers" of data services to query and access the available information on heterogeneous information systems through the exchange of messages. In particular, for the sensor network a form of hardware abstraction is needed, which involves having a custom plugin for each device that will be supported. The architecture of the PERGAMON framework supports the implementation of real-time behavioral change techniques (see Section 2) such as real-time feedback and monitoring of behavior of users.

A typical system created with the PERGAMON framework consists of a web application (website), an Android application for gathering data from sensors, an Android webapp to view the PERGAMON website via an Android device and an Android Unity application for the games. The framework consists of five key components (Figure 1):

- Ground Layer (the central data hub)
- Sensor Network
- Gamification Platform
- Serious Game (the main game and the mini games)
- Virtual Coach

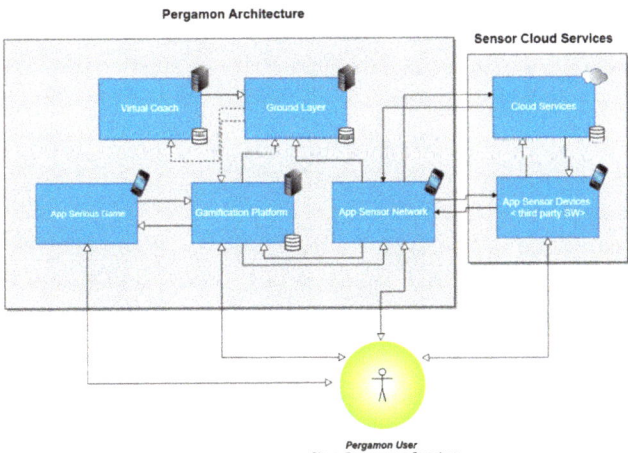

Figure 1. The PERGAMON architecture.

In the following subsections, we will discuss the different components in detail.

3.1. Architecture of the PERGAMON System

Figure 1 presents the architecture of the PERGAMON framework. The Ground Layer has a central place: it stores data from the other components and makes the data available to all connected components via Application programming interfaces (APIs). The connected components are the (i) virtual coach; (ii) serious game(s); (iii) gamification platform; and (iv) the sensor network.

Communication between the different components and the Ground Layer are over secure HTTPS connections and basic authentication is needed to access the RESTful APIs (Representational state transfer (REST) or RESTful web services is a way of providing interoperability between computer systems on the Internet.). The other components in the PERGAMON framework can read, write, update and delete data in the Ground Layer.

3.2. Sensor Network

The Sensor Network component is responsible for the connections between the different sensors used to monitor the users of the system and the PERGAMON framework. The Sensor Network is running on an Android device (smartphone or tablet) and turns it into a sensor hub to which different devices can be connected.

Devices are made compatible with the PERGAMON Sensor Network via a plugin system. Each device must be categorized into a device type, such as "Pedometer", and all devices of that type must use a plugin to provide data to the server to store in the Ground Layer database in a common format. Each plugin written for the Sensor Network can have its own behaviour for obtaining the data from a device. Plugins simply operate via a common request and reply system where the custom behaviour required to interface with each device is contained purely within the plugin and hidden from other PERGAMON components. It is through this plugin architecture that the Sensor Network allows the PERGAMON framework to work with a large range of devices, as well as allowing devices to be easily supported in future. Once data is gathered from the devices connected to the Sensor Network, the data must be pushed up to the cloud once a network connection is available. Data will be held on the device and synchronised with the Ground Layer via a connection to the servers when possible, in order to allow the PERGAMON app to gather data while offline. Once the data is confirmed to be stored in the Ground Layer, the Sensor Network's role in the PERGAMON framework is complete until more data is gathered. Figure 2 presents a schematic overview of the data flow of the Sensor Network.

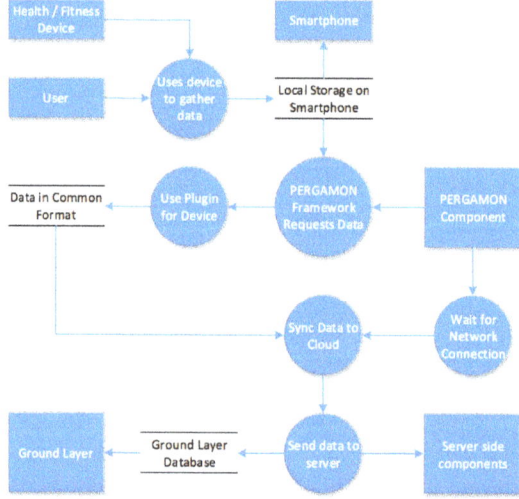

Figure 2. The data flow of the Sensor Network.

The architecture of the Sensor Network will follow a classic object oriented approach (see Figure 3). Every device will be a "PERGAMON Device" in the system, and as such all devices will have the common functionality associated with it. PERGAMON Devices will implement the very basic behaviour of request and reply handling, as well as containing the identifier for which device this class represents. On the next level in the architecture, different types of devices can be found. The three initial types are "Pedometer", "Glucometer" and "Insulin Pen". These classes define in which data format the devices will be expected to return data. Every device will fit one of these categories and more categories can be added if needed.

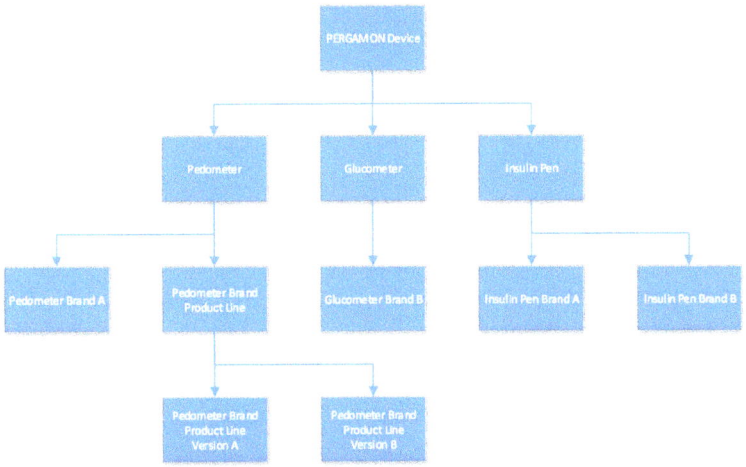

Figure 3. The architecture of the Sensor Network.

The lowest levels in the class hierarchy will be the individual device plugins. They represent actual physical devices instead of categories into which they should fit. They will define the actual behaviour that is executed when the functions defined by parent classes are called.

The architecture of the Sensor Network makes it possible to add new devices and services in an easy and modular way. Compatible sensors and services (currently the Google Fit service, Mi Fit band and Mi Fit band 2 and Menarini blood glucose sensors are supported) connected to the Sensor Network will automatically record data. The Sensor Network will gather the recorded data, process the data and push it to the Ground Layer component. The Sensor Network also provides the possibility for users to enter data manually, such as food intake, mood or sleep.

3.3. Gamification Platform

The third component of the PERGAMON framework is the Gamification Platform. Goals in the platform can be defined and created by a game designer using a platform designer's interface. The main gamification elements in the PERGAMON platform are Tasks and Goals. A task is the basic unit, and corresponds to a single action that can be performed by the user. When a task is complete, the user will receive a certain number of points. A goal is a set of different tasks. The completion of a goal will give the user a bonus score, translated into points. Tasks can belong to the following activities:

- System's activity, i.e., all the activities concerning the PERGAMON framework (User Profile, Social Hub, Food Diary, and so on).
- Sensor Network, i.e., all the activities concerning the use of the glucometer and pedometer.

All the activities in the PERGAMON framwork are gamified, e.g., each interaction with the system will be associated with a score. Users will receive immediate feedback by completing tasks, and gaining scores. A progress bar will indicate the goal percentage of accomplishment showing the progress the user has made (see Figures 4 and 5). The difficulty of the goals will increase when the user advances in using the system. Goals can be mono-thematic (e.g., all about diet or physical activity) or multi-thematic (e.g., "A perfect healthy day", that includes diet, physical activity, and therapy management).

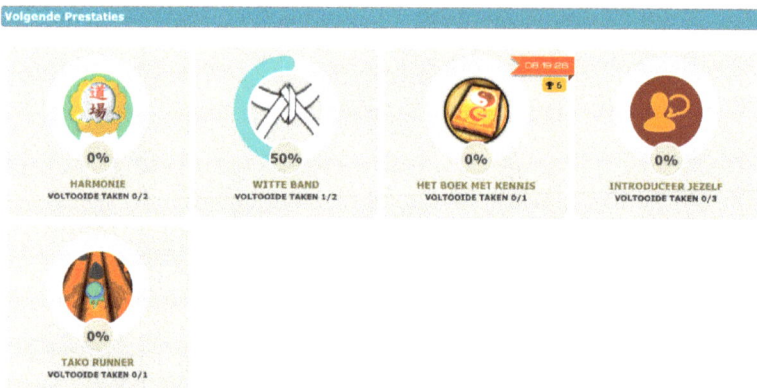

Figure 4. Gamification platform, Goals.

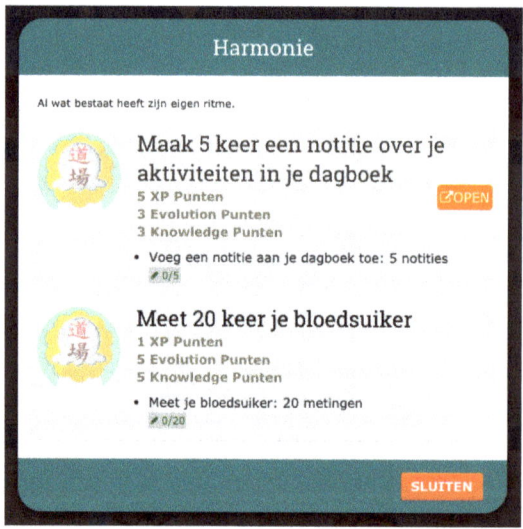

Figure 5. Gamification platform, Tasks.

Users can challenge themselves, deciding to accomplish a task within a certain period of time, receiving, as a consequence, a bonus score, or they can simply conduct their normal life, and accomplish tasks unintentionally as part of their daily routine, while their accomplishments are recorded by the sensor devices from the Sensor Network. Points are associated with both tasks and goals; each task will have its corresponding score, while a goal will give a bonus score as reward. In fact, once a goal is accomplished, users will receive a bonus percentage of points. The gamification platform manages three kind of points:

1. Experience: this type is associated with the general leader board, and allows unlocking special objects in the serious games.
2. Knowledge: this type is associated with the serious game environment and allows skipping between levels
3. Evolution: this type is associated with a specific instance in the gamification.

These three different kinds of points are needed to continue playing the game and are used to create a leader board to share this with friends.

3.4. Games

The PERGAMON framework supports two different kinds of games, the main game (called *Tiki Tako*) and mini games. The main game is an adventure/puzzle game that can be played over a longer period of time. Users have to solve puzzles and levels to make progress in the game. Points (experience, knowledge and evolution points) earned by completing tasks and goals, either in the real world or in the game world, are needed to continue the main game. In this way the main game is linked to the tasks and goals from the real world and to the other components of the PERGAMON framework. Mini games are played in a shorter timespan than in the main *Tiki Tako* game. They are designed to communicate certain educational objectives related to the chronic condition by means of game metaphors. Users are required to play the mini games that are played outside the *Tiki Tako* game to make progress in the main game. The games in the PERGAMON framework are developed in the Unity game engine using the PERGAMON API.

3.5. The Mystery of TIKI TAKO

The TIKI TAKO system for young T1D patients is an instantiation of the general PERGAMON framework. The characteristics of the TIKI TAKO system are presented in Figure 6 and Table 1. The Ground Layer of the TIKI TAKO system supports the storage of data and measurements about physical activity, glucose measurements, insulin intakes, and food. The Sensor Network of the TIKI TAKO system supports different channels and devices that are able to collect information about daily life activities via sensors. It supports the Google Fit service which collects information about physical activity (number of steps and activity intensity). Other sensors compatible with the Google Fit service could be used in the TIKI TAKO system to also collect data about physical activity. We used the Google Fit ©Pedometer (as a service on the smartphone itself, or on an Android Wear smartwatch) and the Xiaomi Mi Fit Band ©(in combination with the Mi Fit app) as sensors. Also the services and devices of iHealth are supported to collect physical activity or blood glucose measurements. Menarini ©blood glucose sensors are also supported to measure blood glucose. The Sensor Network also allows for manual input of information about diet, insulin and sleep.

Within the Gamification Platform five types of goals and tasks for young T1D patients have been implemented:

- "My Sugar" tasks relate to measuring blood glucose, reinforcing the relationship between diet and glucose levels, education about hypo and hyperglycemia or taking notes regarding insulin use.
- "Physical activities" are tasks related to diabetes and physical activity and sports such as setting a number of steps as a daily goal or learning about how to prepare to engage in sports.
- "Active life" tasks support the user to self-manage their diabetes in a more introspective way rather than overtly directing their activities. Examples are writing a to-do list to plan activities in a day or reviewing one's activity or BG data.
- "Website Activities" are tasks related to the use of the system and the website such as creating a profile or installing applications on the smartphone.
- "Mystery of TikiTako" tasks are related to the main game of the TIKI TAKO system such as how to continue in the game or how to finish a mini game.

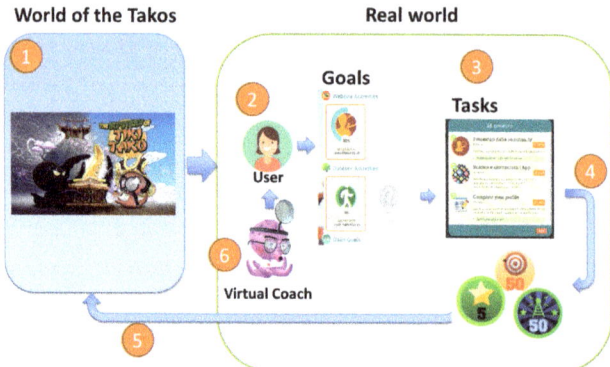

Figure 6. Main characteristics of the *Tako Game* (see Table 1 for explanation).

Table 1. Main characteristics and game elements of the *Tako Game* for diabetic children (see Figure 6).

1	Theme: in the world of the Takos, an evil monk has stolen the sacred tentacle from the Temple. T-Shan is called in by the Great Red Tako to retrieve it. In order to accomplish his mission, T-Shan must overcome a series of challenges, helped by the player (the patient), who can guide T-Shan and obtain precious suggestions and points in the Real World.
2	In order to gain points to help T-Shan in the world of the Takos, the player had to accomplish the empowerment goals in his/her game dashboard. The empowerment goals were related to the following activities: • Monitoring blood glucose levels (diary entries, use of a sensor device such as glucometer) • Acquiring skills and knowledge (learn carbohydrate counting, how to balance a healthy meal, etc.) • Social activities (set up a personal profile, use the wall) Other goals are also directly linked to the game itself e.g., requiring the player to play a mini game to be able to proceed to another scene in the temple. Players are never alone in their quest: they are helped by the Great Red Tako (i.e., the virtual coach), who supports and provides motivational messages to help them in accomplishing the set goals.
3	Each therapeutic goal is made up of several tasks that are rewarded with points when completed. Some can be carried out online (e.g., take an "educational candy", i.e., view a learning resource, watch a video, read a document; or "fill in the diary"); others may be carried out by the user in their daily activities and tracked thanks to wearable sensor devices (glucometer and pedometer) that automatically detect and synchronise data about blood glucose level and physical activity, so that the PERGAMON system knows that a task has been carried out.
4	Points are of three types and each type is linked to a specific type of action: • Experience: gained through the game to contribute to the player's ranking in the general leaderboard • Knowledge: used in the world of Tako to unlock some locations • Evolution: used to make the Tako avatar grow and acquire graphical assets
5	Points are used to get suggestions (and thus solve a riddle or overcome an obstacle), or get an object that can be used later on to do something in the game in the world of the Takos.
6	The virtual coach, situated in the real world, can affect the game world of the Takos by providing suggestions on some tasks particularly helpful for the users that can help them gain points advising players to complete a goal related to the levels in the game.

The Serious Game component of the TIKI TAKO system consists of the main "Mystery of TikiTako" game and seven mini games. The main game is an adventure and puzzle game in which the player takes on the role of an investigator who tries to solve a mystery. The investigator, the main character in the main game, also has T1D. The player progresses in the game by successfully directing the main character to control his diabetes and solve puzzles through the mini games that have educational goals, such as how to do insulin injections or how to balance blood glucose levels. Table 2 provides an overview of the seven different mini games and their learning objectives.

Table 2. Overview of the mini games in the *Tiki Tako Game*. In the left colom the name of the game and a screen capture, on the right side the learning objective related to this mini game.

Mini Game		Learning Objective
Ramen Master		The objective is to teach and test the knowledge of the player about the types of food to eat according to the blood glucose levels.
Tako Maze		The objective of the game is to teach and test the knowledge of the player about the carbohydrates amount present in different food items.
Tako Doctor		To reinforce the best practice around the stages necessary in administering an insulin injection. Players will solve a simple drawing puzzle alongside each key step of the injection process, with the theory that the repetition of playing the game will begin to ingrain the steps in memory.
Tako Chef		Tako Chef aims to increase awareness of how certain foods and diabetic items affect blood glucose levels. The player must learn to quickly identify an item that is suitable (among unsuitable items) for a given blood glucose level.
Tako Runner		Tako Runner aims to help the player understand how exercise and diet affect blood glucose levels, and that exercise should stop when those levels are too low or high.
Tako Swimmer		Tako Swimmer aims to help the player understand how exercise and diet affect blood glucose levels, and that exercise should stop when those levels are too low or high.
Tako Explorer		Tako Explorer aims to familiarize the player with key terminology used when talking about diabetes.

3.6. Virtual Coaching

The Virtual Coach component of the PERGAMON framework is designed to keep track of the personal objectives of each of the users as well as their achievements in the real world and in the game world. The coach uses this information to assist the users in achieving their objectives by processing collected data and offering guidance in the form of reminders, notifications and suggestions about certain actions and events.

Figure 7 presents an overview of the virtual coach component. The data for the virtual coach comes from the Ground Layer. Data from the sensor network and data from the games can be accessed by the virtual coach component. Knowledge for the virtual coach is gathered from rules for self-management of T1D in cooperation with healthcare professionals. Personalization and tailoring of these self-management rules is done by defining personal goals between the client and the healthcare professionals (shared decision making). The Virtual Coach component consists of a coaching engine and a graphical representation of the virtual coach [16]. Coaching rules are defined in the coaching engine and allow for the analysis of data available in the Ground Layer derived from other components of the PERGAMON framework. The coaching engine is a rule- based engine based on the ECA (event, condition and action) engine developed at the University of Twente [16]. A typical coaching rule looks like the one in Figure 8. The rule (named 'glucose_hyper' in this example) is executed based on an event (in this case the event 'glucose_update'), triggered by an event from the Ground Layer (in this case a trigger from the sensor network of a new measure of value 13.0). The rule is only executed when the value of the new measurement is greater than 10.0 (a blood glucose level of 10 or higher is called a hyperglycemia). Conditions can be general fixed values (such as hypoglycemia or hypoglycemia) or personals goals (such as the number of steps or the number of times a user wants to measure their blood glucose levels). The action of this coaching rule is a suggestion to play a mini game.

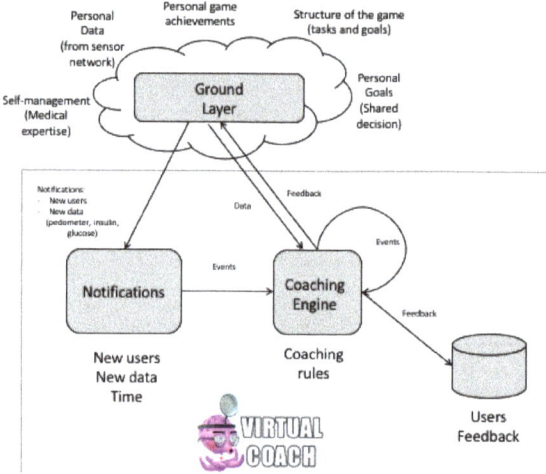

Figure 7. The coaching engine of the Virtual Coach of the PERGAMON platform depicting the knowledge and data source components used by the Virtual Coach.

```
fire('glucose_update', {'value': 13.0})

@event('glucose_update')
@condition(lambda c,e: c.value > 10.0)
def glucose_hyper(ctx, e):
    #Play the Tako Maze mini game}
```

Figure 8. An example of coaching rule

The coaching rules are executed by triggers that are event- or time-based. Event based triggers are notifications from the sensor network or other components of the PERGAMON framework via the Ground Layer. Examples of triggers for coaching events are the creation of new users, data from sensors or achievements in the game(s). Time based triggers are based on the time of day and related to self-management (e.g., measuring glucose levels before dinner or before sleeping). All events are processed by the coaching engine and the result of these coaching rules can be a dialogue act of several kinds such as a *suggestion* (e.g., to play mini games where the user can meet educational objectives), a *reminder* or a *notification* (e.g., when personal goals are reached or users forget to do their measurements) or *hints* about how to continue in the main game. The Virtual Coach is able to send text messages and notifications to the website and to the Android application. By presenting the Virtual Coach as a cartoon-like character from the main game world, the coach connects the in-game world with the primary world of the user's daily care activities. Figure 9 gives an example of a coaching message presented on the website including an educational movie with extra background information.

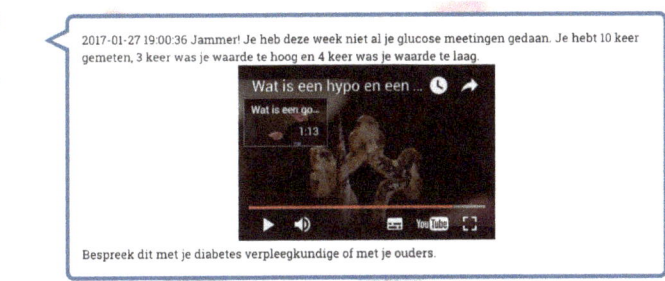

Figure 9. Example of a coaching message on the PERGAMON website. The message is in Dutch (English: *"Too bad! This week you did not do all your glucose measurements. You measured 10 times, 3 times your level was too high and 4 times your level was too low. Please, discuss this with your diabetes nurse or with your parents."*).

4. User Evaluations

After a two week pilot test with seven patients with T1D another group of 14 patients from the participating hospital in Ede tested the system over 6–8 weeks.

4.1. Goals

The user evaluation aimed to see how patients with T1D experience the game, a core element of gaming [57]. We used a mixed methods approach (i.e., direct observation, questionnaires, and semi structured interviews) to answer the following questions: Do players like to step into the "magic circle" [58] and does striving for progress in the game motivate healthy behaviours? Do users appreciate the coaching messages? Do users find the educational films useful? Do users find it difficult to use the system? Do users encounter any technical problems they cannot solve?

4.2. Materials and Methods

4.2.1. Participants

Twenty-one adolescents with Type 1 diabetes participated in a pre-pilot (n = 7) and pilot study (n = 14). Participants were registered patients at the pediatric diabetes department from the Gelderse Vallei Hospital in Ede (the Netherlands). The first group of participants was allocated to a pre-pilot study in September 2016 and the second group of participants was allocated to a subsequent pilot study performed during October–December 2016. Participants were included if they fulfilled the following inclusion criteria: (a) diagnosis of Type 1 diabetes for at least six months; (b) between 12 and 18 years of age; (c) written informed consent provided by adolescents themselves and one of their parents (or legal guardians); (d) availability of an Android smartphone with an internet/data connection and (e) a reasonable level of understanding of the Dutch language. If the adolescent did not have an Android smartphone available, they were provided with a phone that satisfied system requirements.

4.2.2. Design

The first group ($n = 7$) pre-pilot tested the PERGAMON platform for two weeks at home. Based on the results several suggestions were made and implemented to improve the platform. The second group ($n = 14$) pilot tested the adjusted PERGAMON platform for six to eight weeks at home. Both studies used a pre-post test design with a mixed-method approach in which questionnaires as well as open-ended interview questions were used.

4.2.3. Procedure

Adolescents and their parents were contacted and informed about the study by their pediatrician or specialized diabetes nurses working at the pediatric diabetes department of Gelderse Vallei Hospital in Ede (the Netherlands) where both studies were performed. Adolescents who expressed their interest in participating in the study and fulfilled the inclusion criteria were sent an information letter including an informed consent form. After two weeks, participants were contacted to see if they had any further questions and to plan the first hospital visit. During the first hospital visit, participants were informed about the specific components of the PERGAMON platform (i.e., sensor network, virtual coach and serious game) in more detail and were offered support with downloading and installation of the applications on their Android device. The pre-pilot group participants evaluated the platform for two weeks at home and the subsequent pilot group participants were allowed to use the PERGAMON platform for six to eight weeks at home. No instructions were given for doing specific tasks. This was done to stimulate the report of technical or other issues naturally encountered during use in real life. A technical help desk, covered by the nurses and researchers involved, was available during the study period through contact by email or phone during office hours. Apart from the online questionnaires filled in during the pre- and post-test hospital visits, participants had the opportunity to share their experiences concerning usability and acceptability in a focus group during the second hospital visit.

The focus group was guided by a short outline presented through PowerPoint and ended with an open discussion about suggestions on how to improve the performance and adequacy of the platform. The focus group was moderated by a researcher experienced in usability research and testing. A second researcher (i.e., nurse) was present and made field notes.

All participants and one of their parents (or legal guardians) gave their informed consent for inclusion before they participated in the study. Both studies were conducted in accordance with the Declaration of Helsinki, and the protocol was approved by the Ethics Committee of the Gelderse Vallei Hospital (BC/1606-383) on 1st of August 2016 and by Coventry University (P45142) on 29th of June 2016.

4.2.4. Measures

Socio-demographic questionnaire—A self-constructed socio-demographic questionnaire was used to collect socio-demographic information (e.g., gender, age, ethnic background) and general information concerning participants' previous smartphone use.

Problem Areas in Diabetes Questionnaire [59]—The Dutch translation of the Problem areas in Diabetes (PAID) was used to examine diabetes related emotional distress. It consists of 20 items on a 5-point Likert scale. An example item is "Feeling scared when you think about living with diabetes". In the current study, the total PAID score was used as an indication of the patient's diabetes related emotional distress before and after using the PERGAMON platform. A score of 40 or higher is considered to be an indication of "emotional burnout". This questionnaire demonstrates good psychometric characteristics and the Dutch version used has been validated with patients in the Netherlands [59].

System Usability Scale (SUS; Dutch translation [60])—The Dutch translation of the SUS was used to measure usability of the PERGAMON platform. This questionnaire consists of 10 items on a 5-point Likert scale ranging from strongly agree to strongly disagree. An example item is "I thought the system was easy to use". A score above 68 is interpreted as above average usability and below 68 is interpreted as below average. This questionnaire is internationally acknowledged as a reliable questionnaire to measure system usability [60].

Semi-structured interview—A semi-structured interview was used during group discussions (focus groups) to explore user experiences of the PERGAMON platform with regard to design, enjoyment, storyline, ease of use, educational value, engagement and innovative aspects of the platform (e.g., the virtual coach, sensors, serious games), as well as their overall judgment about the PERGAMON platform.

5. Results

Background characteristics and smartphone use of both study groups are presented in Table 3. We asked participants "Do you expect that the PERGAMON platform will support you in your diabetes management?". Of the 21 participants in the pre-pilot and the pilot groups 7 (33.33%) answered positively; 1 (4.76%) answered negatively, and 13 (61.90%) said they did not know.

Table 3. Socio-demographic characteristics and smartphone use in both study groups ($N = 21$).

	Total ($N = 21$)	Pre-pilot ($n = 7$)	Pilot ($n = 14$)
Male	10 (48%)	2 (29%)	8 (57%)
Female	11 (52%)	5 (71%)	6 (43%)
Age (years), mean	13.90	14	13.86
Smartphone use in general? n (%)			
Social media	3 (14.29%)	1 (14.29%)	2 (14.29%)
Search information	2 (9.52%)	2 (28.57%)	0 (0%)
Call/Text/Whatsapp	8 (38.09%)	3 (42.85%)	5 (35.7%)
Listen to music	5 (23.81%)	0 (0%)	5 (35.7%)
Other	3 (14.29%)	1 (14.29%)	2 (14.29%)
Smartphone use for health? n (%)			
Monitoring physical activity	2 (9.52%)	1 (14.29%)	1 (7.14%)
Monitoring nutrition	1 (4.76%)	1 (14.29%)	0 (0%)
Monitoring blood glucose	1 (4.76%)	0 (0%)	1 (7.14%)
No monitoring	17 (80.95%)	5 (71.42%)	12 (85.72%)
Favourite computer genre? n (%)			
Puzzle	2 (9.52%)	1 (14.29%)	1 (7.14%)
Action	8 (38.09%)	4 (57.14%)	4 (28.57%)
Racing	1 (4.76%)	0 (0%)	1 (7.14%)
Multi-player	4 (19.04%)	0 (0%)	4 (28.57%)
Other	6 (28.57%)	2 (28.57%)	4 (28.57%)

In total, 71 adolescents with T1D were approached to take part in the pilot study, of which 30 patients met the inclusion criteria and indicated their interest to participate in the pilot study. Sixteen participants (7 males/9 females) withdrew their consent because of delayed study start date (13%), time constraints due to school activities (56%), time constraints due to activities outside school hours (13%), low motivation to participate (6%), low expectations regarding the game format (6%) and worries about their diabetes condition (6%).

During the pre-pilot study there was one drop-out during the second hospital visit due to academic under achievement at school.

5.1. Problem Areas in Diabetes Questionnaire

Participants in the pre-pilot study demonstrated a mean PAID score of 21.25 (SD = 21.21; range = 0.00–55.00) at the first hospital visit and a mean PAID score of 10.63 (SD = 8.62; range = 0.00–22.50) at the second hospital visit after two weeks. Furthermore, participants in the pilot study showed a mean PAID score of 16.52 (SD = 14.17; range = 0.00–52.50) at the first hospital visit and a mean PAID score of 12.95 (SD = 9.84; range = 0.00–31.25) at the second hospital visit. Results indicate that participants did not experience a great deal of diabetes related emotional distress (score < 40) at baseline or after using the PERGAMON platform.

5.2. System Usability Scale

After using the PERGAMON platform, participants from the pre-pilot study group demonstrated a mean SUS index of 44.58 (SD = 21.18; range = 25.00–82.50) which indicates a below average usability score. Almost all participants indicated that they found the PERGAMON platform unnecessarily complex (statement 2) and not easy to use (statement 3). Half of the participants felt that they needed assistance to be able to use the PERGAMON platform (statement 4; Table 1). In the pilot-study, group participants had a mean SUS index of 50.18 (SD = 13.71; range = 35.00–90.00) which indicates a below average usability score. As can be seen in Table 4, although 50% of pilot study participants thought the PERGAMON platform was easy to use after playing it for two weeks (statement 3) and 57% did NOT think (disagreed) they would need assistance when using the system (statement 4); 57% did NOT think (disagreed) that they would like to use the system frequently (statement 1).

Table 4. Pre-pilot and pilot study usability (SUS) questionnaire scores (in %).

	Disagree (1–2)		Neutral (3)		Agree (4–5)	
	Pre	Pilot	Pre	Pilot	Pre	Pilot
Positive items						
1: I think that I would like to use this system frequently	50.0	57.1	33.3	21.4	16.7	21.4
3: I thought the system was easy to use	66.7	28.6	33.3	21.4	0	50.0
5: I found the various functions in this system were well integrated,	33.3	50.0	33.3	35.7	33.3	14.3
7: I would imagine that most people would learn to use this system very quickly	50.0	57.1	16.7	14.3	33.3	28.6
9: I felt very confident using the system	33.3	42.9	50.0	35.7	16.7	21.4
Negative items						
2: I found the system unnecessarily complex	16.7	35.7	0	28.6	83.3	35.7
4: I think that I would need assistance to be able to use this system	50.0	57.1	16.7	28.6	33.3	14.3
6: I thought there was too much inconsistency in this system	33.3	50.0	33.3	28.6	33.3	21.4
8: I found this system very cumbersome/awkward to use	33.3	42.9	33.3	35.7	33.3	21.4
10: I needed to learn a lot of things before I could get going with this system	33.3	50.0	0	28.6	66.7	21.4

5.3. Semi-Structured Interview

PERGAMON platform—One participant in the pre-pilot study group indicated that he never used the platform. Three participants (43%) indicated that they used the PERGAMON platform a couple of times a week and the remaining participants said that they used the platform (almost) every day. The average usage time was 10 h (ranging from 10 min to 40 h). Four participants from the pilot study group indicated that they never used the platform. However, most of the participants (57%) indicated that they used the PERGAMON platform once a week and two participants used the platform more often. The time that they used the platform ranged between 10 min and 18 h. On average, participants from the pre-pilot group rated the game ("How would you rate the game on a scale of 1 to 10?") with a

6.83 (SD = 0.98; on a 10-point scale), whereas the pilot study group participants rated the game with a 6.07 (SD = 1.44). Overall, most participants (except for five) in both study groups encountered technical problems such as failures in transfer of blood glucose values to the PERGAMON platform, or low performance of the game. In total, only four participants felt the PERGAMON platform supported them in their diabetes management. Suggestions to improve the platform include making the game less complex/difficult to play, change the appearance of the game to fit with its target group and better communication between the different components of the platform. Most participants appreciated that the game set real-world goals.

TikiTako adventure game—Three participants (43%) indicated that they played the game a couple of times a week and the remaining participants indicated they played the TikiTako adventure game (almost) every day. The average playtime was 8 h (ranging from 15.00 min to 40.00 h). Four participants (29%) indicated that they played once a week and another four participants (29%) indicated they played once a month. One participant played the adventure game almost every day. The time that they played the game ranged between 15 min and 9 h. On average, participants from the pre-pilot group rated the game with a 5.67 (SD = 2.34; on a 10-point scale), whereas the pilot study group participants rated the game with a 6.07 (SD = 1.98). Both groups rated the game as difficult to play (>8.00 on a 10-point scale) as there was not enough explanation given or explanations were too cryptic. Participants from the pre-pilot study group scored 8.50 on average (SD = 1.38) whereas participants from the pilot study scored 8.43 on average (SD = 0.65). In total, four participants (19%) in both study groups indicated that they learned from the game, namely refreshing diabetes knowledge. Also more than half of the participants in the pre-pilot group (57%) and in the pilot group (50%) want to get access to this game once it has been fully developed. Moreover, a large part of the pre-pilot group (57%) and of the pilot group (64%) would recommend the game to other participants with T1D, because "you can acquire diabetes knowledge" and "because you become more motivated concerning self-management". Suggestions to improve the game include the appearance, the look-and-feel, the solving of technical issues, more interesting mini games and making it less difficult to finish levels.

Mini games—Overall, participants rated the seven mini games for likability in a range from 4.42 (SD = 2.78) to 7.33 (SD = 2.52; on a 10-point scale) with Tako Maze indicated as the most popular mini game in the pre-pilot study group and Ramen Master as the most popular in the pilot study group. Participants from the pre-pilot study group indicated that the mini game could be improved by offering more explanation for certain mini games or that the difficulty level should be adaptive and set by the user themselves. Furthermore, participants from the pilot study suggested that there should be a better technical performance of the mini games (e.g., response time to tapping the screen) and a more mature look-and-feel of the game.

Virtual coach—All participants in the pre-pilot study (except for one) indicated that they received messages from the virtual coach, ranging from 3 to 8 messages. Almost all participants (except for one) understood the virtual coach messages that were mainly focused on blood glucose measurement. Participants indicated on a 7-point Likert scale to which degree the coach was up-to-date (mean = 4.67; SD = 2.58), supportive (mean = 3.50; SD = 2.07), friendly (mean = 5.33; SD = 1.63) and pleasant (mean = 4.67; SD = 1.21). Almost all pilot study participants (except for three) indicated that they received messages from the virtual coach, ranging from 2 to 10 messages. All participants understood the messages of the virtual coach and indicated on a 7-point scale that the coach was up-to-date (mean = 4.21; SD = 1.72), supportive (mean = 3.79; SD = 1.81), friendly (mean = 5.07; SD = 1.39) and pleasant (mean = 4.50; SD = 1.79). According to the participants in the pre-pilot study, the virtual coach could be improved by adding the capability of answering their questions and by appearing less often on their phone screen as an overlay. Participants in the pilot study group suggested that the virtual coach could be improved by decreasing the frequency of messages and by offering the user to turn the virtual coach's messages on or off.

5.4. Focus Groups

TikiTako adventure game—With regard to the adventure game, participants from the pre-pilot study indicated that they got stuck after a few levels. It was too difficult for them to continue the game and therefore they stopped playing. Several participants said that the hints in the game were too cryptic and that advice from the virtual coach (as a game guide) was difficult to understand. Furthermore, they said the look and feel of the game was childish and did not match the difficulty level of the game. Even after in-game feedback was simplified and made less cryptic, participants from the pilot study generally indicated that the TikiTako adventure game was too childish in terms of its graphics and storyline and this simplicity did not match with the difficult and highly complex puzzles.

Mini games—Participants from both study groups indicated that the interface was not user friendly as users did not know they could use the "help" button to get more information about how to play the game. One participant suggested that it might be good to receive information about this before or during the mini game. In addition, participants found the (menu) buttons too small. Mini games about food and intake of insulin were seen as more useful for children recently diagnosed with diabetes. Furthermore, the look and feel of the mini games was described as childish and did not match with the difficulty level of the mini games. Even after the number of points needed to reach the goal at the end of the games was lowered, puzzles remained highly complex according to the pilot study participants.

Virtual coach—Participants in both study groups were positive about the timing of messages and the number of reminders sent. Participants also provided positive feedback about the weekly overview messages given by the virtual coach, although they were not noticed by all participants. One participant from the pre-pilot study explained that receiving messages (or notifications) from the virtual coach helped to support their self-management. Participants in the pre-pilot group indicated that an overlay image of the virtual coach on their screen was annoying when they received a message from the coach. Therefore, the interface of the virtual coach was revised for the pilot study (i.e., messages were made clickable so that the whole message was visible at first instance) so that participants could be aware that more content was available than just the label text on the message box. Participants in both the pre-pilot and the pilot study said that educational movies presented by the virtual coach about diabetes were nice but became boring after multiple viewings. During both studies participants said that because of synchronization problems and requirements to enter data on a daily basis (and not after each measurement), feedback from the virtual coach was not up-to-date and therefore perceived as incorrect. More importantly, the coach was not developed to respond immediately to high or low glucose readings leading participants to suggest that it would be good if the virtual coach could send messages when measurements differed from normal values.

Sensors—Participants from both study groups liked the idea that sensor data can automatically be sent to the PERGAMON platform. However, not every participant was enthusiastic about wearing a Mi-Fit band or changing their trusted blood glucose meter for a new meter that automatically sends the glucose data to the platform (i.e., most participants used a pump and other glucose monitors). Entering the glucose measurements by hand was perceived as a lot of extra work and a hurdle with this technology.

6. Discussion

This report presented a proof of concept of a pervasive gamified platform framework that is a unique combination of integrated sensors (wearables), a virtual coach and serious games in healthcare. This description of this platform contributes to research on pervasive technology approaches in healthcare [49,61]. Behaviour change theories and game design principles underpinning the framework were presented with particular attention to how these theories and principles were combined and applied to develop content across the technology components to promote positive health behaviours among young people with T1D. This work contributes to efforts to link theories more closely to interventions in the research literature [62]. This report also presented the results of pilot tests of early prototypes of the framework. Consistent with previous literature documenting issues that often arise in early evaluations of prototypes, [18,61,63,64], we found that similar issues of usability and technical quality assurance presented challenges for users. We received several comments that the games were difficult to play and were "overly complex" due to design issues and should be more simple and straightforward to play. At the same time, participants commented that the "look and feel" of the games seem to be targeted to a much younger audience and should be designed for a more mature audience. These issues made it difficult to answer some of the original questions of the research (e.g., Do players like to step into the "magic circle", and Does striving for progress in the game motivate healthy behaviours). In addition, we were unable to evaluate fundamental questions about use of the platform and engagement in health behaviours because our findings did not confirm a widespread assumption in the literature that users carry their mobile platforms with them "everywhere" and that the platforms are constantly connected to data networks [61,63,65]. Specifically, we found that because of the central server architecture, progress in the game and coaching critically depended on the user being continuously connected. What became clear from the evaluation "in the wild" is that we incorrectly assumed that users would be continuously online, they would wear their physical activity wrist band all day and they would consistently send their BG data to the sensor network immediately after measuring. Some carried their own mobile phone (not the phone provided) and used the phone provided for gaming only at home. This led to a less than optimal user experience. Thus, the prototype we evaluated was not truly "pervasive" in practice given technology constraints and individual differences in user preferences for using the technology. Finally, the variation in use and feedback of the platform also supports claims that simply applying gamification principles to an intervention does not guarantee increased engagement with a technology, much less, increased motivation to engage in health behaviours targeted by the intervention [49]. The games, and the platform overall, could be improved by simplifying the interface so that it is more intuitive and easy to use, reducing the difficulty of the games for increased playability, modifying the look of the game so that it is more appealing to the target users, and addressing technical issues reported so that the platform is free of major technical bugs that inhibit enjoyment and prevent use of the technology. The implementations of these improvements should be further evaluated because recent research suggests that participatory design processes do not always lead to positive effects on health behaviours [66].

The results from the pilot study contribute to and further the literature on challenges faced when deploying pervasive technologies in healthcare [61]. The negative feedback we report in particular is significant because it presents a more balanced report of technologies (reporting negative as well as positive findings) that contribute to theoretical and practical progress in the field. This addresses a pervasive problem that negative reports of findings including negative user feedback of new technologies are not reported [23,61,67]. The findings from the pilot study also contribute to research on the state of information technologies that suggest that more reliable technology systems should be developed and deployed in healthcare [68]. In sum, the balanced reviews provided in this report not only contribute to scientific efforts to understand the application of technology to healthcare but may also be of practical value for informing the strategic planning of technology development efforts to improve healthcare. Specifically for the latter, in the future, evaluations of similar prototypes such as ours should consider the current findings that suggest specific areas of challenge (e.g., usability, acceptability of look and feel, technical performance) should be addressed before evaluating the impact of the prototype on health outcomes.

The pilot studies show the importance of finding a good balance between flawless and non-obtrusive technology, between challenging but not too difficult game play, and the relevance of designing and fine-tuning to the age group as well as to the level of knowledge and experience of the individual user. Furthermore, the use of mobile technology in combination with web-based elements has been shown to be feasible with potential to change healthcare by supporting a vulnerable group of patients in self-managing their chronic disease. We emphasise the value of mixed methods long-term user studies "in the wild" with patients from the target group in their daily environment, as well as the involvement of the medical team in their role as care providers in these types of user studies.

6.1. Limitations

The current study demonstrates the design and evaluation of a pervasive coaching and gamification platform within a clinical sample of young diabetes patients. However, the findings in this report are limited. The platform evaluated in this research was of a prototype version of the framework. As such, difficulties with usability and seamless functioning of the technology were challenges in evaluating basic research questions regarding user engagement and impact on outcomes. In terms of research design, the small sample size of participants and relatively high attrition rate, seen in similar studies of smartphone apps for health (e.g., [69]), suggest that the results may have limited generalizability to the broad population of potential users. Also, because users of prototypes in our studies were not compared to a control group of users of comparable prototypes, it is not clear how much their feedback was specific to the content and design of the prototypes we tested, or could be attributed to general issues common with early versions of technologies.

6.2. Future Research

Future research efforts to develop complex and integrative platforms such as the platform described in this study should incorporate user input and co-design approaches and rigorous quality assurance testing before being subjected to user evaluation studies. The ideal of a user-centered design process, common to the field of human-computer interaction, that engages target users early and often [46] is sometimes hard to realize but considered necessary for successful design. Future studies should also address issues of deployment by engaging with key stakeholders in healthcare in addition to patients as end-users to facilitate the ultimate success of the technology in "real world" settings. In terms of methodology, future research on platforms such as the PERGAMON platform in this study, should be conducted with larger groups of patients/users (including those recently diagnosed) with rigorous research designs and in a hospital setting over a longer period to see if indeed gamification helps patients to automate self-care behaviours. If proven effective, further studies should aim to examine and clarify which features and game elements contribute to a positive user experience and increase self-care for patients with a chronic condition.

6.3. Implementation Challenges of Serious Gaming and Virtual Coaching in Healthcare

There are various challenges on the way to the implementation of a pervasive integrated system such as the PERGAMON gamification platform into the practice of hospitals in their care for chronic diseases. It is essential that the technology used to enhance self-management, is integrated in the daily routine of the patients in a non-obtrusive way [10–12]. Every step that requires extra actions on top of all obligatory procedures for the user has to be avoided. During the past years some progress has been made in simplifying blood glucose monitoring [5], but these systems are expensive and not-reimbursed. Simplification, unobtrusiveness, safety, reliablity and robustness are prerequisites for introducing new techniques such as the PERGAMON platform.

Prejudice and stigmatization play important roles in the acceptance of tools and devices that support disease management [70,71]. This is not only the case for medical devices, but also when the game, or platform components like an activity tracker, or a sensor look clumsy or childish, they may become objects of mockery [72]. We learned from the user evaluations how essential a good balance is between flawless and non-obtrusive technology, challenging but not to difficult gameplay, and excellent fine-tuning to the age group.

In health care a rather conservative attitude often exists toward new developments. An important reason is that, because of safety precautions, proven technology is preferred above new techniques. So far, proof of the effectiveness of serious gaming is considered insufficient, and privacy issues or cyber-crime are increasingly considered to be a risk. Furthermore, the ICT departments in health care institutions are fully focused on medical systems and do not have the knowledge, the experience or the willingness to deal with other applications before their added value is demonstrated. Research has shown that the perception of facilitators, i.e., the degree to which an individual believes that an organizational and technical infrastructure exists to support the use of the system, is one of the most important variables to consider for increasing doctors' and nurses' intention to use the new technology for telemedicine [73].

A second factor that impedes the introduction of complex digital platforms may be a financial one. Hospitals and other healthcare systems are non-profit organisations and the return on investments for serious gaming and virtual coaching is still very uncertain. Patients on the other hand are used to the fact that the costs of healthcare are largely reimbursed by health insurance companies. Before they are willing to pay for the apps and wearables, they have to be convinced that playing, learning and being coached by a gaming platform offers them great benefits. Health insurance companies will only reimburse the costs of these platforms when there is proof of savings or an explicit and measurable increase in the quality of health care, which is hardly ever the case. Finally, many patients with chronic diseases have long-standing habits of performing their repetitive actions in a certain way and with a particular device. Technology acceptance studies in health care showed that changing to new devices (e.g., blood glucose meters) will only be accepted by the patients if the benefits that they experience are very clear [73].

7. Conclusions

This paper provided an overview of an innovative integrated pervasive gamified platform that combined sensors, mobile technologies, virtual coaching and serious games. The description of the platform provided insight into how theory could be applied to the design of behaviour change technology in healthcare. The findings from the user study contributed to knowledge about challenges faced when developing and testing complex behaviour change technologies in healthcare. They have practical significance for strategic planning for successful technology development of behaviour change interventions in healthcare.

Acknowledgments: This is a product of the PERGAMON consortium. The PERGAMON project received funding from the European Union's Horizon 2020 research and innovation programme under grant agreement No. 644385. We are grateful to all children and their parents and caregivers for participating in the user evaluations.

Author Contributions: These authors contributed equally to this work. P.d.B. designed and implemented the gamification platform. R.K. designed and implemented the virtual coach. K.B., P.K. and G.J.v.d.B. conceived and designed the user evaluations; R.K., R.o.d.A. and G.J.v.d.B. conducted the user evaluations; K.B. analyzed the data; R.K., R.o.d.A., K.B., G.J.v.d.B. and P.K. wrote the paper

Conflicts of Interest: The authors declare no conflict of interest. The founding sponsors, the EU research program, had no role in the design of the study; in the collection, analyses, or interpretation of data; in the writing of the manuscript, and in the decision to publish the results.

References

1. Grady, P.A.; Gough, L.L. Self-Management: A Comprehensive Approach to Management of Chronic Conditions. *Am. J. Public Health* **2014**, *104*, e25–e31.
2. Diaz-Valencia, P.A.; Bougnères, P.; Valleron, A.J. Global epidemiology of type 1 diabetes in young adults and adults: A systematic review. *BMC Public Health* **2015**, *15*, 255.
3. Mauras, N.; Fox, L.; Englert, K.; Beck, R.W. Continuous glucose monitoring in type 1 diabetes. *Endocrine* **2013**, *43*, 41–50.
4. Hood, K.K.; Peterson, C.M.; Rohan, J.M.; Drotar, D. Association Between Adherence and Glycemic Control in Pediatric Type 1 Diabetes: A Meta-analysis. *Pediatrics* **2009**, *124*, e1171–e1179.
5. Markowitz, J.T.; Harrington, K.R.; Laffel, L.M.B. Technology to Optimize Pediatric Diabetes Management and Outcomes. *Curr. Diabetes Rep.* **2013**, *13*, 877–885.
6. Van der Burg, G. mHealth in diabetes management—The BLink experience. In Proceedings of the 39th ISPAD Annual Conference 2013, Gothenburg, Sweden, 16–19 October 2013.

7. Patton, S.R. Adherence to Glycemic Monitoring in Diabetes. *J. Diabetes Sci. Technol.* **2015**, *9*, 668–675.
8. Weinzimer, S.A.; Beck, R.W.; Chase, H.P.; Fox, L.A.; Buckingham, B.A.; Tamborlane, W.V.; Kollman, C.; Coffey, J.; Xing, D.; Ruedy, K.J.; et al. Accuracy of Newer Generation Home Blood Glucose Meters in a Diabetes Research in Children Network (DirecNet) Inpatient Exercise Study. *Diabetes Technol. Ther.* **2005**, *7*, 675–683.
9. Holl, R.; Swift, P.; Mortensen, H.; Lynggaard, H.; Hougaard, P.; Aanstoot, H.; Chiarelli, F.; Daneman, D.; Danne, T.; Dorchy, H.; et al. Insulin injection regimens and metabolic control in an international survey of adolescents with type 1 diabetes over 3 years: results from the Hvidore study group. *Eur. J. Pediatr.* **2003**, *162*, 22–29.
10. Rausch, J.R.; Hood, K.K.; Delamater, A.; Pendley, J.S.; Rohan, J.M.; Reeves, G.; Dolan, L.; Drotar, D. Changes in treatment adherence and glycemic control during the transition to adolescence in type 1 diabetes. *Diabetes Care* **2012**, *35*, 1219–1224.
11. Pyatak, E.A.; Florindez, D.; Weigensberg, M.J. Adherence decision making in the everyday lives of emerging adults with type 1 diabetes. *Patient Preference Adherence* **2013**, *7*, 709–718.
12. Holtz, B.E.; Murray, K.M.; Hershey, D.D.; Dunneback, J.K.; Cotten, S.R.; Holmstrom, A.J.; Vyas, A.; Kaiser, M.K.; Wood, M.A. Developing a Patient-Centered mHealth App: A Tool for Adolescents With Type 1 Diabetes and Their Parents. *JMIR mHealth uHealth* **2017**, *5*, e53.
13. Sabete, E. *Adherence to Long-Term Therapies: Evidence for Action*; World Health Organization; Genève. 2003.
14. Goyal, S.; Nunn, C.A.; Rotondi, M.; Couperthwaite, A.B.; Reiser, S.; Simone, A.; Katzman, D.K.; Cafazzo, J.A.; Palmert, M.R. A Mobile App for the Self-Management of Type 1 Diabetes Among Adolescents: A Randomized Controlled Trial. *JMIR mHealth uHealth* **2017**, *5*, e82.
15. Osborn, C.Y.; Mayberry, L.S.; Mulvaney, S.A.; Hess, R. Patient Web Portals to Improve Diabetes Outcomes: A Systematic Review. *Curr. Diabetes Rep.* **2010**, *10*, 422–435.
16. Op den Akker, H.; Klaassen, R.; Nijholt, A. Virtual coaches for healthy lifestyle. In *Toward Robotic Socially Believable Behaving Systems-Volume II*; Springer: Berlin/Heidelberg, Germany, 2016; pp. 121–149.
17. Ye, X. GlucOnline Coach: A virtual coach app for diabetes patients. Master's Thesis, University of Twente, Enschede, The Netherlands, 2015.
18. Brzan, P.P.; Rotman, E.; Pajnkihar, M.; Klanjsek, P. Mobile Applications for Control and Self Management of Diabetes: A Systematic Review. *J. Med. Syst.* **2016**, *40*, 210.
19. Chomutare, T.; Fernandez-Luque, L.; Arsand, E.; Hartvigsen, G. Features of Mobile Diabetes Applications: Review of the Literature and Analysis of Current Applications Compared Against Evidence-Based Guidelines. *J. Med. Internet Res.* **2011**, *13*, e65.
20. Eng, D.S.; Lee, J.M. The Promise and Peril of Mobile Health Applications for Diabetes and Endocrinology. *Pediatr. Diabetes* **2013**, *14*, 231–238.
21. Boyle, L.; Grainger, R.; Hall, R.M.; Krebs, J.D. Use of and Beliefs About Mobile Phone Apps for Diabetes Self-Management: Surveys of People in a Hospital Diabetes Clinic and Diabetes Health Professionals in New Zealand. *JMIR mHealth and uHealth* **2017**, *5*, e85.
22. Williams, G.C.; Freedman, Z.R.; Deci, E.L. Supporting Autonomy to Motivate Patients With Diabetes for Glucose Control. *Diabetes Care* **1998**, *21*, 1644–1651.
23. Kato, P. Video games in health care: Closing the gap. *Rev. Gen. Psychol.* **2010**, *14*, 113–121.
24. Deterding, S.; Dixon, D.; Khaled, R.; Nacke, L. From Game Design Elements to Gamefulness: Defining "Gamification". In Proceedings of the 15th International Academic MindTrek Conference: Envisioning Future Media Environments, Tampere, Finland, 28–30 September 2011; ACM: New York, NY, USA; pp. 9–15.
25. Baranowski, T.; Buday, R.; Thompson, D.; Baranowski, J. Playing for real: Video games and stories for health-related behavior change. *Am. J. Prev. Med.* **2008**, *34*, 74–82.
26. Thompson, D.; Baranowski, T.; Buday, R.; Baranowski, J.; Thompson, V.; Jago, R.; Griffith, M.J. Serious Video Games for Health How Behavioral Science Guided the Development of a Serious Video Game. *Simul. Gaming* **2010**, *41*, 587–606.
27. Cugelman, B. Gamification: What It Is and Why It Matters to Digital Health Behavior Change Developers. *JMIR Serious Games* **2013**, *1*, e3.
28. Järvinen, A. Games without Frontiers: Methods for Game Studies and Design. Ph.D. Thesis, University of Tampere, Tampere, Finland, 2008.
29. Schell, J. *The Art of Game Design: A book of Lenses*; Morgan Kaufmann Publishers, Burlington, USA: 2008; p. 512.

30. Chomutare, T.; Johansen, S.; Arsand, E.; Hartvigsen, G. Play and learn: Developing a social game for children with diabetes. *Stud. Health Technol. Inform.* **2016**, *226*, 55–58.
31. Lieberman, D. Video games for diabetes self-management: examples and design strategies. *J. Diabetes Sci. Technol.* **2012**, *6*, 802–806.
32. Aoki, N.; Ohta, S.; Masuda, H.; Naito, T.; Sawai, T.; Nishida, K.; Okada, T.; Oishi, M.; Iwasawa, Y.; Toyomasu, K.; et al. Edutainment tools for initial education of type-1 diabetes mellitus: initial diabetes education with fun. *Medinfo* **2004**, *11*, 855–859.
33. Aoki, N.; Ohta, S.; Okada, T.; Oishi, M.; Fukui, T. INSULOT A cellular phone-based edutainment learning tool for children with type 1 diabetes. *Diabetes Care* **2005**, *28*, 760.
34. Pouw, I.H. You are what you eat: Serious Gaming for Type 1 Diabetic Persons. Master's Thesis, University of Twente, Enschede, The Netherlands, 2015.
35. Brown, S.J.; Lieberman, D.A.; Gemeny, B.A.; Fan, Y.C.; Wilson, D.M.; Pasta, D.J. Educational video game for juvenile diabetes: Results of a controlled trial. *Med. Inform.* **1997**, *22*, 77–89.
36. Fuchslocher, A.; Niesenhaus, J.; Krämer, N. Serious games for health: An empirical study of the game *Balance* for teenagers with diabetes mellitus. *Entertain. Comput.* **2011**, *2*, 97–101.
37. Lieberman, D.A. Management of chronic pediatric diseases with interactive health games: Theory and research findings. *J. Ambul. Care Manag.* **2001**, *24*, 26–38.
38. Theng, Y.L.; Lee, J.W.; Patinadan, P.V.; Foo, S.S. The Use of Videogames, Gamification, and Virtual Environments in the Self-Management of Diabetes: A Systematic Review of Evidence. *Games Health J.* **2015**, *4*, 352–361.
39. Charlier, N.; Zupancic, N.; Fieuws, S.; Denhaerynck, K.; Zaman, B.; Moons, P. Serious games for improving knowledge and self-management in young people with chronic conditions: A systematic review and meta-analysis. *J. Am. Med. Inform. Assoc.* **2015**, *23*, 230–239.
40. Johnson, D.; Deterding, S.; Kuhn, K.A.; Staneva, A.; Stoyanov, S.; Hides, L. Gamification for health and wellbeing: A systematic review of the literature. *Internet Interv.* **2016**, *6*, 89–106.
41. Deacon, A.J.; O'Farrell, K. The use of serious games and gamified design to improve health outcomes in adolescents with chronic disease: A review of recent literature. In Proceedings of the International Conference on Successes and Failures in Telehealth, Auckland, New Zealand, 1 November–3 November 2016; pp. 1–3.
42. Sardi, L.; Idri, A.; Fernández-Alemán, J.L. A systematic review of gamification in e-Health. *J. Biomed. Inform.* **2017**, *71*, 31–48.
43. Kumar, V.S.; Wentzell, K.J.; Mikkelsen, T.; Pentland, A.; Laffel, L.M. The DAILY (Daily Automated Intensive Log for Youth) trial: A wireless, portable system to improve adherence and glycemic control in youth with diabetes. *Diabetes Technol. Ther.* **2004**, *6*, 445–453.
44. Cafazzo, J.A.; Casselman, M.; Hamming, N.; Katzman, D.K.; Palmert, M.R. Design of an mHealth App for the Self-management of Adolescent Type 1 Diabetes: A Pilot Study. *J. Med. Internet Res.* **2012**, *14*, e70.
45. Klingensmith, G.J.; Aisenberg, J.; Kaufman, F.; Halvorson, M.; Cruz, E.; Riordan, M.E.; Varma, C.; Pardo, S.; Viggiani, M.T.; Wallace, J.F.; et al. Evaluation of a combined blood glucose monitoring and gaming system (Didget) for motivation in children, adolescents, and young adults with type 1 diabetes. *Pediatr. Diabetes* **2013**, *14*, 350–357.
46. Klasnja, P.; Consolvo, S.; McDonald, D.W.; Landay, J.A.; Pratt, W. Using mobile & personal sensing technologies to support health behavior change in everyday life: Lessons learned. In Proceedings of the American Medical Informatics Association (AMIA) Annual Symposium, San Francisco, CA, USA, 14–18 November 2009; pp. 338–342.
47. Lauritzen, J.; Årsand, E.; Horsch, A.; Fernandez-Luque, L.; Chomutare, T.; Bellika, J.; Hejlesen, O.; Hartvigsen, G. Social media and games as self-management tools for children and adolescents with type 1 diabetes mellitus. In Proceedings of the International Conference on Health Informatics, HEALTHINF 2012, Vilamoura, Portugal, 1–4 February 2012; pp. 459–466.
48. McCarthy, G.M.; Rodríguez Ramírez, E.R.; Robinson, B.J. Letters to Medical Devices: A Case Study on the Medical Device User Requirements of Female Adolescents and Young Adults with Type 1 Diabetes. In *Persuasive Technology: Development and Implementation of Personalized Technologies to Change Attitudes and Behaviors, Proceedings of the 12th International Conference, PERSUASIVE 2017, Amsterdam, The Netherlands, 4–6 April 2017*; de Vries, P.W., Oinas-Kukkonen, H., Siemons, L., Beerlage-de Jong, N., van Gemert-Pijnen, L., Eds.; Springer: Cham, Switzerland, 2017; pp. 69–79.

49. Baranowski, T.; Blumberg, F.; Buday, R.; DeSmet, A.; Fiellin, L.E.; Green, C.S.; Kato, P.M.; Lu, A.S.; Maloney, A.E.; Mellecker, R.; et al. Games for Health for Children—Current Status and Needed Research. *Games Health J. Res. Dev. Clin. Appl.* **2016**, *5*, 1–12.
50. Van Wynsberghe, A. Designing Robots with Care. Ph.D. Thesis, University of Twente, Enschede, The Netherlands, 2012.
51. Burke, S.D.; Sherr, D.; Lipman, R.D. Partnering with diabetes educators to improve patient outcomes. *Diabetes Metab. Syndr. Obes. Targets Ther.* **2014**, *7*, 34–43.
52. Oinas-Kukkonen, H.; Harjumaa, M. Persuasive Systems Design: Key Issues, Process Model, and System Features. *Commun. Assoc. Inf. Syst.* **2009**, *24*, 485–500.
53. Abraham, C.; Michie, S. A taxonomy of behavior change techniques used in interventions. *Health Psychol.* **2008**, *27*, 379–387.
54. Locke, E.A.; Latham, G.P. Building a practically useful theory of goal setting and task motivation: A 35-year odyssey. *Am. Psychol.* **2002**, *57*, 705–717.
55. Patrick, H.; Williams, G.C. Self-determination theory: Its application to health behavior and complementarity with motivational interviewing. *Int. J. Behav. Nutr. Phys. Act.* **2012**, *9*, 18.
56. Oinas-Kukkonen, H. Behavior Change Support Systems: A Research Model and Agenda. In *Persuasive Technology*; Ploug, T., Hasle, P., Oinas-Kukkonen, H., Eds.; Springer: Berlin/Heidelberg, Germany, 2010; Volume 6137, pp. 4–14.
57. Calvillo-Gámez, E.H.; Cairns, P.; Cox, A.L. Assessing the core elements of the gaming experience. In *Evaluating User Experience in Games*; Springer: London, UK, 2010; pp. 47–71.
58. Huizinga, J. *Homo Ludens: A Study of the Play-Element in Culture*; The Beacon Press: Boston, MA, USA, 1955.
59. Snoek, F.J.; Pouwer, F.; Welch, G.W.; Polonsky, W.H. Diabetes-related emotional distress in Dutch and US diabetic patients: Cross-cultural validity of the problem areas in diabetes scale. *Diabetes Care* **2000**, *23*, 1305–1309.
60. Brooke, J. SUS-A quick and dirty usability scale. *Usabil. Eval. Ind.* **1996**, *189*, 4–7.
61. Orwat, C.; Graefe, A.; Faulwasser, T. Towards pervasive computing in health care: A literature review. *BMC Med. Inform. Decis. Mak.* **2008**, *8*, 26.
62. Michie, S.; Prestwich, A. Are interventions theory-based? Development of a theory coding scheme. *Health Psychol.* **2010**, *29*, 1–8.
63. Alemdar, H.; Ersoy, C. Wireless sensor networks for healthcare: A survey. *Comput. Netw.* **2010**, *54*, 2688–2710.
64. Lyles, C.R.; Harris, L.T.; Le, T.; Flowers, J.; Tufano, J.; Britt, D.; Hoath, J.; Hirsch, I.B.; Goldberg, H.I.; Ralston, J.D. Qualitative evaluation of a mobile phone and web-based collaborative care intervention for patients with type 2 diabetes. *Diabetes Technol. Ther.* **2011**, *13*, 563–569.
65. Free, C.; Phillips, G.; Galli, L.; Watson, L.; Felix, L.; Edwards, P.; Patel, V.; Haines, A. The effectiveness of mobile-health technology-based health behaviour change or disease management interventions for health care consumers: A systematic review. *PLoS Med.* **2013**, *10*, e1001362.
66. DeSmet, A.; Thompson, D.; Baranowski, T.; Palmeira, A.; Verloigne, M.; De Bourdeaudhuij, I. Is participatory design associated with the effectiveness of serious digital games for healthy lifestyle promotion? A meta-analysis. *J. Med. Internet Res.* **2016**, *18*, e94.
67. Kato, P.M. Evaluating efficacy and validating health games. *Games Health Res. Dev. Clin. Appl.* **2012**, *1*, 74–76.
68. Bates, D.W. The quality case for information technology in healthcare. *BMC Med. Inform. Decis. Mak.* **2002**, *2*, 7.
69. Allen, J.K.; Stephens, J.; Dennison Himmelfarb, C.R.; Stewart, K.J.; Hauck, S. Randomized controlled pilot study testing use of smartphone technology for obesity treatment. *J. Obes.* **2013**, *2013*, 151597.
70. Vanstone, M.; Rewegan, A.; Brundisini, F.; Dejean, D.; Giacomini, M. Patient Perspectives on Quality of Life With Uncontrolled Type 1 Diabetes Mellitus: A Systematic Review and Qualitative Meta-synthesis. *Ont. Health Technol. Assess. Ser.* **2015**, *15*, 1–29.
71. Browne, J.L.; Ventura, A.; Mosely, K.; Speight, J. 'I'm not a druggie, I'm just a diabetic': A qualitative study of stigma from the perspective of adults with type 1 diabetes. *BMJ Open* **2014**, *4*, e005625.

72. Drummond, D.; Hadchouel, A.; Tesnière, A. Serious games for health: three steps forwards. *Adv. Simul.* **2017**, *2*, 3.
73. Gagnon, M.P.; Orruno, E.; Asua, J.; Abdeljelil, A.B.; Emparanza, J. Using a Modified Technology Acceptance Model to Evaluate Healthcare Professionals' Adoption of a New Telemonitoring System. *Telemed. J. e-Health* **2012**, *18*, 54–59.

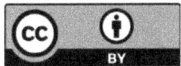

© 2018 by the authors. Licensee MDPI, Basel, Switzerland. This article is an open access article distributed under the terms and conditions of the Creative Commons Attribution (CC BY) license (http://creativecommons.org/licenses/by/4.0/).

MDPI
St. Alban-Anlage 66
4052 Basel
Switzerland
Tel. +41 61 683 77 34
Fax +41 61 302 89 18
www.mdpi.com

Sensors Editorial Office
E-mail: sensors@mdpi.com
www.mdpi.com/journal/sensors

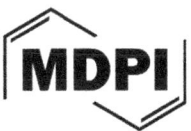

www.ingramcontent.com/pod-product-compliance
Lightning Source LLC
LaVergne TN
LVHW070419100526
838202LV00014B/1486